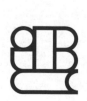

Child Health
Services Research

Elisa J. Sobo
Paul S. Kurtin
Editors

· ·

Foreword by
James M. Perrin

Child Health Services Research

· ·

Applications, Innovations, and Insights

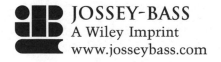

JOSSEY-BASS
A Wiley Imprint
www.josseybass.com

Published by Jossey-Bass
A Wiley Imprint
989 Market Street, San Francisco, CA 94103-1741   www.josseybass.com

Jossey-Bass books and products are available through most bookstores. To contact
Jossey-Bass directly call our Customer Care Department within the U.S. at 800-956-7739,
outside the U.S. at 317-572-3986 or fax 317-572-4002.

Jossey-Bass also publishes its books in a variety of electronic formats. Some content that
appears in print may not be available in electronic books.

Library of Congress Cataloging-in-Publication Data

Child health services research : applications, innovations, and insights / edited by
Elisa J. Sobo and Paul S. Kurtin. — 1st ed.
    p. cm.
  Includes bibliographical references and index.
  ISBN 0-7879-5875-1 (alk. paper)
  1. Child health services—Research—Methodology.   I. Sobo, Elisa Janine, 1963-   .
II. Kurtin, Paul S., 1951-   .
  [DNLM: 1. Child Health Services. 2. Health Services Research—methods.
3. Quality Assurance, Health Care—organization & administration.
WA 320 C53464 2003]
  RJ101.C5257 2003
  362.1'9892'00072—dc21
                                                                              2002008545

FIRST EDITION
HB Printing   10 9 8 7 6 5 4 3 2 1

Contents

Foreword   xi
  James M. Perrin

Preface   xv
  Elisa J. Sobo and Paul S. Kurtin

Note to the Reader   xxi
  Blair L. Sadler

The Editors   xxiii

The Contributors   xxv

Part One: Child Health Services: Setting an Accountability Agenda

1. An Introduction to Applied Child Health
   Services Research: Connecting Knowledge
   and Action   3
   Paul S. Kurtin

2. Laying the Foundation: Identifying Major
   Issues in Applied Child Health Services
   Research   25
   Pradeep Gidwani, Elisa J. Sobo, Michael Seid,
   and Paul S. Kurtin

Part Two: Child Health in Context: Home, Neighborhood, Community, Culture

3. Prevention and Healing in the Household: The Importance of Sociocultural Context   67
    Elisa J. Sobo

4. Documenting Child Health: The Community Indicators Movement   121
    Diana R. Simmes, Lillian F. Lim, and Kimberly Dennis

5. Partnering with the Community: Implementation, Evaluation, and Impact   155
    Kimberly Dennis and Diana R. Simmes

Part Three: Child Health in Conventional Health Care Settings: Improving Organizational Performance

6. Health-Related Quality of Life   209
    Tara Smith Knight, Tasha M. Burwinkle, and James W. Varni

7. Conceptual Models of Quality of Care and Health-Related Quality of Life for Vulnerable Children   243
    Michael Seid, Elisa J. Sobo, Mirjana Zivkovic, Melissa Nelson, and Maryam Davodi Far

8. Standardized Approaches to Clinical Care: Pathways and Disease Management   275
    Patricia J. Richardson, Elisa J. Sobo, and Erin R. Stucky

Part Four: Child Health Outcomes: Broadening the Reach of Applied Research

9. Translating Research into Practice:
    Planning Research to Inform Policy and
    Program Development   313
        Kimberly Dennis

10. Looking to the Future: The Need for Applied
    Child Health Services Research   353
        Paul S. Kurtin and Blair L. Sadler

Glossary   359
Name Index   373
Subject Index   385

Foreword

· ·

The past decade has seen tremendous growth in child health services research. Major new initiatives by the Agency for Healthcare Research and Quality, in collaboration with the David and Lucile Packard Foundation and other groups, have led to substantial new knowledge about the measurement of child health status and health care quality and new efforts to improve child and adolescent health care. Related efforts by the federal Maternal and Child Health Bureau and the Center for Medicare and Medicaid Services (formerly known as the Health Care Financing Administration) have also brought attention to the importance of child health services research. New organizations, such as the Child Health Accountability Initiative and the National Initiative for Child Healthcare Quality, have sprung up, and we have seen new efforts by older groups, such as the Foundation for Accountability, with its Child and Adolescent Health Measurement Initiative, to assess child health care quality. Efforts by a number of federal research agencies to expand inclusion of children in research protocols have also led to better understanding of the health care and health services issues affecting children. Changes in health insurance, with decreasing employer-based dependent coverage and increased public insurance, especially through Medicaid expansions and the new state Child Health Insurance Program (SCHIP), have strengthened research into costs and coverage. And large variations in utilization and outcomes have directed major efforts to understand and improve children's access to health care.

These efforts have provided better documentation of the special needs of children and adolescents and the ways they differ from other populations. These issues include (1) the different epidemiology of childhood illness, with much lower rates of chronic illness and an emphasis on prevention and enhancing growth and development; (2) the dependence of children for their health status and health services on adults (especially, parents, and educators); (3) the dynamics of childhood growth and development, influencing both how illness presents and how it affects growth and development at different ages; and (4) the high rates of child poverty, given the strong interaction between poverty and health status and the use of health services. These issues make clear the importance of focused efforts in child health services research, and of avoiding the assumption that research on adult populations provides sufficient information to explain health care access and services for child and adolescent populations.

This volume pulls together important work in several areas of child health services research, organized by an active and diverse group of researchers at Children's Hospital and Health Center in San Diego. Led by Paul Kurtin, a visionary spokesperson for improving the care of children in different communities and for accountability in health services, this group—the Center for Child Health Outcomes (CCHO)—integrates a multidisciplinary staff with expertise in care organization, hospitals, ambulatory services, measure development, qualitative methods, child behavior, and health care outcomes. Based on a program of services to improve care for children in the diverse communities of San Diego and in the complex health care environment of Southern California, CCHO has pioneered in the development of communitywide assessments of child health, innovative programming to change the services children receive, quality improvement in children's inpatient services, along with a major commitment to development of measures of children's quality of life and health status. Of particular importance are CCHO's community health indicators efforts, establishing workable systems to assess the broad health of children in population-based studies.

This volume describes some of the key efforts of the San Diego group, but it also goes well beyond that to explore key issues in child health services research. It lays out recent highlights in child health services research and indicates research that will be needed in the next several years. It describes methods and findings from studying child health services in culturally diverse communities, a particularly important area given the great and growing diversity of America's children and adolescents. It describes well how good health services research translates directly into programs and interventions to improve care. CCHO's members have also pioneered in the development of measures of care and outcomes. Building on a strong base of methodologically precise measure development, the group's exceptional work, with its careful and sophisticated approach to measurement, has helped countless other investigators.

Child health care has seen recent and dramatic approaches to improving the quality of child health services, partly organized through the new National Initiative for Child Healthcare Quality and the Child Health Accountability Initiative. Both offer great promise for children and their health providers. This volume explores key issues in child health care quality and offers guidance to next steps. Related work addresses clinical management and disease pathways for children's health care. Again, the different epidemiology of childhood disease calls for very different efforts in this area, exploring different units of observation, measurements of outcome, and means of intervention.

In assembling this volume, Elisa Sobo and Paul Kurtin have provided an important service to researchers, child health providers,

and policymakers. The book offers a concise overview of applied
child health services research and should guide many communities
and organizations in their efforts to improve care and health outcomes for children and adolescents.

December 2002   JAMES M. PERRIN
                       Professor of Pediatrics,
                       Harvard Medical School.
                       Director,
                       Center for Child and Adolescent Health Policy,
                       Director, Division of Child Pediatrics,
                       Massachusetts General Hospital for Children.

Preface

· ·

This book began as many books do: with a desire to widely share what has worked for us in meeting the needs of the children and families that we serve here at Children's Hospital and Health Center, San Diego. With funding from the National Library of Medicine (NLM), we set forth to bring together here the core lessons learned through work completed by members of the hospital's Center for Child Health Outcomes (CCHO) over the past eight years. The NLM supported our book project through grant number 1 G13 LM07489-01 as part of its mission to provide information of value to U.S. health professionals.

Why would anyone be interested in our experiences? The Center for Child Health Outcomes has been a critical driving force in Children's transformation into an organization that makes quality its core strategy. CCHO has successfully led a fundamental change in clinical practice throughout our integrated delivery system, beginning with standardizing care to excellence via the use of evidence-based clinical pathways. Our efforts have resulted in the continuous improvement of clinical outcomes as well as the continuous reduction in the costs of providing care. However, CCHO's approach to evaluation and improvement goes beyond clinical care within the hospital-based delivery system to affect child health services in the community and influence health policy even more widely.

While CCHO is certainly not alone in undertaking efforts such as these, very few organizations and investigators are actively engaged in the scale and scope of activities that CCHO is involved in. Based on our experience, then, we seek to broaden and deepen the field of applied child health services research (CHSR) as it is presently practiced by providing those who are new to the area, as well as health care professionals already engaged in this work, with useful information regarding the skill sets and knowledge that researchers interested in conducting applied CHSR should have if they are to be effective in improving child health services and the health and well-being of children. The need for such information is great and growing; for example, the Institute of Medicine's 2001 report on quality in health care (*Crossing the Quality Chasm*) strongly favors increased and better training in quality and systems improvement, and the lessons described in this book help toward that end. The lessons learned that we share here have not been part of most medical, nursing, or other health curricula. The Accreditation Council for Graduate Medical Education recognizes this shortcoming and has mandated that the skills and knowledge needed to rigorously assess and improve clinical practice be taught in all residency training programs; nursing and other health care educational and training programs may shortly follow suit. This book will help support this critical skill-building effort by providing practical knowledge and examples that can be routinely applied in clinical practice as well as in the evaluation and improvement of community-based programs.

The book is intended to demonstrate the beneficial impact that applied CHSR can have when it takes the broad perspective on health that we recommend and when it is conceived and designed in collaboration with end users and other stakeholders. Advice on how to do this is woven throughout the text.

In addition to providing a useful book for individual investigators and practitioners, we want to send a strong, positive message of the value to large health care organizations of having their own internal applied research divisions. CCHO is one such division. Importantly, CCHO's research is not just hospital-based and not just clinically oriented: it pervades the entire continuum of care, takes a holistic perspective, involves both clinical and administrative processes and systems, and extends into the community that Children's serves.

Structure of the Book

While child health services include a broad array and continuum of interconnected services and sites of care, each of the book's chapters can stand on its own, so that chapters may be consulted one at a time when a specific topic is of interest. However, the chapters are arranged in a logical sequence so that the book can be read from front to back by those seeking to acquire familiarity with the field as a whole, such as students, professionals interested in making a transition to the field, or managers interested in learning what applied CHSR may offer their organizations.

The book is divided into four parts; the first relates to accountability; the second, to context; the third, to organizational performance; and the last, to future directions in applied CHSR. We open with an introduction to the field that defines applied research, details the present mission of applied CHSR, and describes the climate in which this mission has evolved. Chapter Two focuses on identifying critical and emerging issues in the field after laying out relevant history, especially in regard to health care oversight. The chapter also discusses important differences between child and adult health services.

Part Two, which concerns the context in which health is created and maintained, begins with a discussion, in Chapter Three, of cultural aspects of child health and related home health practices. Child health is not simply the product of doctor office visits but rather the complex outcome of a host of interlocking forces— some of which may, overtly, seem to have little to do with medical matters but which nonetheless exert a crucial influence on child health. Chapters Four and Five concentrate on community issues, including community-level indicators and report cards, and ways to partner with a community in order to ensure that one's research has the biggest possible impact on child health.

Part Three examines care in conventional settings such as clinics and hospitals. It begins, in Chapter Six, by discussing health-related quality-of-life measures that can supplement our understanding of and inform care in such settings. Chapter Seven extends this discussion by focusing on how health care structures and processes might affect quality of life for vulnerable children. Barriers to care play a large role in this discussion, as do structure, process, and outcome variables that help identify factors associated with poor health outcomes in this population. Clinical pathways and disease management are the focus of Chapter Eight. This chapter includes an examination of how organizational climates can change from being antiguideline to being fully supportive through nonadversarial outcomes research.

In the final part of the book, Chapter Nine discusses methods for translating research into practice, focusing on overcoming communication barriers that can exist between researchers, policymakers, program staff, and community members. It argues that applied CHSR is crucial not only for improvement but also for program survival. Finally, Chapter Ten examines the near- and long-term future of applied CHSR. A glossary is provided at the book's end to help those new to the field in understanding its jargon.

Central Goals

We cover quite a bit of ground in the ten chapters that comprise this volume. Our main goal is to broaden perspectives and teach readers new ways to *think* about applied CHSR. In light of this goal, the remarkably broad array of topics that may be included within CHSR, and the limitations of time and page space, there are certain topics that the book cannot address. For example, we do not cover issues related to secondary data, which we consider important (and recognize as sometimes the only data available) but not as directly useful as primary data collection is to the type of real-time improvement work that we do. Similarly, we do not address macro-level financial questions such as the impact of various reimbursement mechanisms on care. In today's health care world, financial arrangements constantly shift, so although such questions are very important, much of what we describe in this book concerns improvements that can and shall be made independent of specific reimbursement practices.

We also do not provide in-depth methodological information regarding analysis strategies. While we do discuss in great detail many of the issues that should be taken into account when designing applied research projects, the details of an analysis strategy will rest on the particular question investigated. In addition, there are many methods texts available that will be useful in devising specific analytical plans. Finally, we do not cover each and every child health issue in the examples provided; there is very little discussion of, for example, dental health. The unique aspects of older children's health (adolescent health) receive little specific attention due to our decision to focus, in the limited space of this book, on children more dependent on adults for their care. Nonetheless, the reader should come away from the text well prepared to conduct applied research on any aspect of child health; the principles described are applicable to the entire range of child health issues.

Indeed, if our ambitions have been realized, the reader will come away from this book with the knowledge necessary for productive and influential work in the health care systems of the twenty-first century. To best achieve their mission of improving child health, health care organizations will find it absolutely necessary to incorporate and utilize applied health services research that supports a central strategy of continuous, relentless quality improvement. Through this volume, we hope to assist all stakeholders in achieving this imperative.

ELISA J. SOBO
PAUL S. KURTIN

Note to the Reader

. . . .

Why would the senior leadership of any health care organization want to support applied health services research? This book answers that question.

Eight years ago, Children's Hospital and Health Center embarked on a multidisciplinary effort to create the Center for Child Health Outcomes, a center employing applied child health services research (CHSR) with the goal of ensuring that every child we treat receives optimal care. To achieve this goal, we established the following objectives: (1) decrease unnecessary variations in care, (2) improve overall resource efficiency, (3) enhance clinical effectiveness by decreasing the gap between knowledge and practice, and (4) establish a collaborative approach to care delivery. The rationale for this goal and these objectives was born out of our recognition that current practice did not always reflect the latest scientific knowledge, that increased managed care competition was forcing cost reductions, and that our organization was beginning to apply industrial models of variation reduction and continuous improvement to a health care setting.

This book describes the processes we have engaged, the techniques we have used to obtain significant and sustainable results, and the lessons learned by our entire organization. In addition to improving care, applied CHSR has significantly helped transform our culture to one that embraces quality measurement and quality improvement as a core strategy.

Investing in this work requires a significant multiyear commitment of time, talent, and resources. I know that I share the conclusions of our board of trustees, our medical staff, and our management that this investment has paid significant dividends and will continue to do so far into the future.

December 2002   BLAIR L. SADLER
                                   President and Chief Executive Officer
                                   Children's Hospital and Health Center
                                   San Diego, California

The Editors

· ·

ELISA J. SOBO, Ph.D., a medical anthropologist, is a research scientist with the Center for Child Health Outcomes and Trauma Services, Children's Hospital and Health Center, San Diego. She is also an associate clinical professor in the Department of Family and Preventive Medicine at the University of California San Diego School of Medicine. In addition to numerous articles, Sobo has authored, coauthored, or coedited eight books, including *The Cultural Context of Health, Illness and Medicine* (1997), *Using Methods in the Field* (1998), and *The Endangered Self: Managing the Social Risk of HIV* (2000), which received the 2001 Medicine and People award. Sobo is a fellow of the Society for Applied Anthropology and serves on the editorial boards of *Reviews in Anthropology* and *Anthropology and Medicine*. Her present research interests include the rhetorical rationalization of biomedical risk, patient-parent-practitioner communication, patients' and families' experiences of and functional acculturation to the world of biomedicine, and organizational culture.

PAUL S. KURTIN, M.D., is the vice-president for clinical innovations and director of the Center for Child Health Outcomes at Children's Hospital and Health Center, San Diego. For over a decade, he has been involved in designing, implementing, evaluating, and improving health services for children that enhance their health and well-being while also meeting the resource management demands of a highly competitive managed-care environment. He is also the founding medical director of the Child Health Accountability Initiative, a collaborative of fifteen children's hospitals working together to define, measure, and improve health outcomes for hospitalized children.

The Contributors

TASHA M. BURWINKLE, M.A., is a graduate student at the California School of Professional Psychology at Alliant International University in San Diego and a research assistant at the Center for Child Health Outcomes, Children's Hospital and Health Center, San Diego. Burwinkle has coauthored works regarding health-related quality of life in population-based samples and in children with rheumatic conditions, cancer, diabetes, and cardiac conditions, as well as works related to staff, patient, and parent satisfaction with the health care environment. She has also served as a site therapist to investigate problem-solving therapy interventions in mothers of children with cancer and is working on her grant-funded dissertation, titled "The Impact of Health-Related Quality-of-Life Assessment in Pediatric Rheumatology Clinical Practice." Burwinkle is a student member of both the Society of Behavioral Medicine and the American Psychological Association.

KIMBERLY DENNIS, M.P.A., a community analyst at the Center for Child Health Outcomes, Children's Hospital and Health Center, San Diego, received her degree (with a concentration in advanced policy analysis) from Columbia University's School of International and Public Affairs. She has many years' experience as a researcher, analyst, and writer on diverse public issues, including children and families, welfare reform, substance use, and community development. Most of her professional career has been spent in the public sector, working for nonprofit organizations in New York City, Washington, D.C., and California. Dennis is particularly interested in how research can be used to influence public policy and recently coauthored a book, *Responding to Alcohol and Other Drug Problems in Child Welfare: Weaving Together Policy and Practice*, for the Child Welfare League of America.

MARYAM DAVODI FAR, M.H.A., D.P.A., completed her doctoral work at the University of La Verne with an emphasis in health care. She currently serves as the executive director of the San Diego American Indian Health Center. Her areas of research interest include cultural and linguistic barriers in health care and the impact of technology on the patient-physician relationship and communication. While at Children's Hospital and Health Center in San Diego, Far worked in the Marketing and Community Relations departments and for the Center for Child Health Outcomes.

PRADEEP GIDWANI, M.D., M.P.H., a physician scientist at the Center for Child Health Outcomes, Children's Hospital and Health Center, San Diego, completed a Pediatric Health Services Research fellowship at Massachusetts General Hospital in Boston in 2000. He is a board-certified pediatrician. During his fellowship, he earned a master's in public health degree at the Harvard School of Public Health. He completed his residency at Children's Hospital Medical Center in Cincinnati after receiving his doctor of medicine degree from George Washington University in 1995. Prior to medical school, Gidwani worked for the National Commission to Prevent Infant Mortality in Washington, D.C., and for the Centers for Disease Control and Prevention. He received his bachelor of arts degree in anthropology from Northwestern University in Evanston, Illinois. His research focuses on asthma, parents' perceptions of childhood behaviors, and cultural barriers to care.

TARA SMITH KNIGHT, Ph.D., received her doctorate in educational psychology with an emphasis in developmental studies from the University of California, Santa Barbara. She served as a research associate at the Center for Child Health Outcomes, Children's Hospital and Health Center, San Diego, for three years. She has coauthored works regarding health-related quality of life and childhood aggression. Knight is currently conducting health services research in the Department of Pharmaceutical Economics and Policy at the University of Southern California, with a focus on clinical pathway development, disease management program evaluation, and quality-of-life research. Other research interests include the study of at-risk populations, ADHD, and the development and evaluation of prevention programs focusing on adolescents.

LILLIAN F. LIM, M.P.H., a certified health education specialist, received her degree from the Graduate School of Public Health at San Diego State University with a concentration in health promotion. Lim's work at the Center for Child Health Outcomes, Children's Hospital and Health Center, San Diego, includes data-related technical assistance to community-based organizations, the development of a community health report card, and a statewide evaluation of child health insurance programs. Her past experience in community health involves countywide tobacco prevention and cessation for youth and evaluation assistance for various HIV prevention programs. Lim's other interests include the implementation and evaluation of childhood asthma programs.

MELISSA NELSON, M.P.H., a research assistant at the Center for Child Health Outcomes, Children's Hospital and Health Center, San Diego, received her degree from the Graduate School of Public Health at San Diego State University with a concentration in health promotion. While in graduate school, she worked on two federally funded projects. One assessed mental health services used by children and adolescents throughout the county. The other examined the relationship between access to health care and school attendance and achievement. Nelson also worked in the state of California's Department of Health and Human Services' Office of Health Promotion on a number of projects, including the state assembly bill that banned smoking in bars and restaurants.

PATRICIA J. RICHARDSON, M.A.O.M., R.C.P., a clinical researcher at the Center for Child Health Outcomes, Children's Hospital and Health Center, San Diego, earned her graduate degree in organizational management at the University of Phoenix. She is also a licensed respiratory care practitioner in the state of California. Richardson's focus is on clinical improvements and innovations, specifically in the area of clinical pathways, disease management, and clinical systems. She has been responsible for the development of more than fifty-two clinical pathways and disease management programs, as well as the development of a process for unit-specific clinical and financial report cards.

BLAIR L. SADLER, J.D., has been the president and CEO of San Diego's Children's Hospital and Health Center since 1980. He has served as a medical-legal specialist for the National Institutes of Health, on the faculty of Yale University, and as assistant vice president at the Robert Wood Johnson Foundation. Prior to his appointment at Children's, Sadler served as vice president and director of the hospital and clinics at Scripps Clinical and Research Foundation. Sadler chairs the Child Health Accountability Initiative (CHAI), a consortium of fifteen children's hospitals dedicated to improving the quality of health of America's children. He is vice chair of the Center for Health Design and is on the National Quality Forum's steering committee on acute hospital measures. President Clinton appointed him to the U.S.-Mexico Border Health Commission, on which he still serves. Sadler has coauthored three books and has written numerous articles on quality and health care, and he speaks widely on the topic.

MICHAEL SEID, Ph.D., a research scientist and associate director for research at the Center for Child Health Outcomes, Children's Hospital and Health Center, San Diego, received his doctorate in psychology from the University of Illinois, Urbana-Champaign. His areas of expertise include measuring and improving pediatric health care quality, program evaluation, quasi-experimental methods and data analysis, the interface between managed care and child health, and research ethics. He is an expert in using real-time science to generate knowledge for operational and policy decision makers and in understanding the intersection between science and managed care in a pediatric health system. Seid has served as the chair of the Children's Hospital's Institutional Review Board, as a research consultant, and as research adviser to allied physicians and to students at San Diego State University's Graduate School of Public Health. He is on the review board of the *Journal of Clinical Outcomes Management* and has published widely in such journals as *Medical Care*, *Archives of Pediatrics and Adolescent Medicine*, *Pediatrics*, *American Journal of Medical Quality*, and *Milbank Quarterly*.

DIANA R. SIMMES, M.P.H., is a research scientist with the Center for Child Health Outcomes at Children's Hospital and Health Center, San Diego. She received her graduate degree from the Boston University School of Public Health with a concentration in health law. She is a graduate of the Maternal and Child Health Leadership Program funded by the U.S. Department of Health and Human Services' Maternal and Child Health Bureau. Her research interests include community health, maternal and child health policy formation, and design and evaluation of prevention programs, particularly programs targeted toward children and adolescents. Simmes has published in peer-reviewed journals, including the *American Journal of Public Health*, *Millbank Quarterly*, *Archives of Pediatric and Adolescent Medicine*, and *Health Affairs*. Simmes has also been an invited speaker at academic research conferences, San Diego State University, and other children's hospitals.

ERIN R. STUCKY, M.D., F.A.A.P., is a board-certified pediatrician and a practicing pediatric hospitalist at Children's Hospital and Health Center in San Diego. An active member of the National Association of Inpatient Physicians and member of the American Academy of Pediatrics National Committee on Hospital Care, Stucky serves as both physician adviser to medical staff and quality management at Children's as well as its director of education. Her duties include oversight of and educational responsibilities for pediatric and family practice residents and administrative responsibilities for fellowship programs. Stucky is involved in the facilitation and implementation of pathways and algorithms at the medical center. As medical director for children's health care management services, she interacts with health plan medical directors and over 180 primary care and specialty pediatricians. Physician education and patient advocacy are a common part of her daily activities.

JAMES W. VARNI, Ph.D., is a senior scientist at the Center for Child Health Outcomes at Children's Hospital and Health Center, San Diego, and a professor of psychiatry at the University of California, San Diego, School of Medicine. Varni is a Fellow of the American Psychological Association, the Society of Behavioral Medicine, and the Society of Pediatric Psychology and has published over 150 journal articles and book chapters in behavioral medicine and four books on children and families. He is a recipient of the Significant Research Contributions Award from the American Psychological Association. His areas of expertise are measurement instrument development, conceptual models, and cognitive–behavior therapy interventions in pediatric chronic health conditions. During the past fifteen years, he has developed and field-tested the items comprising the PedsQL 4.0 (Pediatric Quality of Life Inventory).

MIRJANA ZIVKOVIC, M.D., Ph.D., a project coordinator at the Center for Child Health Outcomes, Children Hospital and Health Center, San Diego, graduated from Belgrade University Medical

School, Belgrade, Yugoslavia, where she also earned her doctorate. Zivkovic is a health care researcher focusing on children's health, public health, and preventive approaches in general, and she has over twenty years of experience teaching medical students and mentoring graduate students in health promotion, prevention, and health education. She has coauthored or edited three books and has had numerous articles published in peer-reviewed journals such as *Medical Care*, *Quality Assurance in Health Care*, *Health Promotion International*, and *Pediatrics*.

Child Health
Services Research

Part I

Child Health Services

Setting an Accountability Agenda

1

An Introduction to Applied Child Health Services Research

Connecting Knowledge and Action

Paul S. Kurtin

This chapter introduces important trends and conceptual frameworks in the field of **child health services research (CHSR)**. Child health services range from one-child-at-a-time clinical interventions in a clinician's office to regionwide public health and social services and interventions. CHSR examines the **structure**, **processes**, and **outcomes** of health services for children (see Chapter Seven, by Seid, Sobo, Zivkovic, Nelson, and Far) for the ultimate purpose of improving the health and well-being of children.

This volume is specifically concerned with **applied child health services research**, which has a distinctly proactive purpose. The methods used in applied research, and the results of that research, have *immediate* impact on service design, delivery, and outcomes. This requires close collaboration between the investigators, the providers of services, and the end users of the research findings.

One example of applied CHSR is the collaboration, for program design and evaluation, of investigators with a community-based organization providing services for children with asthma. Another is real-time, rapid-cycle program improvement facilitated by investigators working with primary care physicians to increase immunization rates for a defined population of children.

Applied CHSR can take place in at least two different settings. Research findings can lead to actions in organizations separate, distinct, and usually distant from the researchers and the site of the research. Conversely, investigators can generate new information within the same organization that uses the findings to modify service delivery. Most organizations do not have internal applied CHSR capabilities and therefore implement findings from the work of others. Even organizations with active applied CHSR programs make use of both internally and externally derived information.

The concurrent short-cycle-time nature of the evaluations often required in this type of work presents applied CHSR with important challenges. However, we believe that rigorously designed research can be performed, even when many variables cannot be controlled, and the results can be used in real time to inform and improve the services being studied.

While the overarching goal of applied CHSR is to improve health services for children in order to improve their health and well-being, contributing to the accumulated knowledge within CHSR is also critically important. But knowledge not coupled tightly to action, whether that action consists of new policies or improved interventions, has limited ability to improve the health of children.

Complex Adaptive Systems and Applied CHSR

The modern health care industry is widely considered to be the most complex industry in America. For example, delivering the right medication to the right patient at the right time in a single hospital involves many highly trained individuals and many separate steps in several different locations. This seemingly simple yet critically important process is only one of the hundreds of complex activities routinely performed within a hospital, and a hospital is only a small part of the overall health care system providing services to children. Because of the greater availability of data, particularly at the process level, when compared to health services delivered in ambulatory primary care or specialty offices, much more applied CHSR has been undertaken in hospital settings.

In addition to being a complex system, health care can also be described as an **adaptive system.** An adaptive system is one that can learn from its environment and change its behavior based on that new knowledge (Zimmerman, Lindberg, & Plsek, 1998). The constant changes in the science, organization, and delivery of health services demonstrate the adaptability of the health care system. Some of these changes are adaptive; that is, improvements in service delivery are achieved. Other changes are maladaptive and lead to decreased effectiveness and efficiency. Many of the behaviors used by health care organizations to survive in managed care, such as the race to buy physician practices, have in fact led to the financial ruin of significant segments of the system (see Chapter Eight, by Richardson, Sobo, and Stucky).

Complex adaptive systems, such as a health care delivery system, adapt and change in order to increase their likelihood of survival (Stacey, 1996; Zimmerman et al., 1998). Survival for a health care organization can be defined as both financial stability and the ability to achieve its stated mission. Organizations survive by taking in new information, processing that information, and behaving differently due to the knowledge gained from the new information. Applied CHSR works with the system's need to do all those things. Applied CHSR can influence this evolution in organizational behavior by helping to determine how and what health services delivery systems learn. For example, applied CHSR can influence and help shape an organization's improvement efforts by adapting the science and practice of industrial quality improvement to a health care setting.

As survival increasingly hinges on the consistent delivery of high-quality services, health care organizations have much learning and adaptation to do if they are to reliably deliver services that are safe, effective, efficient, child- and family-centered, timely, and equitable (Institute of Medicine, 2001). Investigators engaged in applied CHSR can, and often do, take on the added responsibility of diffusing adaptive innovations throughout the field. Discovering effective practices and publishing results is not sufficient for improving child health. Proven, effective practices must be widely and openly shared so as to positively affect as many children and families as possible.

CHSR'S Broad Mission

Our practice of applied CHSR consists of the design, implementation, evaluation, and improvement of health services for children and families. Evaluation is the essential component of all applied CHSR. The remaining components of service design, implementation, and improvement occur in various frequencies and combinations or may not be present at all in a given project. Applied CHSR investigators and practitioners must be skilled and prepared to use all of these components.

Adding to the challenge of applied CHSR is the complexity inherent in evaluating services for children. Simply defining what services are to be evaluated can be a complex task. For example, children, depending on their age, spend a great deal of time in day care or school, often receiving some type of health services in those settings. But these same children also receive health services in private offices, community clinics, urgent care settings, or the home. Therefore, when planning an evaluation of the impact of health services on specific health outcomes, determining which sites of care and which types of caregivers are included in the evaluation will shape both the methods and the findings of the evaluation.

The fundamental models of health and disease that applied CHSR uses also present challenges to research design and implementation. While much adult-focused health services research (HSR) concerns itself with a particular physical condition or disease, CHSR uses a broad definition of health, best exemplified by the contention that health is not simply the absence of disease; it is a state of complete physical, emotional, and social well-being (World Health Organization, 1948). Such a broad definition of health is necessary because even though most children are physically well, they still have important needs, often unmet, relating to their behavioral, social, and mental health.

Such a broad definition of health makes it difficult to classify and organize outcomes of health services. The Center for Child Health Outcomes (CCHO) at Children's Hospital and Health Center, San Diego, developed and employs the Healthcare Matrix (Seid, Sadler, Peddecord, & Kurtin, 1997) to organize its approach to evaluating the outcomes of health services for children. The matrix shown in Table 1.1 contains three broad categories of health outcomes: clinical, financial, and patient-based. In contrast to clinical and financial outcomes, patient-based outcomes must be assessed by the child or family and include satisfaction, access, and functional status or health-related quality of life. These various outcomes can then be assessed in an individual child, in a group of similar children (such as children with asthma), in a defined population of patients (such as children covered by a particular managed care

Table 1.1. The Healthcare Matrix.

	Individual	Disease Group	Defined Population	Community	Employees
Financial					
Clinical					
Patient-based					

Source: From Accountability: Protecting the Well-Being of America's Children and Those Who Care for Them (p. 10), by M. Seid, B. L. Sadler, K. M. Peddecord, and P. S. Kurtin, Alexandria, VA: National Association of Children's Hospitals and Related Institutions. Copyright © 1997 by Children's Hospital, San Diego. Reprinted with permission.

contract), and in the community at large. Because children are embedded in their families and families are embedded in the community, community outcomes must often be included in an assessment of child health outcomes (see Chapter Four, by Simmes, Lim, and Dennis).

Evaluating Quality

Unfortunately, there remain significant methodological difficulties in rigorously assessing the quality of health outcomes for children. For example, what type and strength of evidence is needed to compare outcomes of different providers when so much is at stake? How does this differ from the type of evidence needed to inform quality improvement projects within an organization? The data needed to compare providers must be very strong conceptually and rigorously measured because the providers held accountable by the results will carefully scrutinize and criticize the results. The concern of providers is valid because of the difficulty in reliably and rigorously measuring quality with methods that are neither too expensive nor burdensome to implement.

Another concern for the field of CHSR is that quality for the full range of child health services has not yet been specifically defined. This makes quality in child health services hard to measure. But when quality is given a conceptual and **operational definition** (that is, when it is defined in a way that can be measured) and that definition is broadly adopted, quality can be evaluated in a manner that will influence the design and delivery of health services for children. In addition, with measures of quality that are both broadly adopted and well understood by the many stakeholders in child health care, it will be possible to adequately inform the choices of purchasers, payers, and consumers. Perhaps most important, with broadly adopted and well-understood quality measures, it is possible to hold providers accountable for their performance. Local improvement efforts, such as at the single clinic or hospital level, can be successful with local definitions of quality. Likewise, all stakeholders in large-scale, communitywide improvement efforts must agree on specific operational definitions of quality to be successful in achieving their goals.

Using Measures to Inform Improvements

Despite the many difficulties, over the past several years, frameworks for quality assessment and specific measures of quality have been established in child health—for example, the Foundation for Accountability, or FACCT (Lansky, 1996), and the Health Plan Employer Data Information Set, or HEDIS (Kuhlthau et al., 1998). While the work of developing quality measures for the full spectrum of child health services is certainly not complete, there is an emerging shift in the focus of applied CHSR from developing appropriate, reliable measures to *using* those measures to inform improvement efforts. This shift, which is new to health care, acknowledges the difference between measures used for accountability and measures used for improvement. The skills, tools, and conceptual approaches needed for health service improvement are being adapted from fields outside of health care, such as the manufacturing and service industries (Berwick, 1996). These approaches to improvement have provided new methods for applied CHSR to shape the delivery of child health services.

Four Challenges

Four significant challenges face health care service delivery:

1. Unnecessary variation (Wennberg, Freeman, Shelton, & Bubolz, 1989)

2. The gap between knowledge and practice (Forrest, Simpson, & Clancy, 1997)

3. The need for systems thinking (Batalden & Mohr, 1997; Institute of Medicine, 2001)

4. Patient safety (Kohn, Corrigan, & Donaldson, 1999)

These challenges have, in many ways, resulted from HSR efforts to identify and document important shortcomings in the provision of health care. The tools and techniques of applied CHSR will be pivotal in addressing these problems.

Almost twenty years of HSR has substantiated the first challenge facing health care, **unnecessary variation,** which means variation in the care of patients with similar conditions that is not due to patient need or preference or science but rather to provider preference and habit. This variation is found between regions of the country (Wennberg et al., 1989), as well as between individual physicians practicing in a single hospital (Kurtin, Richardson, Seid, & Sadler, 2002). Decades of work in the field of industrial quality improvement have shown that unnecessary variation leads to higher costs and lower quality (Deming, 1982/2000). This results in customers (patients) and payers, either commercial insurers or the government, receiving lower value for their health care dollars.

Second is the gap between knowledge and practice, including the gap between best practice and usual practice. The vast majority of routine medical care is not based on rigorous medical science but rather on personal experience, personal discretion, and anecdotes. Unfortunately, even when evidence regarding the most effective practices does exist, clinical guidelines based on that evidence are often not followed (Flores, Lee, Bauchner, & Kastner, 2000). This gap contributes significantly to unnecessary practice variation and is an important contributing factor in the delivery of services that are less than maximally effective.

Third is the need for **systems thinking**. Thinking in terms of processes or systems is essential in health care because no single individual or institution acting alone can provide consistently high-quality services throughout the entire continuum of care. This is especially true for pediatric patients because they receive health services in such unusual sites as the home or school and from a variety of fragmented and uncoordinated programs and providers. Health care services must be designed, implemented, evaluated, and improved with a systems perspective that recognizes the needs and contributions of the many stakeholders in health care and the systems that create it (Institute of Medicine, 2001).

At the level of an organization, systems thinking means creating and providing services based on an understanding of the interrelationships and interactions of its many processes and providers in meeting the needs of its customers. In an organization, a particular group of providers, with their associated technology, information resources, and work processes directed toward meeting all the needs of a group of patients or clients, can be considered a **microsystem** (Nelson et al., 2000). A microsystem can be used as the unit of analysis and improvement for the delivery of health services.

For the individual provider, systems thinking requires shifting the focus from one patient at a time to groups of similar patients. This allows the provider to obtain better and more generalizable outcomes information in order to change practice, if necessary. Systems thinking requires the provider to evaluate his or her own practices and decide how best to deliver care for all patients with similar conditions. Providers must individually take on the task of improving the access to and quality of the services they provide to their patients. This approach forms an intersection between one-patient-at-a-time clinical medicine and population health. It challenges individual providers to develop consistent, effective, and efficient practices for the population of patients they care for.

The fourth challenge is patient safety. The recent Institute of Medicine report *To Err Is Human* (Kohn et al., 1999) clearly demonstrated the need to make safety a fundamental property of the health care system. Systems thinking teaches that safety, like quality, cannot be added onto a process as an afterthought but must be designed and built into the fabric of the process itself. Unnecessary variation within a process, as just described, may exacerbate any tendency toward error. *To Err Is Human* is a national call to action to significantly improve patient safety, first within hospitals and then throughout the continuum of care.

These four challenges to the current health care system are, in large measure, due to increasing demands for demonstrable high-quality, high-value health care from purchasers, payers, and consumers. The Institute of Medicine report *Crossing the Quality Chasm* (2001) offers multiple suggestions for the kinds of transformational changes needed throughout the health care system if we are to dramatically improve health care for all U.S. residents, children included.

What Is Quality Health Care?

In *Crossing the Quality Chasm*, the Institute of Medicine (2001) proposes to begin this transformation by instituting a new and very broad definition for quality health care. As noted earlier, according to this definition, quality health care has six dimensions: it is (1) safe, (2) effective, (3) efficient, (4) patient-centered, (5) timely, and (6) equitable. Further, quality care must be customized, with the needs and preferences of the patient and family placed first, and quality care must actively engage those who are served. That is, care decisions should not be left only to clinicians to make; patients and families should be encouraged to share decision-making responsibilities to the degree they wish to be involved.

Crossing the Quality Chasm also stresses the need for new and more effective ways to implement the necessary improvements to make this type of quality a reality. Lessons learned by individuals and organizations in improving the quality and safety of health care must be quickly and efficiently disseminated in ways that dramatically increase provider and consumer participation as well as significantly decrease time to adoption. Applied CHSR must now include in its toolbox reliable methods to rapidly share and effectively diffuse best practices (Rogers, 1995).

Innovation and Dissemination

One approach to the rapid spreading of best practices is the use of collaboratives such as the Child Health Accountability Initiative (CHAI), a group of fourteen children's hospitals collaborating to improve health care for hospitalized children. CHAI was created in October 1997 to focus attention on the quality of care of hospitalized children and children with special health care needs (Kurtin, Sadler, Payne, & Bates, 2001). These populations of vulnerable children were usually not included in other national efforts to define and improve quality of care for children.

There are several other examples of groups collaborating to improve child health. These include the American Academy of Pediatrics' Pediatric Research in the Office Setting group, the Vermont-Oxford Neonatal Network, the National Initiative for Child Health Quality, and the many groups of providers working on quality and process improvements in short-term collaboratives such as those organized as part of the Institute for Healthcare Improvement's Breakthrough Series. Each of these collaboratives has reported advances in improving health care for children (Bocian, Wasserman, Slora, Kessel, & Miller, 1999; Gardner et al., 2000; Homer, Kleinman, & Goldman, 1998; Horbar, 1995).

As with CHAI, many of these child-focused collaboratives were organized in response to the lack of knowledge on how best to design and deliver high-quality services to children in specific settings such as the neonatal intensive care unit or the private pediatrician's office. This lack of evidence on the effectiveness of child health services also presents barriers to providers of complex pediatric care who are hoping to compete in the marketplace by stressing the quality of the services they provide. For example, children's hospitals and university pediatric programs perform the vast majority of pediatric tertiary care in the United States. However, these sites are also among the most expensive, due to the large amount and wide range of resources needed to care for children of different sizes (from a 1-kg premature infant to a 100-kg adolescent) who present with a large number of relatively rare conditions. Because there are no widely accepted measures of quality for the work done in these specialized sites, the quality of the services provided is difficult to assess. Families often use an organization's local reputation or a recommendation from a friend as surrogate measures in defining a presumed level of quality (Sobo, 2001). It is also easy for payers to assume (and hard to prove otherwise) that quality of care for these conditions is fairly similar among different providers. Because **value** equals *quality per unit cost*, quality is assumed to be equal and held constant among providers, and so the debate between providers and payers over value gives way to a debate over cost. The way for providers to increase their value to payers is then limited to lowering the price of their services. Thus it has been in provider organizations' best interests to form collaboratives in order to develop quality measures and add quality to the value equation.

The Development of CHSR Units Within Organizations

The inability of local and national organizations to define quality and shift the debate toward true value is now coupled with a national demand for **accountability** (Seid et al., 1997). Accountability has become a popular theme in many U.S. business circles. Although the locus of accountability in health care is not clearly defined, consumers, purchasers, and payers for health care services expect it of providers; that is, they expect providers to be able to document the quality of their outcomes with quantifiable and eventually comparable measures. Against this background of increasing demand for accountability, documentation, and improvement in the quality of services, a number of health care organizations have instituted CHSR units. For example, it was this new emphasis on accountability that led Children's Hospital and Health Center in San Diego to establish the Center for Child Health Outcomes (CCHO).

CCHO was conceived as an *applied* CHSR team. That is, like the collaboratives, its goal was to conduct research that directly led to the improvement of health care quality for children served by Children's and its affiliated physicians. Also, like the collaboratives, one of the first tasks faced by CCHO members was to improve the field's tools for quality measurement (some examples are provided in the chapters that follow).

CCHO's first and overarching objective is to help evaluate, design, and improve health services provided by its parent organization. Children's, along with its affiliated medical groups and wide-ranging partnerships, is a natural laboratory for conducting and implementing its own applied health services research as well as applying the research findings of others. CCHO's second objective is to inform consumers and payers on the quality of services provided by Children's and its affiliated physicians. CCHO's third objective is to influence public policy and the practice of pediatrics by sharing its work widely with the field, and its fourth objective is to train future practitioners in the science and practice of quality improvement.

Connections to the Organization

As the need for health care organizations to demonstrably and continuously improve the clinical and financial quality of their performance has grown, a number of models linking organizations with applied CHSR have developed. An important distinction in these models is the degree of connection, if any, between applied CHSR investigators and the day-to-day operations of the organization. CCHO depends on a very close, interactive, iterative relationship with the organization's daily operations. CCHO produces research that is immediately applied; it is conceived as applied from the outset. Other centers are based on a more academic model, in which acting on research results by the parent organization occurs rarely, if at all. Such centers are only loosely connected to their organizations' operations.

Although these models have been in existence for only a few years, early experience suggests that a CHSR unit's ability to affect the quality and nature of health services provided is highly dependent on the closeness of the connection between investigators and front-line operations. In other words, the more directly applied the focus of the research and the more relevance the work is perceived to have by the organization, the more likely the research findings will be incorporated into organizational practice.

Demonstrating CHSR's Value to Organizations

To advance an outcomes and quality improvement agenda throughout the organization, it is critical that an applied CHSR unit demonstrate the value of its work to the various groups of internal stakeholders. At Children's, organizational support grew over time as the research findings of CCHO helped produce sustained improvements in both clinical and financial outcomes. Although clinical quality and social justice are important motivators of much applied CHSR, the bottom line, as demonstrated by cost savings, is a crucial factor when soliciting organizational backing or the support of external grantmaking institutions.

The foundation of CCHO's effort to build support relies on the approach the group has taken toward the science and methods of health services research and quality improvement. The development, implementation, evaluation, and ongoing improvement of **clinical pathways** (see Chapter Eight, by Richardson, Sobo, and Stucky) became the initial means to achieve the goal of improving both clinical and financial outcomes. Pathways also became the means for addressing and reducing both unnecessary variation in care and the gap between knowledge and routine practice. Because pathways are developed using an interdisciplinary approach that takes into account the complexity of health care processes, pathways also help acculturate staff to the systems approach to health care improvement.

Physicians are key stakeholders in any health care organization. In our experience, before physicians will change their practices and adhere to practice guidelines or pathways, they need to understand the health services science behind the pathways, and they need concrete demonstrations that these pathways do improve the care of hospitalized children. For example, the first concept presented to the physicians by CCHO, and supported by internal data, was that great variation in practice existed between and among the physicians caring for similar children and that this variation was driven not by patient need but rather by physician preference and habit. The second concept presented to the physicians and documented with internal data was that there is a substantial disparity between actual practice and what the evidence shows is best practice. The majority of physicians did not follow national practice guidelines, even when these guidelines were created by their own professional societies.

The third concept presented to the physicians was that of clinical **epidemiology** and population health. The physicians were asked to consider several hundred children with asthma as a group rather than to take the one-child-at-a-time approach of routine clinical care. This helped physicians think beyond their own personal preferences and what worked for them (or what they thought worked for them) to appreciate the positive impact that routinized processes of care, when standardized to excellence, could have for all children with a given condition.

The final concept presented to the physicians came from the field of quality improvement and the work of W. Edwards Deming, Joseph M. Juran, and others (Deming, 1982/2000). These applied quality improvement pioneers demonstrated that unnecessary variation in a process leads to two outcomes: higher costs and poorer quality. If variation could be reduced, quality would improve and costs would decrease. This is exactly what was found to occur by CCHO; pathways based on the best available medical evidence reduced unnecessary variation in care, decreased the costs of care, and improved clinical outcomes (see Chapter Eight, by Richardson, Sobo, and Stucky). Due to our pathways work, Children's received the 2002 Ernest A. Codman Award from the Joint Commission on Accreditation of Healthcare Organizations for demonstrating excellence in using outcomes measurement to improve the quality of care.

The overwhelming success of our Pathways Program, as evidenced by eight years of improved quality with reduced costs of care, has helped transform the culture of patient care here at Children's. CCHO's performance improvement record at Children's confirms that an organization can actively seek out and apply the results of

CHSR within its own walls. However, the vast majority of organizations are without internal, applied CHSR capability and must find and apply research results from the outside. By seeking such new information, each organization, being a complex, adaptive system, acquires new knowledge and changes its behavior to enhance its ability to survive and thrive as a health services delivery organization.

It is important to note that this work has taken place primarily in the inpatient setting and in selected specialty clinics. However, the same type of improvement initiative can occur in primary care offices (Bocian et al., 1999; Gardner et al., 2000). Often, in fact, improvement in offices is dependent on improvement in the larger systems they are part of, as with the provision of expensive information technology. Office sites are often too resource-constrained, with inadequate information technology and inadequate staff time, knowledge, and skills to appropriately evaluate their current practices and improve as needed. With the coming changes in residency training that include providing the knowledge and skills needed to evaluate and improve one's own practice (Chesney, 2001), the relatively unmet need to improve care in ambulatory settings will, we hope, begin to be addressed.

CHSR's Methodological Orientation

Working on improvement projects within an organization or on behalf of an organization requires a mixed approach of both qualitative and quantitative methods. The methods selected are dependent not only on the questions asked but also on time constraints. As in international health, which has a long history of rapid method implementation (Nichter & Nichter, 1996; Pelto & Pelto, 1997), applied CHSR has short timelines with multiple and diverse audiences requiring regular communications. The methods used in applied CHSR will also depend on the ultimate use of the obtained information (for example, for internal improvement or for marketplace comparisons of different providers). Because all CHSR methods are heavily dependent on appropriate data and information, which is much more readily available in inpatient settings than in ambulatory settings, it is currently easier to change inpatient care than to change ambulatory care.

Rapid-Cycle Improvement

One method frequently used in CCHO is called **rapid-cycle improvement**. The utility of sequential cycles of improvement has been well described by Tom Nolan and others (see Berwick & Nolan, 1998). Nolan's fundamental improvement method, called **plan, do, study, act (PDSA),** has been modified to fulfill a more rapid-cycle approach emphasizing the importance of thoughtful, quick, incremental improvements.

CCHO has further refined the rapid-cycle approach by adding routine reality checks. If the goals of improvement become too internally focused—that is, if they are of importance to internal audiences but not the marketplace—an organization can become better at things that may not matter and miss opportunities to improve other, more relevant processes. This suboptimization of a process or even of an entire organization can have devastating costs by focusing the organization on the wrong things. In a rapidly shifting marketplace like that of health care, regular checks relating one's work to the real world must be used to shape research design and methods as well as to help in the selection of findings for application. For example, designing care models for a prepayment, capitation model of reimbursement will suboptimize reimbursement if the primary method of reimbursement is fee-for-service or per diem payments.

Applying CHSR in the Real World, in Real Time

Linking applied research to improvement requires a multifaceted, nimble, interdisciplinary team that has the capacity to employ a variety of methods and has the desire to collaborate closely with the end users of the research findings. This requires an explicit acknowledgment of the identity of the end user and how, if at all, the findings are to be applied. This is true whether the findings are to support business decisions in an organization or the policy decisions of local or national governments.

Due to time constraints or the inability to control most variables, the types of research designs needed to improve or make business decisions are often different from those needed to compare providers or prove hypotheses in the usual scientific sense. The health services marketplace does not give time for multiyear randomized controlled trials such as those used to establish the efficacy of a specific medication or intervention. The marketplace does understand, however, rigorous annotated time-series or quasi-experimental designs that suggest, yet may not prove, causality.

Ultimately, applied CHSR seeks information to help answer questions such as these: What are the real-world ramifications of the results of the services being investigated? Is the implementation of recommendations based on the findings even feasible? Will the research questions being asked provide answers that can be used to modify service delivery and organizational thinking? Or will the organization review the findings and say "So what?" because the findings have no obvious operational value? Without answering such questions prior to beginning the investigation, research findings can rarely be applied in real time.

Making the Business Case for Quality

No matter how good the science, important the findings, or responsive the investigators, applied CHSR units cannot expect long-term, ongoing organizational support if no business case is made for keeping them. The inability of an organization to make a business case for quality is one of the biggest impediments to organizational investment in quality improvement (Bringewatt, 2001; Coye, 2001; Galvin, 2001). In today's health care marketplace, with its current reimbursement mechanisms, much of the financial benefit accruing from a provider's quality improvement efforts reverts to the payer and does not benefit the provider. For example, when Children's asthma disease management program significantly reduced emergency department visits and hospital days for children with severe asthma, income was lost due to the decrease in patient days that would have been reimbursed on a per diem or fee-for-service basis. The financial savings went to the payers. The actual financial benefit to providers resulting from their quality improvement work depends on the mechanisms of payment. For example, a provider reimbursed via prepaid capitation will benefit financially by reducing unnecessary utilization, whereas a provider paid via a fee-for-service plan will not. But at least in theory, providers of high-quality care will ultimately benefit by attracting a larger market share.

However, this vision of purchasers and consumers shifting their business to high-quality providers has not yet occurred (Robinson, 2001). Whether payers and consumers do not really understand the types of quality outcome data they are given or whether consumers use other measures (such as personal references) to choose providers, the shift to quality providers has been slow and uneven around the country.

To speed up the public's embrace of the quality agenda, purchasing coalitions such as the Pacific Business Group on Health or the Washington Business Group on Health use quality measures to compare providers. These large health care purchasing groups have also proposed incentives for high-quality providers (Milstein, 1998). The full impact of these efforts remains to be seen.

Because health care in the United States is fundamentally a local or regional business, providers must develop individual strategies to attract business on the basis of demonstrated quality. In CCHO's local marketplace experience, the regular and routine presentation of outcomes data (CCHO's second objective) to purchasers and adult-focused medical groups, highlighting the quality of Children's programs, has been very successful. This is evidenced by Children's significant increase in market share over the past several years.

Maintaining an Applied CHSR Focus

Informing the regional managed care marketplace of the outcomes of services at Children's and of how those services have improved over time expanded the audience for the types of information generated and communicated by CCHO. Even as the areas of child health in which CCHO works have extended beyond the boundaries of Children's to include regional, statewide, and national health services for children, two practices remain firm. First, the prime objective of improving organizational performance in order to improve the quality and value of its services is always given priority within CCHO; the organization's goals are always the first to be met, and CCHO's close connection to the organization is maintained. Second, CCHO remains committed to the approach of applying the results of its investigations firsthand with close collaborators and partners, both inside and outside Children's.

In the rapidly changing, complex, and competitive world of health care, where organizations struggle to survive and thrive, CCHO tries to keep in mind the advice of Albert Einstein: "Out of clutter find simplicity; from discord, make harmony; in the middle of difficulty lies opportunity." These three rules for work represent a worldview from which all who would productively engage in applied CHSR might benefit.

References

Batalden, P. B., & Mohr, J. J. (1997). Building knowledge of health care as a system. *Quality Management in Health Care, 5*(3), 1–12.

Berwick, D. M. (1996). A primer on leading the improvement of systems. *British Medical Journal, 312,* 619–622.

Berwick, D. M., & Nolan, T. W. (1998). Physicians as leaders in improving health care: A new series in *Annals of Internal Medicine. Annals of Internal Medicine, 128,* 289–292.

Bocian, A. B., Wasserman, R. C., Slora, E. J., Kessel, D., & Miller, R. S. (1999). Size and age-sex distribution of pediatric practice: A study from Pediatric

Research in Office Settings. *Archives of Pediatric and Adolescent Medicine*, 153, 9–14.

Bringewatt, R. J. (2001). Making a business case for high-quality chronic illness care. *Health Affairs* (Millwood), 20(6), 59–60.

Chesney, R. W. (2001). Joseph W. St. Geme Jr. Address, 2001: Can one have a successful academic career in 2001? *Pediatrics*, 108, 1349–1352.

Coye, M. J. (2001). No Toyotas in health care: Why medical care has not evolved to meet patients' needs. *Health Affairs* (Millwood), 20(6), 44–56.

Deming, W. E. (2000). *Out of the crisis: Quality, productivity, and competitive position*. Cambridge, MA: MIT Press. (Original work published 1982)

Flores, G., Lee, M., Bauchner, H., & Kastner, B. (2000). Pediatricians' attitudes, beliefs, and practices regarding clinical practice guidelines: A national survey. *Pediatrics*, 105, 496–501.

Forrest, C. B., Simpson, L., & Clancy, C. (1997). Child health services research: Challenges and opportunities. *Journal of the American Medical Association*, 277, 1787–1793.

Galvin, R. S. (2001). The business case for quality. *Health Affairs* (Millwood), 20(6), 57–58.

Gardner, W., Kellcher, K. J., Wasserman, R., Childs, G., Nutting, P., Lillienfeld, H., & Pajer, K. (2000). Primary care treatment of pediatric psychosocial problems: A study from pediatric research in office settings and ambulatory sentinel practice network. *Pediatrics*, 106, E44.

Homer, C. J., Kleinman, L. C., & Goldman, D. A. (1998). Improving the quality of care for children in health systems. *Health Services Research*, 33, 1091–1109.

Horbar, J. D. (1995). The Vermont-Oxford Neonatal Network: Integrating research and clinical practice to improve the quality of medical care. *Seminars in Perinatology*, 19, 124–131.

Institute of Medicine, Committee on Quality of Health Care in America. (2001). *Crossing the quality chasm: A new health system for the 21st century*. Washington, DC: National Academy Press.

Kohn, L. T., Corrigan, J. M., & Donaldson, M. S. (Eds.). (1999). *To err is human: Building a safer health system*. Washington, DC: National Academy Press.

Kuhlthau, K., Walker, D. K., Perrin, J. M., Bauman, L., Gortmaker, S. L., Newacheck, P. W., & Stein, R. E. (1998). Assessing managed care for children with chronic conditions. *Health Affairs* (Millwood), 17(4), 42–52.

Kurtin, P. S., Richardson, P. J., Seid, M., & Sadler, B. L. (2002). *Clinical pathways:*

A quality improvement initiative to provide optimal care. Unpublished manuscript.

Kurtin, P. S., Sadler, B. L., Payne, D., & Bates, J. (2001). Children's hospitals collaborate to improve quality of care. *Journal for Healthcare Quality, 23*, 28–32.

Lansky, D. (1996). The facts about FACCT (Foundation for Accountability). *Clinical Performance and Quality Health Care, 4*, 211–212.

Milstein, A. (1998). Bringing outcome-based quality differentiation to the physician group market. *Medical Outcomes Trust Monitor, 3*(1), 9–11.

Nelson, E. C., Splaine, M. E., Godfrey, M. M., Kahn, V., Hess, A., Batalden, P. B., & Plume, S. K. (2000). Using data to improve medical practice by measuring processes and outcomes of care. *Joint Commission Journal on Quality Improvement, 26*, 667–685.

Nichter, M., & Nichter, M. (1996). *Anthropology and international health*. Amsterdam: Gordon & Breach.

Pelto, P. J., & Pelto, G. H. (1997). Studying knowledge, culture, and behavior in applied medical anthropology. *Medical Anthropology Quarterly, 11*, 147–163.

Robinson, J. C. (2001). The end of managed care. *Journal of the American Medical Association, 285*, 2622–2628.

Rogers, E. M. (1995). *Diffusion of innovations* (4th ed.). New York: Free Press.

Seid, M., Sadler, B. L., Peddecord, K. M., & Kurtin, P. S. (1997). *Accountability: Protecting the well-being of America's children and those who care for them*. Alexandria, VA: National Association of Children's Hospitals and Related Institutions.

Sobo, E. J. (2001). Rationalization of medical risk through talk of trust: An exploration of elective eye surgery narratives. *Anthropology and Medicine, 8*, 265–278.

Stacey, R. D. (1996). *Complexity and creativity in organizations*. San Francisco: Berrett-Koehler.

Wennberg, J. E., Freeman, J. L., Shelton, R. M., & Bubolz, T. A. (1989). Hospital use and mortality among Medicare beneficiaries in Boston and New Haven. *New England Journal of Medicine, 321*, 1168–1173.

World Health Organization. (1948). *Constitution of the World Health Organization*. Geneva: Author.

Zimmerman, B., Lindberg, C., & Plsek, P. (1998). *Edgeware: Insights from complexity science for health care leaders*. Irving, TX: VHA.

2

Laying the Foundation

Identifying Major Issues in Applied Child Health Services Research

Pradeep Gidwani, Elisa J. Sobo,
Michael Seid, Paul S. Kurtin

The Institute of Medicine (Field et al., 1995) defines **health services research (HSR)** as a "multidisciplinary field of inquiry that examines the use, costs, quality, accessibility, delivery, organization, financing, and outcomes of health care services to increase the knowledge and understanding of the structure, process, and effects of health services for individual and populations" (p. 17). As such, HSR plays a critical role in assessing, documenting, explaining, and ultimately improving the quality of health care. This ultimate improvement is accomplished through applied HSR, which affects the health care provision, payment, and policy arrangements that shape patient care (see Chapter One, by Kurtin).

Although HSR exists in many countries, including the United Kingdom and Australia, our focus is on efforts in outcomes research and health care oversight in the United States. It describes the formal inception of the HSR field, traces the development of the **child health services research (CHSR)** subfield, and identifies major issues in this subfield's agenda in the United States.

Health Services Research: Early Efforts

Examples of HSR efforts can be found throughout history. Cotton Mather and Benjamin Franklin might have been the first health services researchers in the United States. Their initial forays in the field took place in the 1720s, when smallpox infection reached epidemic status. In cities such as Boston, half of all residents were infected with the disease. Inoculation—the introduction of a small amount of dried matter from a smallpox patient's lesion into a small cut in the skin of an unaffected individual—caused a mild case of the disease. However, physicians of the time were against inoculation, which they considered a dangerous and unproven technique (King, 1993).

Cotton Mather, a Puritan preacher in Boston, advocated for the procedure (even inoculating his own son, Samuel) and for the compilation of outcome statistics. These results showed that five to twenty times as many individuals who did not receive inoculation died from smallpox as individuals who received inoculations. Mather's views were so strongly opposed by the citizens of Boston that he received death threats (Mather, 1911–1912).

In Philadelphia, after his own son, who was not inoculated, died of smallpox, Benjamin Franklin expanded Mather's work on the outcomes of inoculation. Franklin tracked the successes and failures of the smallpox inoculation not just in Philadelphia but throughout the North American colonies. In 1759, Franklin and William Heberden, an English physician, wrote *Some Accounts of the Success of Inoculation for the Small-Pox in England and America*. This pamphlet, aimed at both physicians and the public, used outcomes data to support the idea of smallpox inoculation (King, 1993).

Overcoming strong initial resistance, Mather's and Franklin's evidence and actions eventually led to widespread acceptance of inoculation and improved general health. Their efforts may even have had an impact on the outcome of the Revolutionary War: U.S. soldiers suffered fewer deaths from smallpox than the British soldiers, who were less frequently inoculated. The work of Mather and

Franklin was evidence that reason, systematic observation, and statistical compilation can serve as a means to controlling disease (King, 1993).

Although Mather and Franklin are among the first U.S. HSR investigators, the physician Ernest A. Codman is most often cited as the founder of modern outcomes assessment in the United States. During the early twentieth century, Codman systematically tracked the outcomes of patient treatments, with the goal of using results to improve the care of future patients. He called his approach the "end result idea," explaining this approach as "the common sense notion that every hospital should follow every patient it treats, long enough to determine whether or not the treatment has been successful, and then to inquire 'if not, why not?' with a view of preventing similar failures in the future" (Codman, 1934, p. vi). He also believed that outcomes data should be made public so that patients interested in what modern medicine could offer might use the data to guide their choices of physicians and hospitals (Codman, 1914).

Like Mather and Franklin, Codman used reason, systematic observation, and statistical compilation to guide his efforts, but he focused on the delivery of medical services in the hospital setting. Also like Mather and Franklin, Codman's work was not immediately appreciated. Once a prominent surgeon on the staff of the Massachusetts General Hospital, he was forced to establish his own hospital so that he could freely pursue performance measurement and outcome improvement work. His hospital was successful until the First World War, when Codman left his hospital to serve as senior surgeon in Delaware. When he returned to Boston in June 1919, he found his hospital closed and in debt, and he was unable to borrow the money to reopen it (Kaska & Weinstein, 1998).

Trends in the Oversight of Health Care

Until recently, seeking professional biomedical care involved a highly calculated risk: even though several states eventually passed perfunctory licensing laws, "in 1846 almost any man with an elementary education could take a course of lectures for one or two winters, pass an examination and thereby automatically achieve the right to practice medicine by state law" (Shryock, 1966, p. 152). Due in part to the overproduction of physicians in a variety of poorly run proprietary medical schools and in part because science had not yet progressed as far as it has now, few people had much faith in physicians' abilities.

Standardization of Biomedical Education and Hospitals

At the same time as Codman was studying patient outcomes, the biomedical community began an emphasis on standards for medical education, licensure, and certification. By 1904, the American Medical Association (AMA) had created the Council of Medical Education, which surveyed and rated the nation's schools. The concern for the quality of U.S. medical education prompted the Carnegie Foundation to commission Abraham Flexner, an administrator and educator, to conduct a comprehensive independent study of the nation's medical schools. Published in 1910 as *Medical Education in the United States and Canada,* the Flexner Report revealed the discrepancies between school catalogue descriptions of courses, clinical opportunities, and the realities of medical training in individual medical schools throughout the nation. Flexner argued to remove medical education from the control of practitioners and place it within the structure of U.S. universities, and he advocated for the closure of substandard schools. The Flexner Report led to the reform of medical education and paved the way for state licensure boards for physicians and other health care professionals.

During the 1930s, in addition to the standardization of medical education and licensure, the leaders of the American College of Surgeons (including Ernest Codman) developed the Hospital Standards program—the forerunner of the Joint Commission on Healthcare Organizations (JCAHO). Over time, the JCAHO, as well as case law and Medicare regulations, led to the development of state agencies to license hospital and professional organizations and governmental agencies to ensure that minimal quality standards were met. Until the 1960s, the medical system was regulated through standardization of training and hospital facilities.

Quality Standards and Measurement

The federal government's role in health care was greatly expanded with the enactment of Medicare and Medicaid in 1965. Medicare originally provided health care coverage to Americans over the age of sixty-five, while Medicaid, a joint federal-state program, provides health care coverage to low-income families with children under twenty-one. The Medicare and Medicaid legislation fueled a rapid growth in access to care, number and types of health care facilities, physician specialization and training programs, the development of a myriad of allied health specialties, and medical technology. In order to more effectively monitor this rapidly changing system, it was necessary to move beyond simply identifying who provided care and in what settings to assess how care was actually delivered (Kessner, Kalk, & Singer, 1973; Starfield & Scheff, 1972; Williamson & Wilson, 1978).

During the 1960s and 1970s, the evaluation of how care was delivered was primarily through informal review by professional peers. Subsequently, techniques such as medical audits were developed to determine if accepted standards were met (Waldman, 1973). In a medical audit, a medical chart is reviewed by a medical professional who checks to see if specific actions have been documented. Most audits focused on very well-defined hospital procedures (such as an appendectomy). This evaluation of process was an adaptation of quality control methods that had been used in manufacturing industries since the 1930s (Deming, 1982/2000).

During the 1970s and 1980s, many industries in the United States, such as the auto industry, faced international competition that forced them to undertake radical improvements in quality while also lowering costs. They had embraced total quality management

(TQM) or **continuous quality improvement (CQI)** philosophies and tools in the 1970s. The philosophy of continuous quality improvement is data-driven, taking a scientific approach to quality improvement. Large corporations began using data to guide their decision making in all facets of business, including health care expenditures. Data-driven decision making focuses on decreasing unnecessary variation, thus leading to improvements in quality while reducing costs.

In response to increased interest in data-driven decision making, the federal government attempted to provide outcome information for consumers and purchasers. In 1986, it began publishing its highly controversial Medicare hospital death rates. Many health care providers immediately attacked the validity of the mortality data (Berwick & Wald, 1990). For example, one of the organizations lambasted in the first report for such high mortality rates was actually a hospice in Nevada. Although health care providers were resistant to reports of outcome information, they foresaw the pivotal role that outcomes data, whether clinical, financial, or patient-based, might play in their future.

Health care providers are often resistant to outcome measurements because such measures do not account for differences in individual patients' illness severity and other risk factors such as comorbidity. The Medicare hospital death rates have led to patient risk adjustment. **Risk adjustment** is a method to systematically modify data in order to better compare the outcomes of patients with differing levels of illness severity. Risk adjustment mathematically levels the playing field, providing clinicians with meaningful comparisons of outcomes such as mortality or length of stay for groups of patients that might otherwise not be comparable (Iezzoni, Ayanian, Bates, & Burstin, 1998). However, risk adjustment methods are controversial, and the link between risk adjustment and reimbursement for services heightens this controversy.

Throughout the 1980s and most of the 1990s, the cost of health care continued to spiral upward, and contracts for health services went overwhelmingly to the low-cost provider, with managed care emerging as a dominant cost containment strategy (see Chapter Eight, by Richardson, Sobo, and Stucky). The government, purchasers, and consumers began demanding both cost containment and more information on performance. Aggressive business cooperatives such as the California Public Employee Retirement System (CalPERS) began requiring increasing amounts of information on the costs and nature of many of the health care services they purchased for their employees (Brennan & Berwick, 1996).

Large national employers were made aware of marked regional variations in both the costs of care and the clinical outcomes of care for their employees (Wennberg, Freeman, Shelton, & Bubolz, 1989). These employers began to hold providers accountable for the costs and quality of care they were purchasing. As stockholders and boards held CEOs accountable for costs and profits, senior management in turn demanded accountability for one of the most expensive costs, health benefits (Milstein, 1997). In effect, this meant a shift to considering the overall value of the services provided. **Value** can be defined as quality per unit of cost. High value can therefore be delivered by maintaining quality while lowering costs or by improving quality at the same or lower costs. However, before a valid comparison of quality between health plans could occur, a common set of quality and performance measures or **indicators** was needed.

Employer purchasing collaboratives and health care plans tend to be concerned about population-based measures of quality and organizational performance. This common concern has resulted in cooperative efforts, through the National Committee for Quality Assurance (NCQA) and other groups, to develop standard measures that can be used by purchasers to compare the performance of health care plans and the providers. These measures could then be used to accredit providers and to compare quality between providers. The latter information would, in theory, be useful to employers and consumers making health care purchasing decisions.

NCQA, a private, not-for-profit organization, was established in 1990 with support from the Robert Wood Johnson Foundation. NCQA requires health care plans seeking accreditation to provide an extensive list of performance measures (National Committee for Quality Assurance, 1993). For example, NCQA manages and continues to develop the Health Employers Data and Information Set (HEDIS), a set of indicators for measuring how well health plans achieve patient satisfaction, provide access to care, and deliver a wide variety of well-accepted preventive, ambulatory, and disease management services. HEDIS is designed to permit purchasers and consumers to make valid comparisons across health plans. Employers may distribute these performance measures directly to employees on report cards that provide information to employees making their choice of health plans during open enrollment periods.

The Foundation for Accountability (FACCT), a nonprofit organization, was founded in 1995 to provide the consumer's perspective on health care plans and has been developing health care measures for clinical conditions and outcomes. The federal government has also sponsored activities to monitor health plans and provide the consumer's perspective. One example is the Consumer Assessment of Health Plans Study (CAHPS), sponsored by the Agency for Healthcare Research and Quality (AHRQ) (2001). CAHPS is a survey tool used to assess consumer experience in health plans. CAHPS developers hope that patient-centered measures can be used along with other process and outcome measures to help inform patients and purchasers.

In summary, as health care has grown more complex, multiple public and private organizations have been involved in assessing health services. The demand for more performance information has been met with resistance. However, although public and private organizations have worked together, duplication of efforts and gaps in measurement continue to exist. Much like the health care system itself, information from the various efforts remains fragmented and incomplete.

Health Services Research: Inception of the Field

Research in the area of health care delivery is nothing new. However, the codification of theories and methodological discussions under the rubric of health services research is a relatively recent development in the United States, traced by McCarthy and White (2000) to the middle of the twentieth century. U.S. HSR, they argue, emerged in 1960 as the result of a merger of the Public Health Research and Hospital Facilities Research study sections of the National Institutes of Health. A series of fourteen papers was commissioned, and these papers defined the field as it stood at that time. They were published together as a book-length volume in 1966 (Mainland, 1966).

About the same time (1965), the Hospital Research and Educational Trust was considering topics around which to organize a journal. It eventually agreed to sponsor the journal *Health Services Research,* which is in its thirty-seventh year. The journal's inception contributed greatly to the development of the HSR field, providing a medium for disseminating information to colleagues and serving as a symbol of the field's scholarly legitimacy.

HSR got another boost from the expansion of health care programs such as Medicare and Medicaid. Interest in health care utilization, cost, and variations in services grew at a faster rate than the HSR study section could handle. The Office of Research and Statistics in the Social Security Administration, who originally administered Medicare and Medicaid, also developed an extensive body of research that was continued by the Health Care Financing Administration (HCFA) when it took over responsibility for the Medicare and Medicaid programs. HCFA, recently renamed the Centers for Medicare and Medicaid Services, continues to play many roles in health care delivery: payer of services, determination of benefits package, and research.

In 1966, Avedis Donabedian developed a conceptual framework for health services that viewed care as a production system. This simple system model defined the components of **structure**, the **process**, and the resultant **outcomes**. This model of structure, process, and outcomes continues to provide the basic paradigm for assessing and improving the quality of care and can be applied to the care of individual patients, patient groups, special populations, or the community at large (see Chapter Seven, by Seid, Sobo, Zivkovic, Nelson, and Far).

In 1967, prior to the creation of the Department of Health and Human Services (HHS), the secretary of the Department of Health, Education and Welfare (HEW) authorized the National Center for Health Services Research (NCHSR). NCHSR consolidated the health research activities in various HEW departments. NCHSR also established HSR centers at sites such as Harvard University, the University of North Carolina–Chapel Hill, the University of California–Los Angeles, and Kaiser Permanente in northern California.

The growth of HSR was marked by the inception, in 1984, of an academic association, the Association for Health Services Research, or AHSR (McCarthy & White, 2000). AHSR later merged with the Alpha Center to form the Academy for Health Services Research and Health Policy (AHSRHP), which in 2002 became simply AcademyHealth.

In 1989, NCHSR was absorbed into the Agency for Healthcare Policy and Research (AHCPR), a public health service agency in HHS. The legislation that established AHCPR (P.L. 101-2399) mandated that the agency support research, data development, and activities that will enhance the quality, appropriateness, and effectiveness of health services. This focus represents lawmakers' frustration with escalating health care costs and their awareness of documented unnecessary variation in medical practice (Wennberg, 1984–1985). AHCPR was reauthorized in 1999 as the Agency for Healthcare Research and Quality (AHRQ).

In addition to the federal government, private foundations have contributed to the development of HSR. The National Library of Medicine maintains a database that provides some information on the foundation's funding of health services research. Six private foundations (the Robert Wood Johnson Foundation, W. K. Kellogg Foundation, Pew Charitable Trusts, John A. Hartford Foundation, Commonwealth Fund, and Henry J. Kaiser Family Foundation) have provided 20 percent of the funding listed, with the federal government providing the other 80 percent (Institute of Medicine, 2001).

Emergence of the Subfield of Child Health Services Research

Adult health services researchers generally have not included children in their work. For example, when the first version of the Health Employers Data and Information Set (HEDIS 1.0) was established, no pediatric indicators were included. In subsequent versions, indicators for immunizations and asthma were included.

Scholars from many disciplines have discussed children's exclusion from most models of health and behavior (for example, Beuf, 1989; Mayall, 1996; Scheper-Hughes & Sargent, 1998). For various reasons, researchers who do the model building either forget that children need to be taken into account or intentionally exclude them as irrelevant to the models. In HSR in particular, Forrest, Simpson, and Clancy (1997) identify five contributing factors underlying children's invisibility: (1) a disease orientation, (2) the overall low costs of child health care, (3) a lack of trained researchers, (4) meager funding, and (5) limited methodological and conceptual foundations.

The disease orientation of HSR has limited applicability when it comes to children because they are generally healthy. The disease orientation has little room for broader issues related to quality of life, injury prevention, or enhancing developmental potential and therefore leaves most children out. In addition, limiting the scope of inquiry to disease leads most health service researchers to prioritize high-cost, chronic conditions of high prevalence. But as Forrest and colleagues (1997) note, children account for only 15 percent of all medical expenditures. The lack of cost associated with child health helps explain their exclusion from the HSR agenda.

Few researchers are trained specifically in child HSR because until recently, little funding had been made available for HSR with a pediatric emphasis. Because few researchers had focused on child HSR, the field has suffered from a lack of well-developed method-ological or theoretical frameworks. Forrest and colleagues' (1997) opinions reflect the proceeding of an expert panel convened by AHCPR in May 1996.

An expert panel meeting of over one hundred participants was convened in May 1997 and titled "Improving the Quality of Healthcare for Children." This expert panel led to a special issue of *Health Services Research* dedicated to child HSR (Halfon, Schuster, Valentine, & McGlynn, 1998). The meeting represented one of the first efforts to bring experts together to chart future directions for the emerging field of child HSR, or CHSR. In the special issue's introduction, Halfon and colleagues described the rationale, development, content, and results of the meeting, which included a research agenda. This agenda focused specifically on monitoring child health, evaluating service efficacy and effectiveness, assessing the quality of care, improving the quality of care, economic modeling, and the development and dissemination of clinical practice guidelines and other information for physicians and consumers. This expert panel called for an expansion of the CHSR workforce: the development of CHSR centers focusing on specific high-priority areas and concentrating on vulnerable populations; improving national child health data collection systems and community health monitoring; building and supporting research networks; and developing a coordinated intra-agency federal effort to move the CHSR agenda forward.

Building on the expert panel meeting's momentum, the National Association of Children's Hospitals and Related Institutions (NACHRI), the Agency for Healthcare Policy and Research (now the Agency for Healthcare Research and Quality, AHRQ), the American Academy of Pediatrics (AAP), the David and Lucile Packard Foundation, the Association for Health Services Research (now AcademyHealth), the Robert Wood Johnson Foundation, and Data Harbor, Inc., jointly sponsored a special one-day meeting in June 1999 in Chicago to bring active proponents of CHSR together. The meeting, called "Improving Children's Health Through Health Services Research," explored the science of CHSR, public and private funding opportunities, networks for conducting research, and the translation of research into policy and practice. The meeting continues annually and has proved to be a valuable source of intellectual stimulation and scholarly connectivity for the growing field.

The Four Ds

In addition to identifying the reasons that children have been ignored, researchers have argued that because childhood is a unique period of life with unique health care needs, certain key concepts related to the difference between children and adults must inform HSR for children (Forrest et al., 1997; McGlynn, Halfon, & Leibowitz, 1995; Perrin, 1985). Differences between children and adults can be summarized by the "four Ds": developmental change, dependence, differential epidemiology, and demographics (Forrest et al., 1997; Jameson & Wehr, 1993; McGlynn et al., 1995; Perrin, 1985). **Developmental change** means that children grow and change rapidly and that their development in numerous areas (cognitive, emotional, social, physical) affects their ultimate health status. **Dependence** means that children are dependent on parents and other adults and on systems (school, social services) for accessing and receiving care. When studying children's access and use of services, a family systems perspective is required. **Differential epidemiology** refers to the fact that most children are free from disease and that in contrast to the epidemiological profile in adults, children are affected by a large number of low-prevalence conditions. Also, because of their epidemiological profile, children require different medical services than adults, such as immunization and developmental screening. **Demographics** refers to the fact that children are disproportionately poor, uninsured, and otherwise vulnerable.

Developmental Change

Children's development is a dynamic process marked by rapid growth and change. Their dynamic development occurs in multiple domains: physical, cognitive, and emotional. In the first year of life, a child will triple his birthweight. By age five, he will be able to tell a simple story. As children grow, they are constantly changing in their physical, cognitive, and emotional development, and measures of child health must account for this dynamic process. For a specific preventative health service such as immunization, the outcome is relatively simple to measure. However, measuring a child's overall health while accounting for developmental change is more difficult. An outcome measure for a child's overall health needs to address physical, cognitive, and emotional functions and must move beyond simple categorical measures to a noncategorical approach. **Health-related quality of life (HRQL)** is one example of a noncategorical outcome measure of health while accounting for developmental change (see Chapter Six, by Knight, Burwinkle, and Varni).

Dependence

Parents are involved in almost all interactions between their child and health care providers, except in the case of adolescent patients, who may interact directly with the provider. Because in most cases parents influence all aspects of a child's health care, including potential access to care, health care utilization, perception of care, and adherence with care, the parents' ability to successfully negotiate the health care system influences a child's health outcomes (see Sobo & Seid, 2001; see also Chapter Seven, by Seid, Sobo, Zivkovic, Nelson, and Far). A four-year-old girl with moderate persistent asthma needs her parents to take her to doctor's appointments, eliminate her environmental triggers, and administer preventive and acute medications to control her disease; she cannot self-manage her asthma. Indeed, much of her health care will occur outside the formal health care system; the majority of child health care occurs in the home setting (see Chapter Three, by Sobo) or in other community settings such as schools (see Chapter Five, by Dennis and Simmes).

The practice of **biomedicine** today generally casts health as an individual state accomplished through the health-seeking partnership of a patient and a physician (nurses and other health care workers are seen as essential support for this dyad, but the physician retains prominence) (Hahn, 1995). This dyadic, two-person model underpins much recent research on patient-clinician interaction (Kravitz, Cope, Bhrany, & Leake, 1994; Roter et al., 1997) and on the modern biomedical enterprise as a whole (Bell, Wilkes, & Kravitz, 1999; Hunt, 1998). However, because of children's dependence and developmental immaturity and their legal status as minors, children's relation to the health service system is overseen not by themselves but by their parents (Forrest et al., 1997; Korsch, 1968). Communication about child health must be analyzed as the outcome of the negotiations of a triad composed of dependent patient (child), empowered intermediary (parent), and authoritative practitioner.

The literature on physician-patient interaction is vast, and the earliest studies took place in pediatric settings (Korsch, 1968). Nonetheless, Tates and Meeuwesen (2001), in their recent review of the literature on the pediatric triad of patient, parent, and physician, found that the implications of the child's presence has received remarkably little attention. Indeed, even Korsch (1968), the progenitor of study in this area, examined the parent-physician dyad, not the pediatric triad.

However, several important findings regarding the pediatric triad have been made. For example, physicians sometimes criticize parents through comments made to children, physicians generally address

parents and children through different speaking frames (consulta-
tive or instrumental, joking or affective), and parents frequently answer questions that physicians have directed toward their children
(Tates & Meeuwesen, 2001). This last pattern of interference has
also been identified in children's guardian-assisted dietary recall interviews (Sobo & Rock, 2001; Sobo, Rock, Neuhouser, Maciel, &
Neumark-Sztainer, 2000). Parents and children may have competing agendas and may therefore relate differently to the interviewer
and have different strategies for aligning themselves with the interviewer. These findings are important because the socioculturally
engendered interpersonal dynamics of the pediatric triad may compromise child health goals by leaving parent, practitioner, or child,
for example, with incomplete or biased information.

Differential Epidemiology

Most children are healthier than adults according to traditional
measures of morbidity and mortality (see Tables 2.1 and 2.2). A large
percentage of the adult population is affected by high-prevalence
chronic conditions such as heart disease and diabetes. In contrast,
a large percentage of children will experience frequent but self-
limiting conditions that decrease in frequency as they reach adoles-
cence (Schor, 1986). These self-limiting illnesses make up a majority
of the acute care visits for children, whereas the majority of acute
visits for adults are attributed to the high-prevalence chronic conditions. In addition to these self-limiting illnesses, children receive
acute care for injuries, the leading cause of morbidity in children
aged seventeen and under (Rivara, Grossman, & Cummings, 1997;
see also Chapter Three, by Sobo).

In addition to acute care visits, children also require extensive preventive services. Where adult preventive services focus on disease
screening and health maintenance, children's preventive services are
broader; they include these activities as well as frequent immunizations and developmental surveillance over time. The latter is essential: 12 to 16 percent of American children have developmental or
behavioral disorders (Boyle, Decoufle, & Yeargin-Allsopp, 1994).

Table 2.1. Causes of Childhood Death at Various Ages.

Rank	Age Under One Year (Rate 875)[a]	Age One to Four Years (Rate 38)	Causes Age Five to Fourteen Years (Rate 22)	Age Fifteen to Twenty-Four Years (Rate 90)
1	Perinatal conditions	Injuries	Injuries	Injuries
2	Congenital anomalies	Congenital anomalies	Malignant neoplasms	Homicide
3	Sudden infant death syndrome	Malignant neoplasms	Homicide and legal interventions	Suicide
4	Accidents and adverse events	Homicide and legal intervention	Congenital anomalies	Malignant neoplasms
5	Infections (respiratory)	Diseases of the heart[b]	Diseases of the heart[b]	Diseases of the heart[b]
6		Respiratory infections	Suicide	

Source: Data from National Center for Health Statistics. Figures are for 1996.
[a]Rate per 100,000 population.
[b]Excludes congenital heart anomalies.

Table 2.2. Utilization of Health Care by Children Aged Seventeen Years and Under.

	Office Visits		Hospital Outpatient Visits		Inpatient Hospital Stays		Emergency Department Visits		Prescription Medicines	
	Children with Any Visits (percentage)	Average Number of Visits	Children with Any Visits (percentage)	Average Number of Visits	Children with Any Stays (percentage)	Average Number of Stays	Children with Any Visits (percentage)	Average Number of Visits	Children Receiving Any Prescription (percentage)	Average Number of Prescriptions
Total	71.5	3.9	7.2	2.0	2.9	1.3	12.9	1.3	58.3	5.4
Health insurance coverage										
Any private	76.2	4.2	7.8	2.0	2.4	—[a]	12.5	1.2	61.4	5.7
Public only	66.8	3.5	7.3	2.0	5.4	—[a]	15.5	1.4	56.0	5.6
None	50.7	2.7	3.7	—[a]	1.9	—[a]	10.8	—[a]	42.8	3.1
Age										
0–4 years	82.9	4.3	9.7	1.8	—[b]	—[b]	15.9	1.3	69.9	6.2
5–9 years	72.2	3.4	6.2	1.8	2.1	—[a]	11.2	1.2	61.3	4.8
10–14 years	64.2	3.5	5.9	1.7	1.0	—[a]	11.7	1.2	47.8	5.4
15–17 years	63.7	4.7	7.2	—[a]	3.8	—[a]	13.2	1.3	51.3	5.1

Source: Data from Medical Expenditure Panel Survey, Agency for Healthcare Research and Quality. Figures are for 1996.

[a]Sample size was too small to provide reliable estimates.

[b]Estimates of inpatient stays are excluded for children under four years of age because data on inpatient stays for newborns were not consistently reported separately from their mothers' stay.

However, developmental surveillance in the physical, cognitive, and emotional domains requires a great deal of clinical attention and effort. It must be "a flexible, continuous process whereby knowledgeable professionals perform skilled observations of children during the provision of health care. The components of developmental surveillance include eliciting and attending to parental concerns, obtaining a relevant developmental history, making accurate and informative observations of children, and sharing opinions and concerns with other relevant professionals" (Dworkin, 1993, p. 532). Because children develop skills variably and show a new skill inconsistently when first mastering it, a single test at one point in time gives only a snapshot of the dynamic process, making periodic screening necessary to detect emerging disabilities as a child grows. Early identification of children with developmental delays or disabilities can lead to treatment and intervention that can lessen the impact on the functioning of the child and the family.

Whereas most children will require only preventive and acute care, a growing number of children experience chronic conditions. In 1994, some 18 percent of U.S. children under eighteen years of age had a chronic physical, developmental, behavioral, or emotional condition that necessitated the use of health and related services of types or amounts beyond those generally required by children (Newacheck et al., 1998). Providing optimal medical care to **children with special health care needs (CSHCN)** requires greater time on the part of health care providers. Such children often require service coordination, lengthy counseling, and an increased number of visits and referrals to medical subspecialists, hospitals, and community resources (see Tables 2.3 and 2.4). In addition to these extra responsibilities, health care providers must ensure preventive care for children with special needs.

Demographics

Children are much more likely than adults to be poor, of minority status, uninsured, and otherwise vulnerable (see Chapter Seven, by Seid, Sobo, Zivkovic, Nelson, and Far). In 1999, one in

Table 2.3. U.S. Children with Special Health Care Needs.

Characteristic	Cases per 100	Estimated Population (in thousands)
All children	18.0	12,608
Age		
0–2 years	9.1	1,085
3–5 years	15.3	1,914
6–10 years	21.0	4,043
11–14 years	21.0	3,222
15–17 years	21.5	2,343
Gender		
Male	20.9	7,482
Female	15.0	5,125
Race		
White, not Hispanic	18.6	8,552
African American, not Hispanic	19.8	2,162
Other, not Hispanic	13.0	402
Hispanic	15.0	1,490

Source: National Health Interview Disability Survey, 1994.

Note: Children with special health care needs are those who have a chronic physical, developmental, behavioral, or emotional condition and who also require health and related services of a type or amount beyond that required by children generally.

six U.S. children lived in poverty. Living in poverty has a significant negative impact on a child's health: "Poor children are more likely to become ill, and when they do become ill they get sicker and die at higher rates than do non-poor children" (Starfield, 1992, p. 17). Minority children are most likely to be poor: one-third of all African American and Latino children live in poverty.

Children of minority background are a fast-growing segment of the U.S. population (see Table 2.5). In 1970, non-Latino European Americans made up 84 percent of the nation's population. By 1990, this number had dropped to 76 percent, and according to U.S. Cen-

Table 2.4. Health Needs of U.S. Children.

	All Children	Children with Special Health Care Needs	Children Without Special Health Care Needs
Health status			
Average annual bed days due to illness	2.8	6.1	2.0
Average annual school absences due to illness	3.6	7.4	2.8
Percentage of children with one or more unmet health needs	7.6	12.9	6.4
Use of health services			
Average annual physician contacts	3.3	6.4	2.6
Percentage hospitalized in past year	3.1	7.4	2.2
Average annual hospital days per 1,000 children	225.0	691.0	122.0

Source: National Health Interview Disability Survey, 1994.

sus Bureau projections, by 2020, non-Latino European Americans will comprise only 64 percent of the population. Latinos will account for 15.2 percent, African Americans 13.3 percent, and Asians and Pacific Islanders 6.8 percent (Charney & Hernandez, 1998).

In 1997, fully 25 percent of all children under the age of five were from minority backgrounds, and this is expected to rise to 48 percent by the year 2025. Populations from Latin America and Asia represent the fastest-growing segments of minority children, with diverse sets of languages and cultures (U.S. Bureau of the Census, 1997). While much growth will be among U.S. citizens, immigrants and refugees will also contribute. The latter are likely to be poor and to experience more cultural and linguistic barriers to health care (Aday, 1994); they also are less likely to be insured (Weinick, Zuvekas, & Cohen, 2000).

Table 2.5. Total U.S. Population by Age and Race or Ethnicity, 2000.

Age	Total Population	White	African American	Native American and Alaska Native	Asian	Pacific Islander	Some Other Race	Two or More Races	Hispanic or Latino (of any race)
Total population	281,421,906	211,460,626	34,658,190	2,475,956	10,242,998	398,835	15,359,073	6,826,228	35,305,818
Under 18 years	72,293,812	49,598,289	10,885,696	840,312	2,464,999	127,179	5,520,451	2,856,886	12,342,259
Under 1 year	3,805,648	2,535,928	548,955	42,167	129,803	6,464	338,786	203,545	771,053
1–4 years	15,370,150	10,323,964	2,255,831	170,885	540,603	26,927	1,307,270	744,670	2,946,921
5–13 years	37,025,346	25,411,015	5,727,934	436,694	1,227,263	65,181	2,755,002	1,402,257	6,185,947
14–17 years	16,092,668	11,327,382	2,352,976	190,566	567,330	28,607	1,119,393	506,414	2,438,338
Percentages									
Total population	100.0	100.0	100.0	100.0	100.0	100.0	100.0	100.0	100.0
Under 18 years	25.7	23.5	31.4	33.9	24.1	31.9	35.9	41.9	35.0
Under 1 year	1.4	1.2	1.6	1.7	1.3	1.6	2.2	3.0	2.2
1–4 years	5.5	4.9	6.5	6.9	5.3	6.8	8.5	10.9	8.3
5–13 years	13.2	12.0	16.5	17.6	12.0	16.3	17.9	20.5	17.5
14–17 years	5.7	5.4	6.8	7.7	5.5	7.2	7.3	7.4	6.9

Source: U.S. Bureau of the Census, Census 2000, Summary File 1.

Although poverty, minority status, and health insurance status all affect child health, these socioeconomic characteristics interact in a complex manner with other characteristics such as those identified by Lu Ann Aday (1993): demographic (age, sex, ethnicity), **human capital** (socioeconomic status, language ability), and **social capital** (family, community, culture) factors. Vulnerability to poor health outcomes is the result of this interaction. Because children are dependent on their parents and other institutions for access to health services, the application of Aday's model to children must include the demographic, human, and social capital characteristics of their families (see Chapter Seven, by Seid, Sobo, Zivkovic, Nelson, and Far).

The Fifth D: Disparities

Although health disparities are implied in the four Ds construct, disparities in health care and health outcomes may warrant its own D, which we call the "fifth D." American society is becoming increasingly diverse, and there is compelling evidence that minority populations suffer from increasing differences in the incidence, prevalence, mortality, burdens of disease, and other adverse health conditions. Health disparities for minority children include high rates of low birthweight, asthma, birth defects, obesity, type II diabetes, exposure to hazardous substances, childhood injury, and death. Minority children are also at greater risk for developmental and learning delays and for social, emotional, and behavioral problems (National Institutes of Health, 2000). In addition, despite a significant decline in the overall infant mortality rate in the 1990s, the infant mortality rate remains twice as high among African Americans as among whites, even when controlling for socioeconomic factors (National Center for Health Statistics, 2000). Native American and Alaskan Native infants also have a death rate almost double that of whites (National Center for Health Statistics, 2000). Untreated dental caries and periodontal disease provide another example: they are twice as prevalent in African American and Latino adolescents as in white youth (McCormick, Kass, Elixhauser,

Thompson, & Simpson, 2000). Despite the fact the asthma is only slightly more prevalent in African American than in white children, African American children experience greater morbidity and mortality due to the disease (Newacheck & Halfon, 2000; Ray, Thamer, Fadillioglu, & Gergen, 1998).

By specifically addressing the fifth D, research and health resources may be directed to reduce and eventually eliminate health disparities; efforts to this end are currently under way at the federal level. For example, the National Institutes of Health have launched the *National Strategic Research Plan to Reduce and Ultimately Eliminate Health Disparities* (2000). Furthermore, the goals of *Healthy People 2010* (U.S. Department of Health and Human Services, 2000) include eliminating health disparities.[1] The Department of Health and Human Services has also launched an initiative to address this problem and improve the prevention of disease, promotion of health, and delivery of health care to minority populations. We are hopeful that these federal efforts will also stimulate activities at the state, regional, and local levels. The elimination of health disparities is a necessary investment for the health and well-being of our nation's children.

Child Health Services Research: Moving the Agenda Forward

The agenda for CHSR generated at the expert panel meeting of 1997 included monitoring child health, evaluating service efficacy and effectiveness, assessing the quality of care, improving the quality of care, performing economic modeling, and developing and disseminating clinical practice guidelines and other information for physicians and consumers (Halfon et al., 1998). In the years since this agenda was first published, much more has been learned about what is needed if applied CHSR is to move forward. We will focus on the ongoing need for monitoring efforts and quality research and discuss the challenges future applied CHSR investigators will face.

Monitoring Child Health

Child health monitoring has generally focused on costs related to how children and their families use the health care system. For example, using the Medical Expenditure Panel Survey (MEPS), McCormick and colleagues prepare an annual report that provides an update on insurance coverage, use of health care services, and health expenditures for children and youth in the United States. In addition, from the Health Cost and Utilization Project (HCUP), the report provides information on variation in hospitalizations for children from a new twenty-two-state hospital discharge data source (McCormick et al., 2000). These efforts mark an impressive start to monitoring child health.

Because many factors influence the health of a child, monitoring child health is a broad undertaking (see Chapter Three, by Sobo, and Chapter Seven, by Seid, Sobo, Zivkovic, Nelson, and Far), and more needs to be done to monitor health-related quality of life (see Chapter Six, by Knight, Burwinkle, and Varni). Communities greatly influence their children's health, so monitoring the child-health-related strengths and weaknesses (such as childhood poverty) of communities is essential. The **community health report card** is a tool that has emerged as a mechanism to monitor the well-being of a community (see Chapter Four, by Simmes, Lim, and Dennis).

Access to Care

Access to care bridges the areas of monitoring child health to other aspects of the CHSR agenda (Halfon et al., 1998), which focus on improving the quality of child health care. Without access to care, children have to forgo care, delay care, or receive it only from urgent care centers or emergency rooms. Whether children are publicly or privately insured, having insurance coverage has been shown to improve their access to care (Weinick, Weigers, & Cohen, 1998). Yet as we write, one in seven children is without health insurance (Henry J. Kaiser Family Foundation, 2001). Medicaid covers one child in five. Despite efforts at expanding this number, Medicaid coverage declined from 21.6 million children in 1995 to 21 million children in 1997—even as the number of children eligible for Medicaid increased. This reduction has been associated with the decoupling of Medicaid and other aid programs after the 1996 Welfare Reform Act as well as confusion about eligibility requirements for immigrant children (Government Accounting Office, 1998). Fully explaining this reduction and understanding how best to increase access for the high numbers of uninsured children remains a challenge in applied CHSR.

In 1997, Congress enacted the Children's Health Insurance Program (CHIP) to expand health insurance coverage for low-income children. CHIP represents the largest investment in children's health insurance since the enactment of Medicaid in 1965. States must supply matching funds, but the required matching rates are lower than Medicaid rates. In addition to lower-rate state matching rates, CHIP benefits packages are not required to be as extensive as Medicaid. Medicaid's benefit package is called Early and Periodic Screening, Diagnosis and Treatment (EPSDT) services, which includes physician, hospital, dental, and vision visits with no cost sharing. Some states elected to require copayments for CHIP based on family income.

CHSR investigators, including individuals at HFCA and AHRQ, have been studying the impact of CHIP, Medicaid, and welfare reform (Agency for Healthcare Research and Quality, 2001). After a slow initial start, CHIP appears to have improved health insurance coverage for children (Cunningham & Park, 2000). However, many questions remain. In some states, more children lose public health insurance coverage than are enrolled each month. This disenrollment problem is beginning to draw attention from applied CHSR investigators, as is ethnoracial variation. Latino children, for example, continue to have lower rates of health care coverage than non-Latinos for reasons that are unclear (Flores, Bauchner, Feinstein, & Nguyen, 1999). Research focusing on barriers to enrollment or disincentives perceived by end users as well as program-level roadblocks is essential (see Chapter Five, by Dennis and Simmes).[2]

Quality of Care

The remaining aspects of the original CHSR agenda—evaluating service efficacy and effectiveness, assessing the quality of care, improving the quality of care, performing economic modeling, and developing and disseminating clinical practice guidelines and other information for physicians and consumers—fall under the rubric "quality of care." *Efficacy* of health care services focuses on the results obtained in ideal settings, while *effectiveness* focuses on results obtained in real-world settings of usual care. The ideal settings of efficacy are often **randomized controlled trials (RCTs)**, in which the outcomes for an experimental group are compared with the outcomes of a nonexperimental or control group. In pediatrics, however, RCTs are relatively rare. This is due in part to the differential epidemiology of childhood illness and the related problem of small samples. It is also due to ethical concerns about informed consent for children. Often the standard of care for children is consensus-driven, using expert panels; the National Heart, Lung, and Blood Institute (NHLBI) guidelines on asthma care (1997) were devised in this way.

The gap between efficacy and effectiveness can be seen as the gap between knowledge of state-of-the-art health care and actual health care practice. While efficacy sets the standard for the best possible care, effectiveness reflects what happens in actual practice. Quality improvement efforts seek to decrease the gap between knowledge and practice, creating the most effective health care and services (see Chapter One, by Kurtin, and Chapter Eight, by Richardson, Sobo, and Stucky).

Assessing the quality of care requires attention to three types of problems: overuse (too much care), underuse (too little care), and misuse (errors in technical and interpersonal aspects of care)

(Chassin & Galvin, 1998; Schuster, McGlynn, & Brook, 1998). Examples of overuse include excessive or unnecessary diagnostic tests, unnecessary surgical procedures, and the overprescribing of antibiotics. Underuse may refer to a lack of immunization and of mental health services, among other things. Misuse, or shortcomings in the technical and interpersonal aspects of care, results if the performance of health care professionals or support systems is inadequate. Misuse also occurs when practitioners cannot communicate well with their patients and when providers fail to account for patient preferences or to include patients in decision making. Assessing overuse, underuse, and misuse is an important first step in improving the quality and safety of care (see Chapter One, by Kurtin).

In addition to technical aspects of care, quality of care includes the interpersonal aspects of care. A link between improved quality of provider-patient communication and improved outcomes exists (Kaplan, Greenfield, & Ware, 1989; Roter et al., 1997; Stewart, 1995). According to the Institute of Medicine (IOM) report *Crossing the Quality Chasm: A New Health System for the 21st Century* (2001), the health system can enhance the provider-patient relationship by supporting patients and their families in what can best be summarized as active, informed engagement. Such engagement, which includes shared decision making when possible, is especially important for patients with chronic diseases, such as asthma, for which care extends over time. Concurrent with IOM recommendations, as part of the Robert Wood Johnson Foundation's national Improving Chronic Illness Care program, Edward Wagner and colleagues developed a guide for chronic care improvement called the Chronic Care Model (CCM). The CCM incorporates patients as "active, informed participants" in their own care and calls for a "prepared, proactive practice team" that supports this (see www.improvingchroniccare.org). Therefore, providers feel more prepared to handle their patient's engagement, and patients are more open to discussing their problems and needs related to their disease. This relationship makes for better communication between the patient and provider and in turn enables the patient to have improved self-management.

Economic modeling related to quality is another challenging area. Because health care is provided by and paid for by multiple entities, understanding the financial incentives for providing quality care is complex. For example, if a hospital implements successful quality improvement for asthma, as with clinical pathways, the cost of hospital admissions and the average length of stay can be reduced (see Chapter One, by Kurtin, and Chapter Eight, by Richardson, Sobo, and Stucky). Urgent care and emergency room visits may also be reduced. Tracking the possible financial benefits of such improvements is an important undertaking because such information may be used to create a business case for quality (Commonwealth Fund, 2001).

The final item on the original CHSR agenda, developing and disseminating clinical practice guidelines and other evidence-based and quality-related information for physicians and consumers, is also of continued importance. NCQA and FACCT are among the organizations that have worked to establish reporting mechanisms so as to better inform consumers about quality health plans. Although these efforts are a step in the right direction, their applied value is undermined by the mistaken assumption that consumers choose health plans based on quality. Research shows that cost plays a greater role than quality of care in health plan choice (Tumlinson, Bottigheimer, Mahoney, Stone, & Hendricks, 1997). Furthermore, consumers' choice of health plans for their children (and themselves) is limited by their employers (Herzlinger, 1997) and by other sociocultural and politicoeconomic factors (see Landsverk et al., 2001).

Another factor limiting the value of consumer-oriented reporting mechanisms is the complexity of their present formats. Much of this has to do with the complexity of health plans themselves, at least from the consumer perspective (Tumlinson et al., 1997). A key factor to the success of a consumer-driven health care quality improvement movement is the easy availability of child-relevant

information on both health plans and specific providers that is easily understandable by children's parents or guardians. Applied
CHSR investigators have only begun to address this challenge.

Adding Diversity to the Agenda

As discussed earlier, the United States is becoming increasingly diverse, and this diversity is growing fastest among young children
(Charney & Hernandez, 1998). Minority children rate lower than
nonminority children on use of and satisfaction with health care,
adherence to treatment regiments, and health outcomes (Flores et
al., 1999; Pachter & Weller, 1993; Weinick et al., 2000). These differences are more marked for families and children with limited English proficiency. Indeed, Brach and Fraser (2000) have shown that
language barriers are at the heart of health care disparities (but see
Clark, de Baca, Reidy, & Turner, 2002).

Even English-speaking minority children and families face potential cultural barriers to care. Cultural sensitivity and culturally
appropriate care may help here. Central to this is a real understanding of the concepts of **culture, ethnicity**, and **race**. An understanding of related provider-patient communication issues is important,
as is the appreciation that health care providers have their own
health belief systems. Indeed, each interaction between health care
providers and patients (even those from similar ethnic and class
backgrounds) can be seen as the interaction of two cultures.

Culture and its relation to child health is discussed at length by
Sobo in Chapter Three (see also Loustaunau & Sobo, 1997; Sobo
& Seid, 2001). The practice of cultural sensitivity and the delivery
of culturally appropriate care are sometimes glossed as **cultural competence**. Cultural competence curricula, developed to improve multicultural care, often use medical cases, literature reviews, the
recounting of personal experiences, and examinations of feedback
from support staff, patients, and practitioners to help health care
workers elucidate and understand their biases before they adversely
affect clinical care (Carrillo, Green, & Betancourt, 1999). Role-

playing solutions to difficult cultural problems can extend awareness and enhance conflict resolution skills.

One of the problems with cultural competence initiatives is that
they leave little room for intracultural variation, which can be
greater than intercultural variation. A wide variety of unique health
beliefs exists within a single group; no one individual can be familiar with all relevant cultural practices. There is a great need for applied research to identify the most crucial aspects of health-related
cultural variation for child health.

Another problem with competence initiatives is that they often
target only first-generation or immigrant families and members of
minority groups. This means that cultural differences based on other
factors (class, occupation, education, geography, lifestyle, and so on)
are ignored in favor of those associated with ethnicity or race—two
technically separate constructs that are often confused both with
each other and with culture.

Ethnicity is a facet of the self that is tied to notions of shared origins that contrast with those of people with whom one shares borders. *Race* is a narrower construct, technically defined as persons with
a relatively homogeneous biologic inheritance. In health practice
and research, as in other spheres, race and its categorization are based
on assumptions about the meaning of a patient's skin color and facial features; *ethnicity* and *race* are often used as synonyms. Some
scholars now use the term *ethnoracial* to signify this conflation.

Because racial categories are socially constructed, they have little significance in terms of biological realities, and so race cannot
serve as a **proxy** measure for biological difference (Goodman, 2000).
Ethnicity may mark certain epidemiological risk factors, as it is generally more narrowly defined than race—but even here, because
people often have multiple ethnicities and may participate only
partly, if at all, in their ethnic traditions, great care must be taken.
Race and ethnicity are, however, important markers of political and
economic inequality in the United States. More applied CHSR that
accounts for the influence of ethnoracially related social prejudice,

political exclusion (or inclusion), and social marginalization (or privilege) on health and well-being is sorely needed.

Ethnoracial background and immigrant status should not be the only criteria taken into account when considering the need for culturally sensitive or appropriate care, as is apparent in the frequency of differences between a health care provider's and a family's view of a child's health problem—even when provider and family are ethnoracially similar. Such differences may result in decreased family satisfaction with clinical interactions, decreased adherence to prescribed therapy, decreased future use of care, and potentially poorer child health outcomes.

The first step in addressing the cultural gap that underlies such differences is having health care practitioners examine their own assumptions, biases, and beliefs when making diagnostic and therapeutic decisions; applied CHSR might help identify the most efficacious ways for doing this. It is also essential that health care providers who work in communities of cultural backgrounds that differ from their own learn as much as possible about their patients by reviewing the literature and by talking with members of the community about their health care preferences for their children's health care. Increasing staff diversity at all levels of patient care sends a strong message to patients about an institution's or practice's commitment to providing culturally appropriate care.

Research has established a link between improved quality of health care provider–patient communication and improved outcomes (Kaplan et al., 1989; Roter et al., 1997; Stewart, 1995). Enhancing provider-patient communication is one of the most important challenges for applied CHSR today. Although translator services may decrease communication barriers—and research is under way to assess its effectiveness—nonverbal communication and body language, such as eye contact, are poorly understood and receive little research attention. Fully understanding and optimizing all types of communication is essential to increasing not only family satisfaction but also adherence; problems with adherence have been generally viewed in terms of a patient's or parent's inability to follow instructions rather than a health care provider's difficulty in supplying an appropriate care plan suited to a family's preferences and means. Applied CHSR must help providers plan for patient-centered care, one of the six dimensions of quality care highlighted in *Crossing the Quality Chasm* (Institute of Medicine, 2001).

Applied CHSR must help health care providers understand the effect that larger societal problems play in the lives of families; this is essential to developing a realistic and therapeutic relationship. English proficiency, educational background, financial limitations, experiences of prejudice in the health care setting, family and household structure, child-rearing practices, and facility in navigating the formal health care system all affect health care decisions. Recent immigrants may have experienced persecution, separation from family and friends, and the loss of livelihood, home, and language. Some investigators have suggested that families be screened for these stressful social circumstances, so long as pediatricians explain the medical reasons for asking sensitive and personal questions (Pachter, 1994).

Health care providers have often been reluctant to focus on the challenges of cross-cultural care because of the perception that such an approach is costly and time-consuming. However, ignoring cultural issues may lead to conflicts, inappropriate testing, inadequate therapy, multiple consultations, and fragmented care, which can drain resources and waste time. Applied CHSR can not only document this but also generate models for providing the best-quality care to children of all cultures.

Conclusion

An interest in health care has existed since the early days of the Republic; however, this interest has often been met with resistance. In the past several decades, efforts by the federal government, businesses, and private foundations have helped overcome this resistance, leading to the birth of the field of health services research. This chapter has traced the emergence of HSR within the context of larger trends in the U.S. health care system and discussed the development of child health services research as a distinct subfield of HSR. CHSR is a growing field that shares many of the challenges of adult HSR but also has its own unique challenges. The following chapters demonstrate the broad range of possibilities within applied CHSR and its goal of improving child care.

Notes

1. *Healthy People 2010* updates the 1979 Surgeon General's Report, *Healthy People*, and *Healthy People 2000: National Health Promotion and Disease Prevention Objectives*. The Healthy People reports establish national health objectives (see www.health.gov/healthypeople).

2. Further discussion of children's health insurance can be found in general pediatrics textbooks and at the Web sites of the Centers for Medicare and Medicaid Services (www.cms.gov), the Henry J. Kaiser Family Foundation (www.kff.org), and the Children's Defense Fund (www.cdf.org).

References

Aday, L. A. (1993). *Evaluating the medical care system: Effectiveness, efficiency, and equity*. Ann Arbor, MI: Health Administration Press.

Aday, L. A. (1994). Health status of vulnerable populations. *Annual Review of Public Health, 15*, 487–509.

Agency for Healthcare Research and Quality. (2001, February). *The child health insurance research initiative*. Retrieved from http://www.ahrq.gov/about/cods/chiri.htm

Bell, R. A., Wilkes, M. S., & Kravitz, R. L. (1999). Advertisement-induced prescription drug requests: Patients' anticipated reactions to a physician who refuses. *Journal of Family Practice, 48*, 446–452.

Berwick, D. M., & Wald, D. L. (1990). Hospital leaders' opinions of the HCFA mortality data. *Journal of the American Medical Association, 263*, 247–249.

Beuf, A. H. (1989). *Biting off the bracelet: A study of children in hospitals* (2nd ed.). College Park: University of Pennsylvania Press.

Boyle, C. A., Decoufle, P., & Yeargin-Allsopp, M. (1994). Prevalence and health impact of developmental disabilities in U.S. children. *Pediatrics, 93,* 399–403.

Brach, C., & Fraser, I. (2000). Can cultural competence reduce racial and ethnic health disparities? A review and conceptual model. *Medical Care Research and Review, 57*(Suppl. 1), 181–217.

Brennan, T. A., & Berwick, D. M. (1996). *New rules: Regulation, markets, and the quality of American health care.* San Francisco: Jossey-Bass.

Carrillo, J. E., Green, A. R., & Betancourt, J. R. (1999). Cross-cultural primary care: A patient-based approach. *Annals of Internal Medicine, 130,* 829–834.

Charney, E., & Hernandez, D. J. (1998). *From generation to generation: The health and well-being of children in immigrant families.* Washington, DC: National Academy Press.

Chassin, M. R., & Galvin, R. W. (1998). The urgent need to improve health care quality. Institute of Medicine National Roundtable on Health Care Quality. *Journal of the American Medical Association, 280,* 1000–1005.

Clark, L., de Baca, R. C., Reidy, K., & Turner, M. (2002, November 20–24). *Is cultural competence all about language? Data from two Medicaid managed care systems serving Latinos.* Paper presented at the 101st annual meeting of the American Anthropological Association, New Orleans.

Codman, E. A. (1914). The product of a hospital. *Journal of Surgery, Gynecology, and Obstetrics, 18,* 491–496.

Codman, E. A. (1934). *The shoulder: Rupture of the supraspinatus tendon and other lesions in or about the subacromial bursa.* Boston: Todd.

Commonwealth Fund. (2001). New initiative weighs "business case" for quality. *Commonwealth Fund Quarterly, 7*(2). Retrieved from http://www.cmwf.org/publist/quarterly/sum01qrt.asp

Cunningham, P. J., & Park, M. H. (2000). Recent trends in children's health insurance coverage: No gains for low-income children. *Issue Brief (Center for Studying Health System Change), 29,* 1–6.

Deming, W. E. (2000). *Out of the crisis: Quality, productivity, and competitive position.* Cambridge, MA: MIT Press. (Original work published 1982)

Donabedian, A. (1966). Evaluating the quality of medical care. *Milbank Memorial Fund Quarterly, 44*(Suppl. 3), 166–206.

Dworkin, P. H. (1993). Detection of behavioral, developmental, and psychosocial problems in pediatric primary care practice. *Current Opinion in Pediatrics, 5,* 531–536.

Field, M. J., Feasley, J. C., Tranquanda, R. E., & Institute of Medicine (U.S.) Committee on Health Services Research: Training and Work Force Issues.

(1995). *Health services research: Work force and educational issues.* Washington, DC: National Academy Press.

Flexner, A. (1910). *Medical education in the United States and Canada: A report to the Carnegie Foundation for the Advancement of Teaching.* New York: Carnegie Foundation.

Flores, G., Bauchner, H., Feinstein, A. R., & Nguyen, U. S. (1999). The impact of ethnicity, family income, and parental education on children's health and use of health services. *American Journal of Public Health, 89,* 1066–1071.

Forrest, C. B., Simpson, L., & Clancy, C. (1997). Child health services research. Challenges and opportunities. *Journal of the American Medical Association, 277,* 1787–1793.

Goodman, A. H. (2000). Why genes don't count (for racial differences in health). *American Journal of Public Health, 90,* 1699–1702.

Government Accounting Office. (1998). *Medicaid: Demographics of nonenrolled children suggest state outreach strategies* (GAO/HEHS-98-93). Washington, DC: Government Printing Office.

Hahn, R. A. (1995). *Sickness and healing: An anthropological perspective.* New Haven, CT: Yale University Press.

Halfon, N., Schuster, M., Valentine, W., & McGlynn, E. A. (1998). Improving the quality of healthcare for children: Implementing the results of the AHSR research agenda conference. *Health Services Research, 33,* 955–976.

Henry J. Kaiser Family Foundation. (2001). *Health coverage for low-income children.* Retrieved March 31, 2001, from http://www.kff.org/content/2001/2144–02/2144–02.pdf

Herzlinger, R. E. (1997). *Market-driven health care: Who wins, who loses in the transformation of America's largest service industry.* Reading, MA: Addison-Wesley.

Hunt, L. (1998). Moral reasoning and the meaning of cancer: Causal explanations of oncologists and patients in southern Mexico. *Medical Anthropology Quarterly, 12,* 298–318.

Iezzoni, L. I., Ayanian, J. Z., Bates, D. W., & Burstin, H. R. (1998). Paying more fairly for Medicare capitated care. *New England Journal of Medicine, 339,* 1933–1938.

Institute of Medicine, Committee on Quality of Health Care in America. (2001). *Crossing the quality chasm: A new health system for the 21st century.* Washington, DC: National Academy Press.

Jameson, J., & Wehr, E. (1993). Drafting national health care reform legislation to protect the health interests of children. *Stanford Law and Policy Review, 5,* 152–176.

Kaplan, S. H., Greenfield, S., & Ware, J. E., Jr. (1989). Assessing the effects of physician-patient interactions on the outcomes of chronic disease. *Medical Care, 27*(Suppl. 3), S110–S127.

Kaska, S. C., & Weinstein, J. N. (1998). Historical perspective: Ernest Amory Codman, 1869–1940: A pioneer of evidence-based medicine: The end result idea. *Spine, 23,* 629–633.

Kessner, D. M., Kalk, C. E., & Singer, J. (1973). Assessing health quality: The case for tracers. *New England Journal of Medicine, 288,* 189–194.

King, C. R. (1993). *Children's health in America: A history.* New York: Twayne.

Korsch, B. M. (1968). Insights into interpersonal relations: Parent groups. *Nursing Clinics of North America, 3,* 751–754.

Kravitz, R. L., Cope, D. W., Bhrany, V., & Leake, B. (1994). Internal medicine patients' expectations for care during office visits. *Journal of General Internal Medicine, 9*(2), 75–81.

Landsverk, J., Kurtin, P. S., Connelly, C., Simmes, D. R., Sobo, E. J., & Seid, M. (2001). *Evaluation of Outreach and Education Campaign for Healthy Families and MediCal for Children.* Sacramento: California Department of Health Services.

Loustaunau, M. O., & Sobo, E. J. (1997). *The cultural context of health, illness, and medicine.* Westport, CT: Bergin & Garvey.

Mainland, D. (1966). *Health services research.* New York: Milbank Memorial Fund.

Mather, C. (1911–1912). *Diary of Cotton Mather* [1681–1724]. Boston: Peabody Fund/Massachusetts Historical Society.

Mayall, B. (1996). *Children, health and the social order.* Buckingham, England: Open University Press.

McCarthy, T., & White, K. L. (2000). Origins of health services research. *Health Services Research, 35,* 375–387.

McCormick, M. C., Kass, B., Elixhauser, A., Thompson, J., & Simpson, L. (2000). Annual report on access to and utilization of health care for children and youth in the United States, 1999. *Pediatrics, 105,* 219–230.

McGlynn, E. A., Halfon, N., & Leibowitz, A. (1995). Assessing the quality of care for children: Prospects under health reform. *Archives of Pediatric and Adolescent Medicine, 149,* 359–368.

Milstein, A. (1997). Managing utilization management: A purchaser's view. *Health Affairs* (Millwood), *16,* 87–90.

National Center for Health Statistics. (2000). Births, marriages, divorces, and deaths: Provisional data for January 1999. *National Vital Statistics Report, 48*(1), 1–2.

National Committee for Quality Assurance. (1993). *Health plan employer data and information data set and user's manual.* New York: Author.

National Heart, Lung, and Blood Institute. (1997). *Guidelines for the diagnosis and management of asthma* (NIH Publication No. 97-4051). Washington, DC: U.S. Department of Health and Human Services, National Institutes of Health.

National Institutes of Health. (2000). *National strategic research plan to reduce and ultimately eliminate health disparities*. Retrieved from http://www.nih.gov/about/hd/strategicplan.pdf

Newacheck, P. W., & Halfon, N. (2000). Prevalence, impact, and trends in childhood disability due to asthma. *Archives of Pediatric and Adolescent Medicine, 154*, 287–293.

Newacheck, P. W., Strickland, B., Shonkoff, J. P., Perrin, J. M., McPherson, M., McManus, M., et al. (1998). An epidemiologic profile of children with special health care needs. *Pediatrics, 102*, 117–123.

Pachter, L. M. (1994). Culture and clinical care: Folk illness beliefs and behaviors and their implications for health care delivery. *Journal of the American Medical Association, 271*, 690–694.

Pachter, L. M., & Weller, S. C. (1993). Acculturation and compliance with medical therapy. *Journal of Developmental and Behavioral Pediatrics, 14*, 163–168.

Perrin, J. M. (1985). Chronically ill children in America. *Caring, 4*(5), 16–22.

Ray, N. F., Thamer, M., Fadillioglu, B., & Gergen, P. J. (1998). Race, income, urbanicity, and asthma hospitalization in California: A small area analysis. *Chest, 113*, 1277–1284.

Rivara, F. P., Grossman, D. C., & Cummings, P. (1997). Injury prevention (Pt. 1). *New England Journal of Medicine, 337*, 543–548.

Roter, D. L., Stewart, M., Putnam, S. M., Lipkin, M., Stiles, W., & Inui, T. S. (1997). Communication patterns of primary care physicians. *Journal of the American Medical Association, 277*, 350–356.

Scheper-Hughes, N., & Sargent, C. (Eds.). (1998). *Small wars: The cultural politics of childhood*. Berkeley: University of California Press.

Schor, E. L. (1986). Use of health care services by children and diagnoses received during presumably stressful life transitions. *Pediatrics, 77*, 834–841.

Schuster, M. A., McGlynn, E. A., & Brook, R. H. (1998). How good is the quality of health care in the United States? *Milbank Quarterly, 76*, 517–563.

Shryock, R. H. (1966). *Medicine in America: Historical essays*. Baltimore: Johns Hopkins Press.

Sobo, E. J., & Rock, C. L. (2001). "You ate all that?" Caretaker-child interaction during children's assisted dietary recall interviews. *Medical Anthropology Quarterly, 15*, 222–244.

Sobo, E. J., Rock, C. L., Neuhouser, M. L., Maciel, T. L., & Neumark-Sztainer, D. (2000). Caretaker-child interaction during children's 24-hour dietary recalls: Who contributes what to the recall record? *Journal of the American Dietetic Association, 100,* 428–433.

Sobo, E. J., & Seid, M. (2001, November 30). *Cultural issues in pediatric medicine: What kind of "competence" is needed?* Paper presented at the 100th annual meeting of the American Anthropological Association, Washington, DC.

Starfield, B. (1992). Effects of poverty on health status. *Bulletin of the New York Academy of Medicine, 68,* 17–24.

Starfield, B., & Scheff, D. (1972). Effectiveness of pediatric care: The relationship between processes and outcome. *Pediatrics, 49,* 547–552.

Stewart, M. A. (1995). Effective physician-patient communication and health outcomes: A review. *Canadian Medical Association Journal, 152,* 1423–1433.

Tates, K., & Meeuwesen, L. (2001). Doctor-parent-child communication. A (re)view of the literature. *Social Science and Medicine, 52,* 839–851.

Tumlinson, A., Bottigheimer, H., Mahoney, P., Stone, E. M., & Hendricks, A. (1997). Choosing a health plan: What information will consumers use? *Health Affairs* (Millwood), *16,* 229–238.

U.S. Bureau of the Census. (1997). *Statistical abstract of the United States, 1997.* Washington, DC: Government Printing Office.

U.S. Department of Health and Human Services. (2000). *Healthy people 2010: Healthy people in healthy communities.* Washington, DC: Government Printing Office.

Waldman, M. L. (1973). The medical audit study: A tool for quality control. *Hospital Progress, 54,* 82–88.

Weinick, R. M., Weigers, M. E., & Cohen, J. W. (1998). Children's health insurance, access to care, and health status: New findings. *Health Affairs* (Millwood), *17,* 127–136.

Weinick, R. M., Zuvekas, S. H., & Cohen, J. W. (2000). Racial and ethnic differences in access to and use of health care services, 1977 to 1996. *Medical Care Research and Review, 57*(Suppl. 1), 36–54.

Wennberg, J. E. (1984–1985, Winter). Administrators must pursue policies that reduce excess beds, employees. *Health Management Quarterly,* pp. 6–7.

Wennberg, J. E., Freeman, J. L., Shelton, R. M., & Bubolz, T. A. (1989). Hospital use and mortality among Medicare beneficiaries in Boston and New Haven. *New England Journal of Medicine, 321,* 1168–1173.

Williamson, J. W., & Wilson, R. (1978). *Assessing and improving health care outcomes: The health accounting approach to quality assurance.* Cambridge, MA: Ballinger.

Part II

. . . .

Child Health in Context

Home, Neighborhood, Community, Culture

Prevention and Healing in the Household

The Importance of Sociocultural Context

Elisa J. Sobo

This chapter focuses on the household context of children's lives. Child health is not simply an outcome of biomedical health services provision or use; it also and in fact primarily derives from activities undertaken and exposures experienced by children as dependent household members. Accordingly, **child health services research (CHSR)** that limits itself to traditional clinical service provision variables (such as length of hospital stay or cost per case) is of limited utility for the majority of children. Such research fails to account for variability in the degree to which children from different types of households benefit from biomedical care; therefore, it provides no insight into how to decrease household-related variability and concomitant health disparities. This is because it disregards what is crucial to the success or failure of biomedical child health efforts: the *context* in which children and families live their lives and attempt to create and maintain good health.

Appreciation of context is essential for the provision of high-quality health care. It allows for customization of care, which is a key feature in the critical and widely hailed report *Crossing the Quality Chasm* (Institute of Medicine, 2001). Customization is one of the report's "ten simple rules" for the twenty-first-century health care system. A closely related construct, **patient-centered care**, which encompasses responsiveness to the needs and preferences of the patient, is one of the report's "six specific aims for improvement." This underscores the urgency with which child health services investigators must extend their methodological reach to take into account factors that were, until recently, viewed by many as beyond the purview of CHSR.

To aid researchers in identifying salient context variables, which all contributors to this volume see as central to CHSR, this chapter begins by defining *culture* and *household,* two areas in which many key variables are observed. We examine the household production of health and discuss factors associated with safe home environments. Throughout the chapter, we take into account the increasingly multicultural nature of U.S. society today.

This chapter's focus on culture and household is not to deny the power of economic forces. Indeed, aspects of culture and household that encourage or discourage good health are intimately linked to economic (and therefore political) arrangements (Baer, Singer, & Johnson, 1986; Farmer, 1999; Singer, Valentin, Baer, & Jia, 1992). It is precisely because of this fact that a focus on culture and household can serve as a useful starting point for broadening the scope—and usefulness—of CHSR.

What Is Culture?

Culture is a design for living. It is present in all aspects of life. And yet, until we are faced with a contrasting culture that challenges the basis of our beliefs, values, and identities, we generally take our own culture for granted and forget that others may act and understand the world differently.

A **culture**, briefly put, is all the shared, learned knowledge that people in a society hold. A **society** (again, in brief) consists of a group of interdependent people who interact, usually within a specific geographical area. (For a definition of *community,* see Chapter Five, by Dennis and Simmes.)

Culture guides how people in a society interact; it influences and to some degree determines what they believe and value and how they communicate. Culture prescribes rituals, art forms, and customs of daily living—including those related to household structure as well as to health and well-being. It guides the ways in which people meet their society's various needs, including how goods and services (such as health care) are produced and distributed and how children are raised and cared for.

So culture is a kind of knowledge that we use and act on. Importantly, cultural knowledge can be changed or adapted by its users to fit new conditions. A group's culture is always evolving as the life circumstances of the group change.

Although culture is shared, it is not shared equally among all members of a group. Age, gender, and other subcultures exist; they account for much intracultural variation. Intracultural variation would exist even without subcultures, in part because cultural knowledge is distributed unequally—for example, by role—but also because of culture's inherent flexibility. Cultures change all the time, as differences seen over the past few decades in the content of child-rearing advice columns show. Variability can increase when cultures bump up against one another, as they do in pluralistic societies such as our own.

Acculturation

Enculturation entails learning one's native culture; **acculturation** happens when a person learns a new or second culture. Some health services research (HSR) considers acculturation a key variable. However, most researchers actually use the term to mean assimilation to middle-class Anglo-American culture (**assimilation** involves unlearning or rejecting and replacing one's native culture with another, generally the dominant one). For this and other reasons, such as a tendency to conflate linguistic skill with cultural facility, it has been argued that a good acculturation measure does not exist (for a detailed review, see Clark & Hofsess, 1998). Acculturation measures come up short when scrutinized in terms of what they can tell us about people's abilities to navigate the biomedical health care system, and this is the crucial variable for HSR.

The construct of "functional biomedical acculturation" (Sobo & Seid, 2001) refers to learning the skills to move within the health care system and to optimize the health care received. This requires that a person be at least minimally or functionally acculturated to the world (culture) of the health care system (biomedicine). Functional biomedical acculturation is more useful for HSR than "acculturation" as that concept is presently deployed (see Chapter Seven, by Seid, Sobo, Zivkovic, Nelson, and Far; see also Sobo & Seid, 2001).

Ethnicity

Culture is different from **ethnicity**. Culture includes all of our non-biological heritage, including everything socially constructed and learned (Hufford, 1996). Ethnicity is a subset of that. It is a facet of the self that is tied to notions of shared origins that contrast with those of people with whom one shares borders (be they household, neighborhood, or national borders). In the United States, ethnicity is reflected in the classifications of African American, Mexican American, Navajo, and the like. Even without explicit continental, national, or tribal qualifiers, all of us have an ethnic heritage or a mix of ethnic heritages that we may choose to honor.

Many health researchers have erroneously deployed the terms *ethnicity* and *race* as if they were equivalent. However, the concept of "ethnicity" differs from that of "race" in that "race" presumes to sort people into groups on the basis of physical traits, whereas "ethnicity" assumes that groups of people are distinguished by cultural knowledge and practices.

Technically, a **race** is a biological subspecies differentiated by anatomical or physiological characteristics. Historically, however, racial categorizations have focused on traits that are easily seen, such as skin color and facial features; this visual focus has helped groups in positions of power to use racial categorizations oppressively. Research regarding existing racial categories has shown that within-race differences are by far greater than those demonstrated to exist between purported racial groups. In other words, race is a social construct, not a biological fact (see Diamond, 1994; Gould, 1994; Waters, 2000).

Research that lumps all members of a given racial group together leads to spurious conclusions because members can be from completely different backgrounds. For example, the category "Asian" can include people from Korea, Cambodia, and Japan as well as Americans of Asian descent. "Black" can include Somalians, Haitians, Australian Aboriginals, and African Americans. Other racial categories can include equally diverse mixes. Important between-group differences (both biological and cultural) may be masked. Likewise, between-group differences can be erroneously imputed when samples are nonrepresentative for a given racial category, as they normally will be because research is generally geographically limited.

The same caveats hold true for ethnic groupings if too broadly defined. To further complicate matters, people often have multiple ethnicities, and they may participate only partly in their ethnic traditions or not at all. In any case, research groupings based only on "race" or "ethnicity" can lead researchers to overlook other salient differentiating variables, such as gender, income, nationality, migration status, and occupation.

All this notwithstanding, because racial categories are scientifically unsound and because knowledge about learned cultural practices can be applied to decrease health disparities and increase well-being, in this chapter we use the construct of "ethnicity" to denote human diversity associated with notions of shared origins. We recommend the same for CHSR. (An alternative is to acknowledge the common conflation of the terms *race* and *ethnicity* through reference to "ethnoracial" groups; see Chapter Two, by Gidwani, Sobo, Seid, and Kurtin).

Occupation

Like ethnicity, occupation-specific knowledge and patterns of action are sometimes treated as if a culture. Although technically this is not the case, it is true that occupational learning shapes people's habits of thought and action, at least to some degree.

When a person decides to become a physician, for example, he or she acquires not only a new vocabulary but also a way of seeing that goes with that vocabulary. As a Harvard medical student explains, "In a sense we are learning a whole new world . . . because learning new names for things is to learn new things about them. If you know the name of every tree you look at trees differently. Otherwise they're just trees" (Good & Good, 1993, p. 98). Becoming a doctor—or an acupuncturist, a nurse, or any other kind of health worker (researcher included)—is thus a process of acculturation as well as the result of long hours of hard work and study.

The Household and the Health System

Like health workers, pediatric patients and their families have cultural orientations that can influence their encounters with the health system and ultimately their health outcomes. Before discussing these, we must ask about the social settings in which patients and families live their lives. In the case of the pediatric patient, one of the most important settings is the household (another is the school; see American Academy of Pediatrics, Committee on School Health, 2001).

What Is a Household?

A **household** is a group of people who share living space at a given point in time. Household members sleep in the same residence and generally share food. A household is essentially an economic unit; it jointly produces goods or pools money and purchases commodities like power and water or food. As part of this process, households also produce health and illness.

In daily life, people often use the terms *family* and *household* interchangeably. But **family** is a kinship term; it refers to biological (for example, genetic or blood) or legal ties as they relate to descent and ancestry. One of the reasons that the term *household* is confused with *family* in the United States is that households here may be categorized with reference to the contemporary Western kinship arrangements reflected in their makeup: nuclear, extended, blended, joint, and so on (see Gross, 1992). Although a family may live as a household, a household need not contain members of the same kin group. Fewer than one in four U.S. households consists of a two-parent family unit ("At Last," 2001).

The household-family distinction is complicated by the fact that we all know people who are talked about and treated as if kin with the full knowledge that they are related neither biologically nor legally. This is especially relevant to child health research, as people may take responsibility for such things as the socialization, protection, education, and health care of children who are not their biological progeny or legal charges. For efficiency's sake and in honor of the importance of social parenthood, this chapter refers to all primary caregivers of children as "parents"; nevertheless, CHSR investigators collecting kinship data must determine whether the distinction between social kinship and legal or biological kinship is important to the research question at hand.

Moreover, the complexity of the household-family interlink suggests that assumptions or theoretical propositions regarding households may not be generalizable to families, and vice versa. Care should be taken to specify exactly what is under study; the choice to focus on family or household will depend on the needs of the research. Some guidance on what to measure is provided at the chapter's end, after further exploration of context-related issues that CHSR investigators should be aware of.

How Does the Household Intersect with the Formal Health Care System?

The majority of health care is delivered in the household. Much in-home health care is preventive: household members teach children appropriate practices of diet, exercise, dental care, physical maintenance of other kinds, and body awareness. Curative care is proffered when household members are ill or injured.

Although studies of daily health problems in children are still rare, research on suburban Swedish families with young children suggests that children may have at least one health problem (including injuries, infections, skin disorders, allergies, and aches) every three to four days (Dahlquist, Sterky, Ivarsson, Tengvald, & Wall, 1987). Most of these problems are what parents view as mild, but more than 50 percent last for three or more days.

Similar research that focused on families with at least one child aged six to eighteen months (Hojer, Sterky, & Widlund, 1987) had comparable findings: these young children had health problems once every three days (most often respiratory symptoms, followed by gastroenteritis, then rashes or eczema). Perhaps due to increased contact opportunities, significantly more respiratory symptoms were reported for young children who had older siblings or whose parents had relatives or friends living in the immediate vicinity. Parents took some action in response to the symptoms on 70 percent of the complaint days: on 44 percent of the complaint days, they gave the children medicine of some kind; on 13 percent, they altered the children's diets. They consulted biomedical clinicians on only 9 percent of the young children's complaint days.

So most of the time, at least for children without special health care needs, pediatric health services are provided in the household with no reference at all to the formal health care system. This happens, for example, when a parent faced with an ill child decides to wait and watch, prepare a home remedy, procure an over-the-counter remedy, or use drugs prescribed for another purpose. Even when consultations are sought, they may be with care providers who work outside of the formal health care system. Such providers may be professionals, such as herbalists or chiropractors, or nonprofessionals known for their health knowledge or skill, such as a relative or neighbor. Other times, clinicians in the formal health care system may recommend care plans to be carried out at home, such as administering antibiotics and fluids. Home care is indeed the mainstay of child health.

The diversity of sources from which care can come has been mapped in many ways, including Arthur Kleinman's tripartite scheme of *popular, folk,* and *professional* medicine (1978). In this scheme, there are three sectors of health care. The key variables are who provides care and in what context. Popular-sector treatment is based on shared cultural understandings and is provided by nonspecialists: oneself, friends, parents, or other kin and relations. Household health care delivery fits here. Folk-sector healers are specialists whose practice is based on cultural traditions and philosophies, as is the case in the Haitian practice of *vodun* (sometimes called "voodoo"). Legally sanctioned official systems (for example, the biomedical system) make up what Kleinman called the professional sector.

This typology is an advance on simple public-private dichotomizing, in which private or household care is separated from the formal health care system and is discounted. The scheme allows for the interpenetration of these arenas and values care that is given in the home. But the model does have shortcomings; for example, it implies that professional medicine has no cultural traditions. Further, it is not easily applied cross-culturally. Although Kleinman specifically allows that some nonbiomedical practices, such as Ayurvedic medicine, should be classed as professional-sector offerings due to their routinized, formalized, professionalized nature, this is easily forgotten by those who regard those modalities as so-called folk practices.

Bonnie O'Connor's model (1995) has only two parts: *conventional* medicine and *vernacular* medicine. The latter category subsumes Kleinman's (1978) folk and popular sectors and so includes the household; the former consists only of the official health care industry endorsed by dominant Western nations. (It is this authorized, authoritative, dominative (Baer et al., 1986) system referred to in this book as "the health care system.") The contrast in O'Connor's model is simple but important, because it explicitly highlights the authoritative position ascribed to conventional U.S. medicine.

O'Connor's model does not represent conventional medicine as one coherent system. In the United States, conventional systems (hospitals, private practices, rehabilitation centers, school health clinics, and so on) are only loosely systematized. Patient records are not centrally held. And although federal regulations do exist, many areas of practice are subject to local or state standards. Children who receive care from multiple health care subsystems may therefore be challenged by a lack of care continuity.

For example, the child with asthma who is treated at school, by a primary care physician, and in an emergency room may receive three different standards of care. This can be damaging to his or her health, as well as confusing. The child's household standard of care for asthma may differ also, adding to the complexity of his or her medical history, as does consultation with a nonconventional healer.

Despite the fact that the goal of HSR is to understand and assist in the improvement of the formal health services sector itself, a traditional, narrow research mission that concerns only the "professional" or "conventional" sector is no longer tenable. The relationship of care continuity to number and variety of care sources, as well as ways to increase care continuity, are key questions for CHSR investigators. The household is the central node at which the various care systems consulted intersect. Figure 3.1, which combines the insights of both O'Connor and Kleinman, provides a useful heuristic for conceptualizing this intersection.

Figure 3.1. Sources of Pediatric Medical Provision.

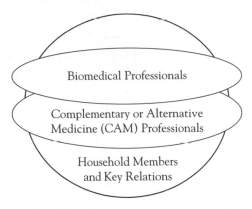

Note: The large circle represents the home; the intersecting ovals represent out-of-household participation. Power relations are represented by vertical stacking; although biomedicine is dominant, the fact that household factors can override biomedical orders is shown in the circle's protrusion over the top of the biomedical oval.

Household Production of (Ill) Health and Injury

Because the household plays such a major role in child health, inclusion of household factors in CHSR efforts is essential. We have already discussed some of the social structural factors that affect child health. To gain insight into what other relevant factors might be, the household production of health, injury, and disease, as well as the cultural understandings that may drive certain responses to the challenge of maintaining children's health, must be discussed, and the articulation of the household with other sectors of health service—that is, the relationship of the home care to other care—must be further examined.

The Health-Producing Household

In an ideal world, all households would be safe, health-promoting places. Children would be given age-appropriate instruction on how to prevent illness and injury and how to promote well-being.

Parents and other household members would watch over children to ensure that they received the nourishment, exercise, and well-child care that they need. However, largely due to macro-level factors, such as those expressed in poverty (see Chapter Seven, by Seid, Sobo, Zivkovic, Nelson, and Far), but for other reasons also, such as habitual or culturally patterned ways of thinking and acting, not all households produce healthy children.

Unintentional Injury

Most childhood injuries happen at home. Now that major infectious diseases are under control in the United States, the major cause of morbidity and mortality among children is injury—primarily unintentional injury occurring from motor vehicle crashes (often due to improperly attached restraints) or from falls. According to the American Academy of Pediatrics (AAP) Committee on Injury and Poison Prevention (2001), falling from a high place is the leading cause of childhood injury.

In urban areas, where many households occupy high-rise apartments, falls from roofs, windows, and balconies are a major source of childhood injury. The AAP committee found that most children injured in long falls are African American or Latino: children in these groups are most likely to be poor, and the poor are more likely to occupy deteriorating housing with no air conditioning and out-of-date safety features. The committee also found that most long falls occur in the summer months, when windows are open and children may play on rooftops, balconies, and fire escapes. The age distribution for long falls is bimodal, with preschool children usually injured by falling out of windows and older children (generally boys) injured by falls from dangerous areas. According to the AAP committee, restricting access to these areas as well as the use of window guards decreases long-fall injuries (2001).

Enacting such safety measures hinges to some degree on landlord cooperation, which may be difficult to come by in low-income housing without legislation and financial support. Education may also help, as many householders may be unaware of the threat. Research can help identify the most vulnerable geographical areas so that education may be targeted. Research can also help determine the best method of intervention delivery as well as the most effective educational content, both of which may vary according to particular household factors.

Even when playing on equipment intended for play, children can get hurt, and again falls are implicated: over 80 percent of injuries on home play equipment are from falls, especially onto hard surfaces. Sharp points, a lack of guardrails, spaces in which children can get trapped, and protruding hardware are also implicated in home play equipment injuries. Death, though not common, can occur, and the lack of protective (soft) surfaces to fall onto contributes to this, as does the presence of loose ropes: almost three-fourths of deaths at home were the result of hanging from ropes, rope swings, and similar play items (U.S. Consumer Product Safety Commission, 2001). Again, safety education is recommended, as well as higher standards for home play equipment. Further, research on how and why children and parents do or do not put recommendations to use is needed; the number of children who know, for example, that bicycle helmets are useful but still do not wear them demonstrates this need.

Patterns of Injury

Injuries may be patterned and predictable. Childhood injuries tend to cluster within sibling groups, at least over brief time spans. Retrospective cohort research conducted in Wisconsin found that children whose siblings were injured were more likely to be injured themselves: 10 percent of all sibling groups identified on the basis of one child's injury experienced injury to a second member within ninety days (Johnston, Grossman, Connell, & Koepsell, 2000).

This research (which included only children and injuries treated in the emergency department or in inpatient settings) calls into question the assumption that children who get injured are intrinsically accident-prone (see also Wazana, 1997). The second sibling's injury suggests that it may be more useful to consider extrinsic, household factors as contributing to childhood injury. Shared social and environmental exposures may explain the clustering. Further, because sibling risk returned to normal after ninety days, it may well be that high-risk households are not permanently so. That is, risk may be a transient phenomenon, associated perhaps with changes in a household's member makeup, pattern of child supervision, or financial status. Life events such as marriage, divorce, death, and birth have been associated with increased morbidity, and the increase in risk of injury to members of sibling groups may reflect such factors (Johnston et al., 2000).

Although this chapter's focus is on household injury, it would be remiss not to acknowledge that many childhood injuries occur at school. School choice is, of course, limited by and related to household location, structure, and income; school is thus in some ways an extension of the household context.

A study conducted in Colorado put the incidence of school injuries at nearly one in ten students (Lenaway, Ambler, & Beaudoin, 1992). Injuries were generally recreation-related. Middle school and junior high school students had the highest injury rate, and boys were about one and one-half more times likely to be injured at school than girls.

Research concerning the social **epidemiology** of injury and the ways this links to household and neighborhood factors is sorely needed. So is research regarding care delivery after an incident has occurred, as well as the ways in which school health systems function and the quality of care they provide. (Regarding the school's role in child health, see American Academy of Pediatrics, Committee on School Health, 2001.)

Risk Perception

The fact that knowledge does not always translate into action suggests that perception of risk is a key factor in the production of injury and avoidable illness. Risk perception is influenced by cognitive biases to which all human beings are prone, as well as by experience and context. Risk perception also is influenced by the cultural value placed on the various anticipated outcomes of the risky action. In some cases, avoiding a health-related risk can put a person at risk for other consequences, such as damage to social or financial status; in this case, health-related risk taking may be viewed as adaptive, at least in the short term (Sobo, 1995). For example, a child's decision not to use a bicycle helmet due to anticipated negative peer response is, at least in the short term, an adaptive and rational plan of action.

Culture also discourages or encourages the view that accidents are unavoidable. Indeed, the term *accident* has been singled out as contributing to this mind-set due to its connotations: an accident is an unintentional event. Many injury prevention specialists therefore avoid using the term. Instead, an event resulting in injury is an *incident*; a motor vehicle collision is a *crash*. Such linguistic switches toward terms that allow for human intentionality make prevention possible—or at least make people more receptive to the preventive approach.

Intentional Injury

One child is killed by a parent every two hours in the United States (Goodman, 1990), and more than one million children are abused each year. About half of these children suffer neglect; one-quarter, physical abuse; one-eighth, sexual abuse (Nair, 1998). These figures are probably low; in many cases, abuse is never reported. When it is not reported—or at least when intervention is not instituted—abuse will recur half of the time. In 35 percent of these cases, a child will be killed or severely injured (Goodman, 1990).

Many parents who kill do not intend to do so. Jill Korbin (1997) found that women incarcerated for fatal child maltreatment all saw themselves as "good" caretakers. Optimistically biased comparisons between themselves and others helped parents maintain the view that they are fulfilling role expectations: they can always find examples of worse parents (Hassin, 1994; Sobo, 1995). This self-perception was, prior to the fatality, supported by health care professionals as well as by friends and relations.

Stressful social circumstances may encourage violent parenting, especially when one's children's behavior is seen to reflect on one's own worth. Poverty is one stressor. However, "any correlation between abuse and poverty is biased by the fact that the behavior of the poor is more likely to be reported in official records than that of members of other classes, who are better equipped to conceal their activities" (Kornblum & Julian, 1995, p. 211). The degree to which one shares personal characteristics such as skin color with potential reporters also seems to be an issue. For example, head trauma is most often missed when parents have characteristics like those of the clinicians performing the evaluations (Leventhal, 1999). The other side of the coin is that because of bias, abuse may be suspected where none occurred: one study showed that 18 percent of children suspected to have been abused were in fact not subjected to maltreatment (Jenny, Hymel, Ritzen, Reinert, & Hay, 1999).

The ways children are treated should always be understood in a cultural context, as should the definition of *harm*. For example, members of various Asian cultures may rub a coin on an ill child's skin to pull the illness out (see the appendix to this chapter). The marks left by coin rubbing might suggest intentional child abuse. This is generally not the case: when seen in context, coin rubbing demonstrates love and caring (Korbin, 1987, p. 28). Clearly, knowledge of the cultural practices common among populations of interest is an essential safeguard against making inappropriate maltreatment assumptions in CHSR.

Several factors placing children at risk for abuse are found across cultures: deformities or handicaps or multiple or difficult births, any of which may be interpreted as malevolent or inauspicious; culturally defined illegitimacy; gender preferences; rapid socioeconomic and sociocultural change; urbanization; unemployment; and poverty. The fact that immigrant children may adjust to a new environment more rapidly than their parents and hence may become less obedient and compliant may also come into play (Korbin, 1987).

Once a child has been abused, a cycle of risk taking and violence may begin. Adolescent males who reported having experienced abuse were also more likely to report risk-taking behavior, such as driving after drinking or committing violent acts (Hernandez, Lodico, & DiClemente, 1993). In contrast, probably for reasons related to how we construct gender roles and expectations, women abused during childhood may be at increased risk for revictimization as adults, for example, through domestic violence or rape (Coid et al., 2001). Experiencing abuse may also be correlated with an increased likelihood of perpetrating child abuse on others. Two-thirds of mothers who kill or attempt to kill their children may have been abused as children (Haapasalo & Petaja, 1999). But not all people who victimize others were abused as children, and not all who were abused as children will become victimizers (Kaufman & Zigler, 1987; Narang & Contreras, 2000). Both the protective factors and the perpetuating factors in the intergenerational violence cycle merit further research.

Disease and Illness

In addition to injury, children may suffer from disease due to household practices. For example, passive smoke inhalation increases children's risk for otitis media, bronchitis, pneumonia, and asthma. Children who live with smokers are more likely to be hospitalized for lower respiratory infections and to receive emergency care for asthma. In addition, they miss more days of school than children who live in nonsmoking households (Emmons et al., 2001). Another negative factor is child exposure to chemicals, often due to aging or poor-quality housing (see Cummins & Jackson, 2001; Landrigan, 2001).

Household dietary practices also influence child health, starting from birth. Children fed more breast milk than infant formula or breast-fed for a longer period of time have significantly lower chances of being overweight as older children or adolescents (Gillman et al., 2001). Regularly eating less nutritious food after weaning also seems to be associated with obesity or "overweight," which affects about one in four U.S. children. (Regarding the related problem of food insufficiency and its effects on child development, see Alaimo, Olson, & Frongillo, 2001.) Overweight does not seem to vary significantly with ethnicity, income, or education, although an inverse relationship between income and weight is noted among non-Hispanic whites, and both Mexican American and non-Hispanic black girls do account for proportionately more overweight children (Troiano & Flegal, 1998).

Being overweight places children at risk for diseases such as diabetes and heart disease as well as sleep apnea. Excess weight also may lead to mental health problems such as depression, low self-esteem, and body image disturbances. A study examining the relationship between weight and self-concept among preschool-aged children found that girls as young as five years old had worse self-concepts if they had higher weights. Parental concern over a child's weight and related food restrictions were also associated with negative self-concepts among the children. The study included only girls because the recent increases in overweight rates are particularly high for them (Davison & Birch, 2001). Gender norms are related to weight issues (Bordo, 1993); how and why they are affecting such young children needs examination.

Quality and quantity of food can foster overweight, but so can eating style. The influence of household norms seems important here. Under laboratory conditions, when parents are present, overweight children eat significantly faster and take significantly larger bites (Laessle, Uhl, Lindel, & Muller, 2001).

Parental factors may also support (or discourage) healthy rates of physical activity among children: in one study that used children's self-reports, children with active fathers engaged in more physical activity themselves (Trost, Kerr, Ward, & Pate, 2001).

Modeling may be impossible in neighborhoods with no parks or recreation spaces or where walking is unsafe due to traffic or discouraged by a lack of sidewalks and an otherwise uninviting environment (as in many commuter suburbs).

Fortunately, adult activity levels and related health outcomes seem to be only modestly correlated with their childhood activity and fitness measures (Leonard, 2001). Nonetheless, more active lifestyles can be more healthful. How and why lifestyle changes happen are questions for future study; the answers might lead to more successful interventions. At present, research has not been able to identify generalizable conclusions regarding how to create successful childhood obesity prevention programs (Campbell, Waters, O'Meara, & Summerbell, 2001).

The Relativity of Health

What is poor health to one person or one culture may be no problem to another, and vice versa. Whereas physician interpretations of body measurements may be that a child is "overweight," parents may not agree. Mothers in one study disagreed with physician labeling of their preschool children as overweight if their children were active and ate diets regarded as "healthy." The mothers viewed their children as overweight if physical activity was limited, diets were "unhealthy," and the children were teased about their weight. Clearly, social norms play a role in health evaluation (Jain et al., 2001).

There are many examples of differences of opinion regarding whether a given condition is a health problem. In some cultures, what many in the United States call mental illness is not only not classified as illness but is interpreted as favor from God that allows an individual to understand or see what others cannot. Another example of dissonant classification occurs in relation to the Navajo, for whom the prevalence of congenital hip disease is relatively high. The Navajo do not regard the condition as significant and so do not consider treatment necessary. The resultant limp carries no stigma for the Navajo, as it might for mainstream U.S. citizens (Adair, Deuschle, & Barnett, 1988).

Disease or Illness?

The Navajo example highlights a technical distinction that should inform HSR. **Disease** is a biomedical phenomenon. A disease is a biomedically measurable lesion or irregularity in a person's physiology or anatomy. It is not disease that spurs a person to seek medical treatment but rather **illness**—the experience of being unwell. As Robert Hahn points out, it is a person's "experience of suffering which engenders the whole medical enterprise. The sufferer's judgment rather than that of biomedicine defines the *underlying problem*" (1984, p.17; emphasis in the original; see also Mechanic, 1962). Although certain conditions will be universally unwanted, one person's major illness may be another's minor annoyance.

People who are biologically diseased may not perceive themselves as ill, and vice versa. Because in most instances disease is self-limiting (it goes away without biomedical intervention), this is not necessarily a bad thing. However, it may pose a problem when children who feel well are labeled as ill or when one feels ill but no disease is found. It may pose financial, health, and other problems for society when individuals with unacknowledged diseases get sicker or pass their diseases to others or when children thought of as not well are prevented from reaching their full potential. Understanding the cultural aspects of illness perception can thus aid in protecting both individuals and society.

In the case of pediatric medicine, the perspectives of children must be explored. Although there are important exceptions (for example, Bibace & Walsh, 1981; Bush et al., 1996; Mayall, 1996), research into children's conceptualizations regarding illness and disease are lacking. We still know very little about how children view their health; this situation must change, and CHSR investigators should be among the vanguard in seeing that it does.

Cultural Understandings of Health

Although we know little about children's views on health, we do know quite a bit regarding what parents think about children's health and well-being. All cultures have ideas about how the body works. Bodies are much the same the world over. Consequently, there are many underlying similarities in different cultures' anatomical and physiological notions.

Familiarity with cross-cultural similarities in ideas about maintaining good health will help researchers incorporate into their studies context variables that are relevant to the HSR questions at hand. For example, a study of chemotherapy outcomes involving care plans that include oral medications must take into account cultural understandings about how the body processes or reacts to the ingestion of pharmaceuticals. In an effort to facilitate informed research design, let us review some basic information about universal themes in cultural understandings of health (further details are provided in the appendix to this chapter).

Many aspects of cross-cultural understandings about the body are simply elaborate abstractions of the basic principles of physics or selective but honest descriptions of basic, universal, embodied experiences (Johnson, 1987; Lakoff, 1987). For example, as shown in the appendix, many health understandings build on knowledge and experience of the hotness or coldness, dryness or dampness, purity or impurity, and heaviness or lightness of substances in the physical world. The flow and blockage of these substances and principles of displacement, imbalance, intrusion, and decay also figure highly in cross-cultural notions regarding health.

In addition to building on basic-level models to create entire health-related explanatory systems, people exposed to different technologies will use different metaphors from these technologies to describe and understand body functions. Martin (1987) demonstrates this in relation to the historical changes our own society has undergone: with industrialization, the body was increasingly imaged as a factory, converting energy into products. Like the factory—indeed, like our society in general—the body was seen as hierarchically organized rather than as made up of systems that functioned as a committee of equals, each exerting mutual influence.

A culture's specific health-related understandings underlie the specific therapies or preventive health practices advocated. While these therapies or practices sometimes make biomedical sense, they always make cultural sense, following a logic for which culture provides the basis.

Caring for the Sick: Patterns of Resort

To serve their patients well, clinicians must understand why parents choose to consult them, know exactly what parents think their children's symptoms mean, and discuss their own inferences before prescribing a treatment regimen. Applied CHSR can support such efforts by developing models for the efficient, valid, and reliable collection of relevant information. Such models must take into account what we already know in regard to the pediatric health-seeking process and practitioner-patient communication.

The Health-Seeking Process

The at-home recognition of symptoms—the first step in what Noel Chrisman (1977) termed the **health-seeking process** and a key factor in realized access to care—depends on cultural definitions of normal health as well as understandings about the causes and contexts of sickness. Some important factors in symptom recognition are the level of danger to life and the interference with lifestyle and function—the disability—engendered. Symptom visibility and frequency are more important still. The visibility and frequency of the symptom in question in other children and the way this compares to its visibility and frequency in a parent's own child is key, for the former provides the parent with a context for evaluating the seriousness of his or her own child's condition.

Most health-seeking theories relate to perception of symptoms and the consequent decision to consult a physician. But symptoms are not always grouped in the same way cross-culturally, and the physician is not always the first or even last provider consulted. Self-care of one's children via home remedies, over-the-counter medicines, or leftover prescription drugs is often the first and only step in dealing with a perceived health problem. As noted by Gidwani, Sobo, Seid, and Kurtin in Chapter Two and by Seid, Sobo, Zivkovic, Nelson, and Far in Chapter Seven, lack of health insurance can affect **patterns of resort** (the patterns people follow when resorting to health care), and self-care may be preferred even when biomedical treatment is free (Demers, Altamore, Mustin, Kleinman, & Leonardi, 1980). In addition to self-care, many people chose to consult alternative practitioners prior to, along with, or instead of physicians. (We shall return to this topic later in this chapter.)

Can the Child Be Cured?

Chrisman's inclusion of the degree to which the individual thinks that something can be done is also a part of the Health Belief Model, a long-standing theoretical framework regarding the likelihood for care seeking (Janz & Becker, 1984; see also Rosenstock, 1966, 1969, 1974, and Becker, 1974, cited in Chrisman, 1977). This model posits that an individual's subjective evaluation of an illness situation, including the value placed on a particular outcome and the belief that a particular action will result in that outcome, becomes the key variable in the utilization of health services. Often the patient's (or, in the case of pediatric care, the parent's) common sense may conflict with clinical judgment (see Becker & Maiman, 1975).

Although cause is not always an issue—in some cases, the cure is not related to perceptions regarding the cause—cause or etiology can be another important driver of care seeking. Health problems can be caused by pathogens, accidents, or physical degeneration; they can also be caused by supernatural means or by relationships that do not meet idealized cultural standards, and they may be treated accordingly. In many cultures, health problems point to social problems. For example, if Jamaican babies fail to thrive—especially if they have trouble walking—observers may assume that "bad" breast milk is the cause. They may attribute a mother's "bad" milk to infidelity—and therefore to the fact that the baby's father has not lived up to expectations to support the child. In a pattern seen universally, the baby's poor health is taken as an indicator of the family's social problems (Sobo, 1993).

Health problems can encompass behavioral or emotional problems, as in the case of attention deficit hyperactivity disorder (ADHD). While research suggests that ADHD is found cross-culturally, the same hyperactive or inattentive behaviors are associated with different degrees of dysfunction in different cultural contexts and may therefore be identified, or not, as a problem in need of biomedical attention. Teachers in Columbia, for example, are more tolerant of ADHD-related behaviors than teachers in the United States. And U.S. teachers are more tolerant of such behaviors in Euro-American and Hispanic American students than in their African American students (Brewis, Schmidt, & Meyer, 2001). Tolerance therefore seems linked not only to cultural context but also to racial and gender stereotypes. Further research is needed in regard to the social and cultural dimensions of diagnosing health problems.

Multiple Treatment Strategies

The concept of the biomedically oriented "lay referral" system originated with Eliot Friedson (1960), who suggested that when people become ill, they first turn to family and friends, then to suggested lay experts, and finally, if nothing works, to a physician and the biomedical system (although lay norms may influence this option).

This behavior is consistent with Romanucci-Ross's still-popular concept, the **hierarchy of resort** (1969/1977). While Romanucci-Ross was concerned with acculturation issues, most scholars who use the phrase today generally mean that people try the most familiar or simplest and cheapest treatment first and then seek more expensive, complex, or unfamiliar treatments if necessary.

Although treatment choice can follow a hierarchical sequence, often patterns of resort are cumulative and pluralistic, involving many treatment modalities at once. People often creatively combine recommendations, coming up with the regimen they feel is right for them. As Chrisman (1977) pointed out, the health-seeking process is dynamic, and people are constantly reevaluating their symptoms and actions and revising their plans.

Procuring Help in the Household Production of Health: CAM Therapies

When parents cannot adequately address a child's health needs through household approaches, professional advice may be sought. Sometimes this entails consulting a practitioner of **complementary or alternative medicine (CAM)**. CAM—medical "interventions neither taught widely in U.S. medical schools nor generally available in U.S. hospitals" (Eisenberg et al., 1993, p. 246)—includes all forms of healing that are not included in the conventional U.S. health system.

The extent of CAM use for children is not yet clear because most CAM use research has focused on adults. Survey data from 1997 indicate that roughly two in five U.S. adults will have used at least one CAM therapy in the past year, with the number of visits to CAM providers far exceeding the number of visits made to all primary care physicians (Eisenberg et al., 1998; Ernst, 2000). As far as children go, we do know that parents who use it for their children may be more likely to use it for themselves and to be better educated than those who do not. This was shown in a survey of parents of children attending a metropolitan ambulatory pediatrics clinic in Canada. Eleven percent of the children had previously seen one or more CAM practitioners (Spigelblatt, Laine-Ammara, Pless, & Guyver, 1994). This figure may be very conservative, as the study focused on children in a hospital outpatient clinic setting and excluded certain forms of therapy that others may consider CAM (such as meditation) as well as self-administered CAM. In comparison, a randomized phone survey of 216 New York adolescents found that more than half (53 percent) of the participants had used at least one CAM therapy (Wilson & Klein, 2000).

CAM and Children with Special Needs

Research suggests that parents of children with special health care needs, such as developmental or other disabilities, are more likely to use CAM. A survey of 455 parents of children with autism found that 50 percent had used at least one "nonstandard" therapy with their autistic child; 32 percent had used two or more (Nickel, 1996). In another study of 401 adults with physical disabilities, 57 percent endorsed using CAM, and 22 percent reported seeing a CAM practitioner (Krauss, Godfrey, Kirk, & Eisenberg, 1998).

Many CAM methods are harmless, and some have proved helpful in small-scale studies, such as acupuncture for drooling problems in children with neurological disabilities (Wong, Sun, & Wong, 2001), constipation (Broide et al., 2001), and cold feet due to cerebral palsy or progressive encephalopathy (Svedberg, Nordahl, & Lundeberg, 2001). Saint John's wort has shown promise for children with symptoms of depression (Hubner & Kirste, 2001), echinacea for preventing recurrent otitis media (Mark, Grant, & Barton, 2001), and the herbal extract combination of *Panax quinquefolium* and *Ginkgo biloba* for improving the symptoms of ADHD (Lyon et al., 2001). Beyond their physiological effects, the interpersonal aspects of many CAM practices can certainly have benefits.

These benefits notwithstanding, some CAM therapies have the potential to interact negatively with biomedical regimes (Lazar & O'Connor, 1997). Children with special health care needs tend to be more highly involved with the health care system than other children (Cohen, 1998) and so may be more likely to be subject to such interactions. Further, many people, including children and the adults who serve as their gatekeepers to the health system, are reluctant to disclose CAM use to their primary care physicians (Cohen, 1998; Eisenberg et al., 1993; Eisenberg et al., 1998; Sibinga, Ottolini, Duggan, & Wilson, 2000; Wilson & Klein, 2000). It is therefore imperative that pediatricians gain a greater understanding of the place CAM therapies hold in the lives of families with children (especially those with special health care needs) and maintain good communication with parents regarding their children's CAM care (LaValley & Verhoef, 1995; Sobo, Walker, & Kurtin, 2001).

The AAP has released recommendations on counseling families regarding CAM (American Academy of Pediatrics, Committee on Children with Disabilities, 2001). Rather than distinguishing between CAM and biomedicine, the guidelines distinguish between "proven" and "unproven" modalities, noting that not all conventional biomedical therapies are scientifically proven and that some unproven CAM therapies may eventually prove, scientifically, to be effective.

Clinical Communication: Building a Better Household–Health System Bridge

The practice of biomedicine today generally casts health as an individual state accomplished through the health-seeking partnership of a patient (one at a time) and a physician; nurses and other health care workers are seen as essential support for this dyad, but the physician retains prominence (Hahn, 1995). This dyadic (two-person) model underpins the modern biomedical enterprise (Bell, Wilkes, & Kravitz, 1999; Hunt, 1998). However, due to children's dependence and developmental immaturity and their legal status as minors, children's relation to the health service system is overseen not by themselves but by their parents (Forrest, Simpson, & Clancy,

1997; Jameson & Wehr, 1993). Because of this, household–health system communication about child health must be analyzed as the outcome of the negotiations of a triad composed of dependent patient (child), empowered intermediary (parent), and authoritative practitioner (see Chapter Two, by Gidwani, Sobo, Seid, and Kurtin).

All three members of the **pediatric care triad** have their own priorities and communication strategies (Sobo & Rock, 2001; Sobo, Rock, Neuhouser, Maciel, & Neumark-Sztainer, 2000; Tates & Meeuwesen, 2001). Still, U.S. parents have a culturally constructed obligation to put the child's best interests first. This includes helping the physician by carrying out aspects of the child's care plan (for example, giving certain pills on a specified schedule).

Parental Competence

Moral judgments about parenting (especially mothering) are implicated, sometimes explicitly, in causal explanations for children's injuries and illnesses (Edwards, 1995; Lock, 1988) and in decisions regarding whether or not a parent can be trusted to help carry out a child's care plan. Identified abuse cases notwithstanding, if physicians do not trust a parent in the intermediary role, they may decide to remove the parent from the care triad. This can be done wholly, through discretionary hospitalization of the child, or partially, through the use of extra medical tests to rule out the risk of progression or degeneration that might go unnoticed by an incompetent parent.

Much of what is known about such competence judgments comes from child abuse research. The bias here is well established and was described earlier. Difficulties in judgment of parental competence also exist with unintentional injury, although this is less well documented. Physicians often misjudge the likelihood of certain gun safety–related behaviors in parents (Becher & Christakis, 1999). They are more likely to have negative perceptions of African Americans and lower-socioeconomic individuals, associating ethnicity with assessments of intelligence, risk behaviors, and compliance patterns (van Ryn & Burke, 2000).

To fairly judge a parent's ability to follow through on a care plan or otherwise competently care for his or her children, a clinician must be able to form an unbiased opinion based on objective parenting competence indicators relevant to the tasks at hand. Letting go of pervasive stereotypes is a first step in this direction; it is imperative if a clinician is to acquire the cultural competence necessary for good household–health system interactions.

Cultural Competence

Cultural competence is a complicated construct. Taken literally, it means competence in the culture in question: complete knowledge of that culture's inventory of understandings and the ability to enact its practice patterns. However, a more limited form of competence may be quite enough to ensure beneficial household–health system interactions.

According to Brach and Fraser (2000), the term **cultural competence**, when deployed in health care settings, may actually function as a gloss for nine separate techniques of promoting patient- or household-clinician communication. These techniques are interpreter services, recruitment and retention policies aimed at enhancing diversity in the workforce, training programs for staff, systems of coordinating with CAM healers, community health workers, culturally relevant health promotion, inclusion of household and community members in health care planning, cultural immersion programs for staff, and administrative and organizational accommodations that allow for diverse cultural needs (for example, in relation to the physical environment or open hours of the clinic).

As Brach and Fraser (2000) note, as yet there is little evidence regarding which techniques are effective and even less evidence regarding when and how to apply the techniques properly. Nevertheless, recent research has shown that language barriers contribute disproportionately to differences in quality of care (Weech-Maldonado,

Morales, Spritzer, Elliott, & Hays, 2001). Better translation leads to better communication, which leads to improved patient satisfaction; satisfaction is correlated with adherence to recommended care plans, which is in turn correlated with better outcomes (Betancourt, Carrillo, & Green, 1999; but see also Clark, de Baca, Reidy, & Turner, 2002).

Adequate translation services rely on trained, professional translators rather than bystanders, family members, or untrained staff who happen to speak the language in question. Nonprofessionals may not actually speak the language as well as necessary and may edit conversations or elaborate on a speaker's message without the speaker's or listener's knowledge. Social closeness with the translator (as when household members are asked to translate) may lead to self-censorship in the patient or family, especially when health information has implications for social standing. Finally, nonprofessionals may lack a background in medical terminology and inadvertently mistranslate, leading to miscommunication.

Miscommunication can occur even with professional translators when linguistic concordance is the only goal. That this is so is seen in the medical miscommunications that occur even between speakers of the same language. The content of what is communicated may be poorly understood if it is not explained in terms that are familiar to the listener. This means that care must be taken to translate technical terms into lay language and that the content of the conversation must be made culturally relevant.

This does not mean adopting a "cookbook" approach to medicine, as so many champions of cultural competence would have clinicians do. Although people who share the same culture generally share certain understandings, immense intracultural variation has been documented. Much of this variation is individual, but it can also hinge on characteristics such as gender and age: although culture is shared, all members do not equally share it, and some will know much more than others about certain cultural domains. Further, many health understandings are flexible and context-dependent (Foster, 1994;

Williams, 2001). Therefore, clinicians should make every effort to understand patients' present understandings of their health concerns, including how and when they came about, what might cause them, what course they might take, and what might be done to help them (Kleinman, 1980). At the same time, information on socioeconomic factors that might make certain treatment courses more realistic than others should be elicited (Betancourt et al., 1999; Carrillo, Green, & Betancourt, 1999).

Such efforts should be undertaken not only with patients and parents who differ culturally from the clinician but also with those who are ostensibly alike. Cultural competence programs that focus only on ethnic diversity only are bound to fail. As Hahn (1995) and others (such as Good & Good, 1993) have demonstrated, the intensive training that the clinician receives creates a gulf between patient and healer. Patients and healers "inevitably conceive of the world, communicate, and behave in ways that cannot be reasonably or safely assumed to be similar or readily compatible"; in other words, *"All medicine is cross-cultural"* (Hahn, 1995, p. 265; emphasis in the original).

The clinician who would practice culturally competent (or culturally appropriate, or really, culturally *relevant*) medicine does well to approach communication as a process that must be tailored to the patient and his or her parents. In individualizing or customizing communications, clinicians will find it helpful to have reflected on their own biases and to have confronted the stereotypes and ethnocentricity that they may bring to clinical encounters (in **ethnocentrism**, one regards one's own culture's values and customs as the only values and customs—or at least the best ones).

Clinicians interested in offering culturally relevant care will also find knowledge about general cultural understandings about health and about proper forms of interaction very helpful. It would be unwise, however, for clinicians to assume that particular cultural understandings apply to all people who share in that culture; informed overgeneralization can have the same effect as uninformed stereotyping. Knowledge of general cultural patterns and common local illness categories should be regarded as a means, not an end (Galanti, 1997).

Through a process of active discussion with patients and parents during which their preferences and views are elicited, clinicians will be better prepared to tailor messages so that they make sense to intended recipients. Patients and parents will be better prepared for shared decision making. The specifics of how to foster collaborative household–health system communication may vary with patient and parent characteristics, household type, and other social factors. Research describing this variation and defining best practices is sorely needed.

Household as Patient

An important premise of this chapter has been that viewing the individual as the unit of care often leads us to ignore the influence of household factors on the person's health. It may also blind us to the reciprocal impact of an individual's health on his or her household and social network. This is especially true where children are concerned, as they are dependent on adult household members for their health care. A child's ill health may affect the entire household. The household must take center stage in CHSR because of its influence on individual child health and the impact that a child's health has on it.

Household Impact of Chronic Illness or Disability in Children

The effect of child health on households is perhaps most severe when children are chronically ill or disabled. Parents have reported frustration in meeting the needs of their sick children as well their healthy ones. They also describe frustration with the perceived unsupportive and unhelpful attitude of many health care providers. They desire practical advice and honest communication (Krafft & Krafft, 1998; Prussing, Sobo, Walker, & Kurtin, 2002).

The day-to-day stress of caring for chronically ill or disabled children can take a negative toll on parental partnerships. Despite the fact that marital distress increases, divorce rates do not seem higher. But as with much other CHSR, studies have generally been conducted with an inadequate **control group** (a group that serves as a point of comparison, having not experienced the condition in question). Most studies are **cross-sectional** (collecting data at one point in time from a cross section of individuals) rather than **longitudinal** (actually tracking variables over time so that change over time is real rather than imputed). Research has focused more on mothers than on fathers, has not distinguished the possibly divergent impacts of different pediatric conditions, and has failed to explore the adaptive function of marital distress. More research is needed in these areas as well as in relation to communication and role flexibility (Sabbeth & Leventhal, 1984).

The self-perceived quality of life of parents of chronically ill or disabled children appears to be intimately linked with the perceived quality of life of the child in question (regarding health-related quality of life, see Chapter Six, by Knight, Burwinkle, and Varni). But other issues, such as opportunities for self-development or for parenting other children, may also influence their perceptions (Canam & Acorn, 1999). Adjustment can entail letting go of certain future plans and going through a grieving process: parents who fail to do so may experience chronic sorrow over missed opportunities or the loss of a "normal" child or "normal" family life (Lowes & Lyne, 2000). Although little research has addressed this aspect of adjustment to a chronically ill or disabled child, it may result in positive emotional or spiritual growth (Prussing et al., 2002).

It is not just parents who must adjust: siblings too must be considered. They may be at higher risk for emotional or psychological disturbance or maladjustment, which has been attributed to parental preoccupation with the ill or disabled child. Siblings themselves have reported feelings of anger, resentment, guilt, and shame. Parents often deny an ill or disabled child's siblings access to full information about the child's condition; siblings thus learn that the topic is not to be discussed. This may result in their being "forced into a peculiar kind of loneliness—a sense of detachment from those they should feel closest to" (Seligman, 1987, p. 1250). Research on sibling resilience and coping in such circumstances, as well as their related quality of life, is sorely needed.

Household-Centered Service Delivery

The worst-case scenario of the chronically ill or disabled child demonstrates clearly the value of adopting the household as the unit of care. This chapter began by defining the household and discussing its articulation with the formal health care system as well as its role in health production and maintenance. The household vantage point was privileged. Here we bring the discussion full circle by examining, this time from the health system perspective, the value of household-centered pediatric health care. Many of the issues covered previously come together in this section, leading to an abundance of questions. Most focus on what we need to know about what health service workers can do to make in-home or household-centered care successful.

Family-Centered Care

In the United States, care that focuses on or actively involves the household is often glossed as "family-centered care." This implies that all members of the family are involved in caregiving when generally they are not. *Family* is often a code word for *women* (Ward, 1993, p. 20). Women bear the principal burden of care delivery for ill or disabled family members. Further, use of the term *family* shifts attention away from structural and material conditions to the affective power of kinship bonds. This shift may lead providers (and researchers) to ignore household variables (such as number and ages of members or access to running water) that mediate a family or household group's ability to respond as directed by biomedical providers. It may also lead providers to accept family-centered care unquestioningly, as rejecting the concept would be seen as antifamily and hence unacceptable in light of the present pervasiveness of profamily rhetoric.

Better Child Health Outcomes Through Household-Centered Service Delivery

Research regarding household-centered care is still limited; the assumption that it leads to better outcomes must be tested further and in multiple contexts (Allen & Petr, 1998). It remains unclear, for example, how best to deal with cultural issues such as the health understandings of a given household (see the appendix to this chapter). It also remains uncertain which members of a household should be included in the unit of caregiving and how much latitude should be given to the household as a consumer and director of care. Within the household, whose wishes should be given priority? Is there information that should be shared with some but not all household members (Allen & Petr, 1998)?

Does offering household-centered care entail any obligations to the well-being of members other than the patient? Sometimes disabled and ill children are the only children in a household with insurance or medical coverage; conversely, sometimes they do not receive the care they might because of a concern over how to spend scarce resources and the perceived return on investment (Scheper-Hughes & Sargent, 1998).

Many other questions arise in this discussion: What types of interventions are best for facilitating household participation in a child's care? Which household types will benefit the most from these? Is household-centered care useful for general prevention or only in cases of chronic conditions? How much of it should be carried out at the home versus at the hospital, clinic, or practitioner's office? What household factors in addition to kinship need to be taken into account to make these decisions? Should patient histories include explicit reference to such factors as number of members; economic arrangements; access to day care; length of time at present address; presence of smokers; use of entitlements; location, age, and size of dwelling; and water and power access so that these variables may be factored into program evaluations?

The literature on home visiting may help in answering some of these questions, as home visiting by definition must take at least a minimum of household variables into account. Home visitors—often nurses or social workers and frequently members of the communities they serve—have direct access to household environments. They aim to provide parents with the support they need to follow through with prescribed treatments or procedures. This support may consist of practical advice, educational intervention, or case management whereby households are linked to community services. In addition, the creation of a trusting, enduring relationship between household members and the home visitor may facilitate change (Gomby, Culross, & Behrman, 1999).

But does home visiting work? Evaluation results are equivocal. Where they are positive, they are generally modest, with benefits concentrated among particular subsets of households. However, there is little consistency for these subsets across programs that have been evaluated—and even, in some cases, across one program's sites (Gomby et al., 1999).

There have been some demonstrated benefits for children whose exposure to abusive parenting was reduced through home visits. For example, Olds and colleagues (1999), reviewing twenty years of research, found fewer emergency department visits for injury and benefits to fifteen-year-olds including less smoking and drinking, less running away, fewer arrests and convictions and parole violations, and fewer sexual partners. But research is needed to determine the specific mechanisms by which home visiting confers benefits and to clarify which households should be targeted. Specifically, threshold levels for home visit intensity and duration should be determined (Gomby et al., 1999), along with who, if anyone in particular, should be the primary subject of the intervention. Methods for ensuring programs' self-sustainability also need to be developed, as even the best home visiting program will cease to be effective without funding.

Besides effectiveness, the costs of household-centered care should be determined. Many people have the idea that care provided by household members is free, saving the rest of society a heavy financial burden. Shifting the care burden to the household by decreasing hospital length of stay has certainly offset certain medical costs for insurance companies and hospitals. But those who temporarily leave the workforce lose wages as well as opportunities for job promotions and pension benefits, and the synergistic effect of all this on household well-being can be dire (Ward, 1993). Even those who remain employed while providing home care incur costs: Forrest and colleagues (1997) report in their review of CHSR challenges that mothers lose at least one week of workdays annually due to child illness; they urge further study of the indirect costs of health care.

Prevention and Healing in the Household: Implications for CHSR Design

Social epidemiologists have long understood that the material conditions of people's everyday lives are among the most important causative factors underlying disease and injury (Waitzkin, 1981). Child health status is also influenced by cultural understandings about family, household, and health provision. Although cultural understandings are certainly at play in the health services system, as the large literature on biomedical culture and the ways that it varies across practices and even states and nations has shown (see, for example, Helman, 1995; Payer, 1989), this chapter has focused on the cultural understandings that underlie the household production of health. It has argued that CHSR would benefit from an expansion of purview to include the household arena.

Much of what this chapter recommends involves **primary data** (data collected in the field, for the project at hand, by and for those who will analyze it) as opposed to existing or **secondary data** (large institutional data sets put together by others, generally from surveillance systems). But even the most traditional HSR projects (those focused on secondary data analysis) can benefit by taking a broader view. For example, severity and **risk adjustment** techniques often used in HSR (mathematical techniques that make comparisons possible across cases despite differences in illness severity) might more accurately predict outcomes if context factors such as those related to household structure, child and parent citizenship, community resources, or parent occupational status were taken into account. Such data might be collected during intake interviews.

A high-level summary of possible categories of variables that will be helpful for broadening the scope of CHSR is provided in Exhibit 3.1. Not all categories listed will be relevant to all research, and not all categories that will be relevant can be listed; the exhibit list is suggestive and not exhaustive.

Some of the variables listed in Exhibit 3.1 can inform more novel research efforts too. One key area for future inquiry is medical choice making, which is increasingly of interest as some parts of the dominant health services system attempt to honor the shared decision-making model, in which patient and parent preferences are paramount and active, informed engagement is encouraged (Institute of Medicine, 2001). We do not presently have a good understanding of the factors that underlie a patient's or parent's preference for shared decision making over the old paternalistic model, nor do we fully understand the costs and benefits that might accrue.

The pediatric triad of patient, parent, and practitioner is also emerging as a central research area because of the important link between good communication and care plan follow-through. More research on the specific approaches that enhance communication within the triad is sorely needed, as is information on which approaches work best with which type of trio; it may be that factors such as educational or cultural background or type of practitioner make a difference. More attention should also be paid directly to the child's own health-related roles and experiences. This and a fuller understanding of the household's central place in pediatric health production and maintenance is especially important in light

Exhibit 3.1. Some Issues to Consider When Designing
Child Health Services Research Projects.

---

1. Household Structure

- Family type (nuclear, joint, extended, blended, adoptive, and so on)
- Number of siblings, number of adults
- Adult availability for child care
- Relationship between child and primary caregiver
- Pets
- Frequent visitors and contacts

2. Household Economy

- Total income; income per occupant
- Occupational class of employed members
- Entitlements in use
- Dwelling size, location, type
- Backyard or playground access
- Neighborhood walkability

3. Household Culture

- Religious beliefs
- Ethnic identity (including number of years or generations in the United States)
- Literacy and primary language
- Health understandings (including acceptability of present care plan)
- Household power structure
- Tobacco, alcohol, and substance use practices; risk perception
- Home remedy use

4. Household Interaction with Various Health Systems

- CAM use
- Biomedical system use
- Quality of interaction with providers
- Continuity of care

of the recent emphasis on customized, patient-centered care (Institute of Medicine, 2001).

Research on household response to children's chronic illness, injury, or disability would benefit from improvements in several areas. First, more representative research is needed; too often, projects are small, and recruitment biases reduce the generalizability of findings. We need more prospective, process-oriented research, and categorical approaches should be complemented by condition-specific studies. Measures should be clinically relevant, and causal pathways connecting household functioning and children's adjustment should be clarified. Research should also be conducted to test interventions modifying risk factors or adding to resilience (Drotar, 1997). For CHSR must focus not only on issues of care, treatment, and safety but also on prevention and the enhancement of children's health and well-being, not only as it is created and maintained during childhood but also as it affects health outcomes and therefore society when children become adults.

Appendix
Cultural Understandings of Health: The Basics

Flow, Blockage, and Cleanliness

Elaborations on a basic spatial, hydraulic model that emphasizes flow and balance and incorporates container and conduit imagery (a "flow model"; see Sobo, 1993) can be found in ethnographic descriptions of a range of cultures (for example, Laguerre, 1987; Meigs, 1983; Snow, 1993) and for biomedical scientists (Martin, 1987, ch. 3). Mexican ideas about *empacho*, in which digestion is blocked and food adheres to intestines or the stomach wall, where it grows moldy, reflect a flow model (Stafford, 1978; Young & Garro, 1982), as does the Chinese concept of life essence energy, *ch'i* or *qi*, which moves through the body carrying warmth, nourishment, and protection (Ergil, 1997).

In a flow system, it is essential that nothing block the body's conduits or channels. To ensure that this does not happen, and for alleviation if it does, people can take occasional purges, as many do with laxatives or emetics. Or they may have other means to regulate flow. For example, in traditional Chinese medicine, *qi* is kept flowing primarily with acupuncture and *moxibustion* (the burning of certain leaves in dry or powdered form on or near the surface of the skin that corresponds to the *qi* channels in question) (Ergil, 1997).

A culture's specific flow-related understandings underlie the specific therapies adopted. Even if such therapy does not make biomedical sense (and sometimes it does), it makes cultural sense, following a logic for which culture provides the basis.

Blocked flow sometimes leads to unrelieved waste, which can build up, fester, and turn septic, releasing toxins into the system. Purges in many cultures are meant to cleanse all bodily systems, including the circulatory, urinary, and respiratory systems. The medicines for these internal cleansings can, but need not be, specialized; for many, bodily systems are interconnected, and waste is eliminated in feces, urine, vomit, or phlegm.

Poisons may also be drawn out through the skin, as with poultices or through cupping or coin rubbing. This last therapy, associated with Asian cultures, involves rubbing a coin on the skin to draw the illness out. In cupping, a heated cup is placed on the skin, creating a vacuum. Both coin rubbing and cupping can leave raised red welts that may concern care providers unfamiliar with the practices.

Keeping Balanced

Not all cultures are so focused on keeping the internal body clean or flow unimpeded. But most do have some notion of equilibrium and strive to maintain some sort of balance. For example, in old Vermont, people used honey and vinegar (acid and alkali) to help maintain bodily balance (Atkinson, 1978). Biomedical practitioners often talk of balance; hormone imbalances, vitamin deficiencies, bacterial imbalances in the gut, and many other problems are conceptualized in terms of an equilibrium model of health.

Hot and Cold

In many cultures, maintaining a balance between hot and cold is essential. Illness happens when the body (which is generally self-regulating) becomes too cool or too hot. A hot body is open or vulnerable to the penetration of cold and other forces in a way that the body ordinarily would not be. Dangerous exposure must be avoided. In a cold body, substances that should run freely may clot and solidify, perhaps leading waste to be reabsorbed into the body. To offset this threat, children may be warmed physically or given heating tonics. A breast-fed child's mother may alter her own intake so that the thermal quality of her breast milk serves as an aid to the child (Helman, 1995).

In some contexts, rather than to counterbalance disequilibria, treatments seek to further heat or cool the body. For example, if the body is heating up in order to melt out some toxin, further heating might help the body accomplish this task and speed recovery. So, for example, a child with diarrhea or a rash might (where these processes are viewed as hot) be given heating foods.

Although sick bodies do feel hot and cold, hot and cold are not necessarily thermal designations but rather symbolic constructions concerning the essential character of an item or state. Classification may be based on color (or darkness or lightness), gender associations (maleness or femaleness), origin (for example, foods from the sea or grown underground may be classed as cold, while foods grown in direct sunlight may be classed as hot), and nutritive value (foods seen as especially nutritious are often classed as hot; Logan, 1969/ 1977). Sometimes the designation of a food, substance, or act as hot or cold is an after-the-fact justification of empirically observed effects (Foster, 1994).

Body Fluids

Thermal systems are sometimes balanced around not only heat and coolness but also dryness and wetness, and specific body fluids can be involved. In French biomedicine, the liver and its bile are central (Payer, 1989), while in African Caribbean and African American medicine, blood is key.

Korbin and Johnston (1982) describe a conflict over blood testing in a pediatric hospital that pitted a mother from Belize against a staff of biomedical clinicians. The mother felt that clinicians were harming her sick daughter with diagnostic blood tests. She was concerned about the loss of blood and the imbalance in her small daughter's already weak body that was bound to result if the drawing of blood did not stop. Accused of "ignorance" and "child abuse" and threatened with legal action, the mother resorted to bringing her daughter herbal teas, to "build her blood back up" (p. 261).

It is worth mentioning that in addition to her worries about blood depletion, the mother feared that hospital staff members were drawing excess quantities of blood so that they could sell it for a profit. Such worries may be common among parents of children from minority groups that have historically been subjected to such maltreatment; it may be a barrier to high-quality care (see Chapter Seven, by Seid, Sobo, Zivkovic, Nelson, and Far).

People may use the word *blood* in various ways. For many Caribbean peoples, blood comes in two types: white and red. When unqualified by adjective or context, the word *blood* in Jamaica means the red kind, built from thick, dark liquid items or reddish edibles such as tomatoes. White blood (*sinews*) comes from light-colored gelatinous foods, such as okra juices. White blood may include pus, synovial fluid, and the vitreous humor that fills the eyes. Both kinds of blood are essential for good health. Consistency as well as sweetness or bitterness of the blood is often a grave concern.

References

Adair, J., Deuschle, K., & Barnett, C. (1988). *The people's health: Anthropology and medicine in a Navajo community* (rev. and expanded ed.). Albuquerque: University of New Mexico Press.

Alaimo, K., Olson, C. M., & Frongillo, E. A. (2001). Food insufficiency and American school-aged children's cognitive, academic, and psychosocial development. *Pediatrics, 108,* 44–53.

Allen, R. I., & Petr, C. G. (1998). Rethinking family-centered practice. *American Journal of Orthopsychiatry, 68,* 4–15.

American Academy of Pediatrics, Committee on Children with Disabilities. (2001). Counseling families who choose complementary and alternative medicine for their children with chronic illness or disability. *Pediatrics, 107,* 598–601.

American Academy of Pediatrics, Committee on Injury and Poison Prevention. (2001). Falls from heights: Windows, roofs, and balconies. *Pediatrics, 107,* 1188–1191.

American Academy of Pediatrics, Committee on School Health. (2001). School health centers and other integrated school health services. *Pediatrics, 107,* 198–201.

Atkinson, P. (1978). From honey to vinegar: Levi-Strauss in Vermont. In P. Morley & R. Wallis (Eds.), *Culture and curing: Anthropological perspectives* (pp. 168–188). Pittsburgh: University of Pittsburgh Press.

At last, good news on the family (probably). (2001, July 28). *Economist,* pp. 29–30.

Baer, H. A., Singer, M., & Johnson, J. H. (1986). Toward a critical medical anthropology. *Social Science and Medicine, 23,* 95–98.

Becher, E. C., & Christakis, N. A. (1999). Firearm injury prevention counseling: Are we missing the mark? *Pediatrics, 104,* 530–535.

Becker, M., & Maiman, L. (1975). Sociobehavioral determinants of compliance with health and medical care recommendations. *Medical Care, 13,* 10–24.

Bell, R. A., Wilkes, M. S., & Kravitz, R. L. (1999). Advertisement-induced prescription drug requests: Patients' anticipated reactions to a physician who refuses. *Journal of Family Practice, 48,* 446–452.

Betancourt, J. R., Carrillo, J. E., & Green, A. R. (1999). Hypertension in multicultural and minority populations: Linking communication to compliance. *Current Hypertension Reports, 1,* 482–488.

Bibace, R., & Walsh, M. E. (Eds.). (1981). *Children's conceptions of health, illness, and bodily functions.* San Francisco: Jossey-Bass.

Bordo, S. (1993). *Unbearable weight: Feminism, Western culture, and the body.* Berkeley: University of California Press.

Brach, C., & Fraser, I. (2000). Can cultural competence reduce racial and ethnic disparities? A review and conceptual model. *Medical Care Research and Review, 57*(Suppl. 1), 181–217.

Brewis, A., Schmidt, K. L., & Meyer, M. (2001). ADHD-type behavior and harmful dysfunction in childhood: A cross-cultural model. *American Anthropologist, 102,* 823–828.

Broide, E., Pintov, S., Portnoy, S., Barg, J., Klinowski, E., & Scapa, E. (2001). Effectiveness of acupuncture for treatment of childhood constipation. *Digestive Diseases and Sciences, 46,* 1270–1275.

Bush, P. J., Trakas, D. J., Sanz, E. J., Wirsing, R., Vaskilampi, T., & Prout, A. (1996). *Children, medicines, and culture.* New York: Pharmaceutical Products Press.

Campbell, K., Waters, E., O'Meara, S., & Summerbell, C. (2001). Interventions for preventing obesity in children (Cochrane Review). *Cochrane Database of Systematic Reviews, 2,* CD001871.

Canam, C., & Acorn, S. (1999). Quality of life for family caregivers of people with chronic health problems. *Rehabilitation Nursing, 24*, 192–200.

Carrillo, J. E., Green, A. R., & Betancourt, J. R. (1999). Cross-cultural primary care: A patient-based approach. *Annals of Internal Medicine, 130*, 829–834.

Chrisman, N. J. (1977). The health seeking process: An approach to the natural history of illness. *Culture, Medicine, and Psychiatry, 1*, 351–377.

Clark, L., de Baca, R. C., Reidy, K., & Turner, M. (2002, November 20–24). *Is cultural competence all about language? Data from two Medicaid managed care systems serving Latinos.* Paper presented at the 101st annual meeting of the American Anthropological Association, New Orleans.

Clark, L., & Hofsess, L. (1998). Acculturation. In S. Loue (Ed.), *Handbook of immigrant health* (pp. 37–59). New York: Plenum Press.

Cohen, W. I. (1998). Atlantoaxial instability: What's next? *Archives of Pediatrics and Adolescent Medicine, 152*, 119–122.

Coid, J., Petruckevitch, A., Feder, G., Chung, W. S., Richardson, J., & Moorey, S. (2001). Relation between childhood sexual and physical abuse and risk of revictimisation in women: A cross-sectional survey. *Lancet, 358*, 450–454.

Cummins, S. K., & Jackson, R. J. (2001). The built environment and children's health. *Children's Environmental Health, 48*, 1241–1252.

Dahlquist, G., Sterky, G., Ivarsson, J. I., Tengvald, K., & Wall, S. (1987). Health problems and care in young families: Load of illness and patterns of illness behaviour. *Scandinavian Journal of Primary Health Care, 5*, 79–86.

Davison, K. K., & Birch, L. L. (2001). Weight status, parent reaction, and self-concept in five-year-old girls. *Pediatrics, 107*, 46–53.

Demers, R., Altamore, R., Mustin, H., Kleinman, A., & Leonardi, D. (1980). An exploration of the dimensions of illness behavior. *Journal of Family Practice, 11*, 1085–1092.

Diamond, J. (1994). Race without color. *Discover, 15*(11), 82–89.

Drotar, D. (1997). Relating parent and family functioning to the psychological adjustment of children with chronic health conditions: What have we learned? What do we need to know? *Journal of Pediatric Psychology, 22*, 149–165.

Edwards, J. (1995). "Parenting skills": Views of community health and social service providers about the needs of their "clients." *Journal of Social Policy, 24*, 237–259.

Eisenberg, D. M., Davis, R. B., Ettner, S. L., Appel, S., Wilkey, S., Rompay, M. V., & Kessler, R. C. (1998). Trend in alternative medicine use in the

United States, 1990–1997: Results of a follow-up national survey. *Journal of the American Medical Association, 280,* 1569–1575.

Eisenberg, D. M., Kessler, R. C., Foster, C., Norlock, F. E., Calkins, D. R., & Delbanco, T. L. (1993). Unconventional medicine in the United States: Prevalence, costs, and patterns of use. *New England Journal of Medicine, 328,* 246–252.

Emmons, K. M., Hammond, S. K., Fava, J. L., Velicer, W. F., Evans, J. L., & Monroe, A. D. (2001). A randomized trial to reduce passive smoke exposure in low-income households with young children. *Pediatrics, 108,* 18–20.

Ergil, M. C. (1997). Chinese medicine. In *Ancient healing: Unlocking the mysteries of health and healing through the ages* (pp. 277–307). Lincolnwood, IL: Publications International.

Ernst, E. (2000). Prevalence of use of complementary/alternative medicine: A systematic review. *Bulletin of the World Health Organization, 78,* 252–257.

Farmer, P. (1999). *Infections and inequalities: The modern plagues.* Berkeley: University of California Press.

Forrest, C. B., Simpson, L., & Clancy, C. (1997). Child health services research. Challenges and opportunities. *Journal of the American Medical Association, 277,* 1787–1793.

Foster, G. M. (1994). *Hippocrates' Latin American legacy: Humoral medicine in the New World.* Langhorne, PA: Gordon & Breach.

Friedson, E. (1960). Client control and medical practice. *American Journal of Sociology, 65,* 374–382.

Galanti, G.-A. (1997). *Caring for patients from different cultures: Case studies from American hospitals* (2nd ed.). University Park: University of Pennsylvania Press.

Gillman, M., Rifas-Shiman, S., Camargo, C. J., Berkey, C., Frazier, A., Rockett, H., et al. (2001). Risk of overweight among adolescents who were breastfed as infants. *Journal of the American Medical Association, 285,* 2506–2507.

Gomby, D. S., Culross, P. L., & Behrman, R. E. (1999). Home visiting: Recent program evaluations—analysis and recommendations. *Future of Children, 9,* 4–26.

Good, B., & Good, M.-J. D. (1993). Learning medicine: The constructing of medical knowledge at Harvard Medical School. In S. Lindenbaum & M. Lock (Eds.), *Knowledge, power, and practice* (pp. 81–107). Berkeley: University of California Press.

Goodman, M. H. (1990). The physical abuse of children: Then and now. *Nurse Practitioner Forum, 1,* 84–89.

Gould, S. J. (1994). The geometer of race. *Discover, 15*(11), 65–69.

Gross, D. R. (1992). *Discovering anthropology.* Mountain View, CA: Mayfield.

Haapasalo, J., & Petaja, S. (1999). Mothers who killed or attempted to kill their child: Life circumstances, childhood abuse, and types of killing. *Violence and Victims, 14,* 219–239.

Hahn, R. A. (1984). Rethinking "disease" and "illness." *Contributions to Asian Studies, 18,* 1–23.

Hahn, R. A. (1995). *Sickness and healing: An anthropological perspective.* New Haven, CT: Yale University Press.

Hassin, J. (1994). Living a responsible life: The impact of AIDS on the social identity of intravenous drug users. *Social Science and Medicine, 39,* 391–400.

Helman, C. G. (1995). *Culture, health and illness* (3rd ed.). Oxford: Butterworth-Heinemann.

Hernandez, J. T., Lodico, M., & DiClemente, R. J. (1993). The effects of child abuse and race on risk-taking in male adolescents. *Journal of the National Medical Association, 85,* 593–597.

Hojer, B., Sterky, G., & Widlund, G. (1987). Acute illnesses in young children and family responses. *Acta Paediatrica Scandinavica, 76,* 624–630.

Hubner, W., & Kirste, T. (2001). Experience with St. John's wort (*Hypericum perforatum*) in children under 12 years with symptoms of depression and psychovegetative disturbances. *Phytotherapy Research, 15,* 367–370.

Hufford, D. J. (1996). Culturally grounded review of research assumptions. *Alternative Therapies in Health and Medicine, 2*(4), 47–53.

Hunt, L. (1998). Moral reasoning and the meaning of cancer: Causal explanations of oncologists and patients in southern Mexico. *Medical Anthropology Quarterly, 12,* 298–318.

Institute of Medicine, Committee on Quality of Health Care in America. (2001). *Crossing the quality chasm: A new health system for the 21st century.* Washington, DC: National Academy Press.

Jain, A., Sherman, S. N., Chamberlin, D. L., Carter, Y., Powers, S. W., & Whitaker, R. C. (2001). Why don't low-income mothers worry about their preschoolers being overweight? *Pediatrics, 107,* 1138–1146.

Jameson, E., & Wehr, E. (1993, Fall). Drafting national health reform legislation to protect the health interests of children. *Stanford Law Policy Review,* pp. 152–176.

Janz, N., & Becker, M. (1984). The health belief model: A decade later. *Health Education Quarterly, 11,* 1–47.

Jenny, C., Hymel, K. P., Ritzen, A., Reinert, S. E., & Hay, T. C. (1999). Analysis of missed cases of abusive head trauma. *Journal of the American Medical Association, 281*, 621–626.

Johnson, M. (1987). *The body in the mind.* Chicago: University of Chicago Press.

Johnston, B. D., Grossman, D. C., Connell, F. A., & Koepsell, T. D. (2000). High-risk periods for childhood injury among siblings. *Pediatrics, 105,* 562–568.

Kaufman, J., & Zigler, E. (1987). Do abused children become abusive parents? *American Journal of Orthopsychiatry, 57,* 186–192.

Kleinman, A. (1978). Concepts and a model for the comparison of medical systems as cultural systems. *Social Science and Medicine, 12,* 85–93.

Kleinman, A. (1980). *Patients and healers in the context of culture: An exploration of the borderland between anthropology, medicine, and psychiatry.* Berkeley: University of California Press.

Korbin, J. (1987). Child abuse and neglect: The cultural context. In R. Helfer & R. Kempe (Eds.), *The battered child* (4th ed., pp. 23–41). Chicago: University of Chicago Press.

Korbin, J. (1997). "Good mothers," "babykillers," and fatal child maltreatment. In N. Scheper-Hughes & C. Sargent (Eds.), *Small wars: The cultural politics of childhood* (pp. 253–276). Berkeley: University of California Press.

Korbin, J., & Johnston, M. (1982). Steps toward resolving cultural conflict in a pediatric hospital. *Clinical Pediatrics, 21,* 259–263.

Kornblum, W., & Julian, J. (1995). *Social problems* (8th ed.). Englewood Cliffs, NJ: Prentice Hall.

Krafft, S. K., & Krafft, L. J. (1998). Chronic sorrow: Parents' lived experience. *Holistic Nursing Practice, 13,* 59–67.

Krauss, H. H., Godfrey, C., Kirk, J., & Eisenberg, D. M. (1998). Alternative health care: Its use by individuals with physical disabilities. *Archives of Physical Medicine and Rehabilitation, 79,* 1440–1447.

Laessle, R., Uhl, H., Lindel, B., & Muller, A. (2001). Parental influences on laboratory eating behavior in obese and non-obese children. *International Journal of Obesity Related Metabolic Disorders, 25*(Suppl. 1), S60–S62.

Laguerre, M. (1987). *Afro-Caribbean folk medicine.* South Hadley, MA: Bergin & Garvey.

Lakoff, G. (1987). *Women, fire, and dangerous things.* Chicago: University of Chicago Press.

Landrigan, P. J. (2001). Children's environmental health: Lessons from the past and prospects for the future. *Children's Environmental Health, 48,* 1319–1330.

LaValley, J. W., & Verhoef, M. J. (1995). Integrating complementary medicine and health care services into practice. *Canadian Medical Association Journal, 153,* 45–49.

Lazar, J. S., & O'Connor, B. B. (1997). Talking with patients about their use of alternative therapies. *Primary Care, 24,* 699–714.

Lenaway, D. D., Ambler, A. B., & Beaudoin, D. E. (1992). The epidemiology of school-related injuries: New perspectives. *American Journal of Preventive Medicine, 8,* 193–198.

Leonard, W. (2001). Assessing the influence of physical activity on health and fitness. *American Journal of Human Biology, 13,* 159–161.

Leventhal, J. M. (1999). The challenges of recognizing child abuse: Seeing is believing. *Journal of the American Medical Association, 281,* 657–659.

Lock, M. (1988). A nation at risk: School refusal syndrome in Japan. In M. Lock & D. Gordon (Eds.), *Biomedicine examined* (pp. 377–414). Boston: Kluwer Academic.

Logan, M. (1977). Humoral medicine in Guatemala and peasant acceptance of modern medicine. In D. Landy (Ed.), *Culture, disease, and healing: Studies in medical anthropology* (pp. 487–495). New York: Macmillan. (Original work published 1969)

Lowes, L., & Lyne, P. (2000). Chronic sorrow in parents of children with newly diagnosed diabetes: A review of the literature and discussion of the implications for nursing practice. *Journal of Advanced Nursing, 32,* 41–48.

Lyon, M., Cline, J., Totosy de Zepetnek, J., Shan, J., Pang, P., & Benishin, C. (2001). Effect of the herbal extract combination *Panax quinquefolium* and *Ginkgo biloba* on attention-deficit hyperactivity disorder: A pilot study. *Journal of Psychiatry and Neuroscience, 26,* 221–228.

Mark, J., Grant, K., & Barton, L. (2001). The use of dietary supplements in pediatrics: A study of echinacea. *Clinical Pediatrics (Philadelphia), 40,* 265–269.

Martin, E. (1987). *The woman in the body: A cultural analysis of reproduction.* Boston: Beacon Press.

Mayall, B. (1996). *Children, health and the social order.* Buckingham, England: Open University Press.

Mechanic, D. (1962). The concept of illness behavior. *Journal of Chronic Diseases, 15,* 189–194.

Meigs, A. (1983). *Food, sex, and pollution: A New Guinea religion.* New Brunswick, NJ: Rutgers University Press.

Nair, P. (1998). Child maltreatment. [Book review]. *Journal of the American Medical Association, 280,* 479–480.

Narang, D. S., & Contreras, J. M. (2000). Dissociation as a mediator between child abuse history and adult abuse potential. *Child Abuse and Neglect, 24,* 653–665.

Nickel, R. E. (1996). Controversial therapies for young children with developmental disabilities. *Infants and Young Children, 8*(4), 29–40.

O'Connor, B. B. (1995). *Healing traditions: Alternative medicine and the health professions.* University Park: University of Pennsylvania Press.

Olds, D. L., Henderson, C. R., Kitzman, H. J., Eckenrode, J. J., Cole, R. E., & Tatelbaum, R. C. (1999). Prenatal and infancy home visitation by nurses: Recent findings. *Future of Children, 9,* 44–65.

Payer, L. (1989). *Medicine and culture: Varieties of treatments in the United States, England, West Germany, and France.* New York: Penguin.

Prussing, E., Sobo, E. J., Walker, E., & Kurtin, P. S. (2002). *Exceptional parenthood and American pediatric care: Illness narratives of Down syndrome in the era of prenatal testing.* Unpublished manuscript.

Romanucci-Ross, L. (1977). The hierarchy of resort in curative practices: The Admiralty Islands, Melanesia. In D. Landy (Ed.), *Culture, disease, and healing: Studies in medical anthropology* (pp. 481–487). New York: Macmillan. (Original work published 1969)

Sabbeth, B. F., & Leventhal, J. M. (1984). Marital adjustment to chronic childhood illness: A critique of the literature. *Pediatrics, 73,* 762–768.

Scheper-Hughes, N., & Sargent, C. (Eds.). (1998). *Small wars: The cultural politics of childhood.* Berkeley: University of California Press.

Seligman, M. (1987). Adaptation of children to a chronically ill or mentally handicapped sibling. *Canadian Medical Association Journal, 136,* 1249–1252.

Sibinga, E. M., Ottolini, M. C., Duggan, A. K., & Wilson, M. H. (2000, October 28–November 1). *Communication about complementary/alternative medicine use in children.* Paper presented at the joint meeting of the Pediatric Academic Societies and the American Academy of Pediatrics, Chicago.

Singer, M., Valentin, F., Baer, H., & Jia, Z. (1992). Why does Juan Garcia have a drinking problem? The perspective of critical medical anthropology. *Medical Anthropology, 14,* 77–108.

Snow, L. F. (1993). *Walkin' over medicine.* Boulder, CO: Westview Press.

Sobo, E. J. (1993). *One blood: The Jamaican body.* Albany: State University of New York Press.

Sobo, E. J. (1995). *Choosing unsafe sex: AIDS risk denial among disadvantaged women.* University Park: University of Pennsylvania Press.

Sobo, E. J., & Rock, C. L. (2001). "You ate all that?" Caretaker-child interaction during children's assisted dietary recall interviews. *Medical Anthropology Quarterly, 15,* 222–244.

Sobo, E. J., Rock, C. L., Neuhouser, M. L., Maciel, T. L., & Neumark-Sztainer, D. (2000). Caretaker-child interaction during children's 24-hour dietary recalls: Who contributes what to the recall record? *Journal of the American Dietetic Association, 100,* 428–433.

Sobo, E. J., & Seid, M. (2001, November 30). *Cultural issues in pediatric medicine: What kind of "competence" is needed?* Paper presented at the 100th annual meeting of the American Anthropological Association, Washington, DC.

Sobo, E. J., Walker, E., & Kurtin, P. S. (2001). Complementary and alternative medicine: What do pediatricians need to know and ask? *California Pediatrician, 17*(1), 20–22.

Spigelblatt, L., Laine-Ammara, G., Pless, B., & Guyver, A. (1994). The use of alternative medicine by children. *Pediatrics, 94,* 811–814.

Stafford, A. (1978). The application of clinical anthropology to medical practice: Case study of recurrent abdominal pain in a preadolescent Mexican-American female. In E. Bauwens (Ed.), *The anthropology of health* (pp. 12–22). St. Louis: Mosby.

Svedberg, L., Nordahl, U., & Lundeberg, T. (2001). Effects of acupuncture on skin temperature in children with neurological disorders and cold feet: An exploratory study. *Complementary Therapies in Medicine, 9,* 89–97.

Tates, K., & Meeuwesen, L. (2001). Doctor-parent-child communication. A (re)view of the literature. *Social Science and Medicine, 52,* 839–851.

Troiano, R. P., & Flegal, K. M. (1998). Overweight children and adolescents: Description, epidemiology, and demographics. *Pediatrics, 101,* 497–504.

Trost, S., Kerr, L., Ward, D., & Pate, R. (2001). Physical activity and determinants of physical activity in obese and non-obese children. *International Journal of Obesity Related Metabolic Disorders, 26,* 822–829.

U.S. Consumer Product Safety Commission. (2001). *Home playground equipment-related deaths and injuries.* Washington, DC: Author.

van Ryn, M., & Burke, J. (2000). The effect of patient race and socio-economic status on physicians' perceptions of patients. *Social Science and Medicine, 50,* 813–828.

Waitzkin, H. (1981). The social origins of illness: A neglected history. *International Journal of Health Services, 11,* 77–103.

Ward, D. (1993). Women and the work of caring. *Second Opinion, 19*(2), 11–25.

Waters, M. (2000). Immigration, intermarriage, and the challenges of measuring racial/ethnic identities. *American Journal of Public Health, 90,* 1735–1737.

Wazana, A. (1997). Are there injury-prone children? A critical review of the literature. *Canadian Journal of Psychiatry, 42,* 602–610.

Weech-Maldonado, R., Morales, L. S., Spritzer, K., Elliott, M., & Hays, R. D. (2001). Racial and ethnic differences in parents' assessments of pediatric care in Medicaid managed care. *Health Services Research, 36,* 575–594.

Williams, B. (2001). Perceptions of illness causation among new referrals to a community mental health team: "Explanatory model" or "exploratory map"? *Social Science and Medicine, 53,* 465–476.

Wilson, K. M., & Klein, J. D. (2000, October 28–November 1). *Adolescents' use of complementary and alternative medicine.* Paper presented at the joint meeting of the Pediatric Academic Societies and the American Academy of Pediatrics, Chicago.

Wong, V., Sun, J., & Wong, W. (2001). Traditional Chinese medicine (tongue acupuncture) in children with drooling problems. *Pediatric Neurology, 25,* 47–54.

Young, J., & Garro, L. (1982). Choice of treatment in two Mexican communities. *Social Science and Medicine, 16,* 1453–1465.

4

· ·

Documenting Child Health

The Community Indicators Movement

Diana R. Simmes, Lillian F. Lim, Kimberly Dennis

With an increasing mandate to demonstrate the value of children's programs and services, the need to document child health outcomes has gained widespread support. Taxpayers, legislators, parents, foundations, and the program staff themselves are demanding to know whether programs and services are actually accomplishing what their proponents promise (Schorr, 1997). The use of community indicators as a tool to document such results is, however, still gaining acceptance. **Community indicators** are measures of child and family well-being that are tied to local community areas (Coulton, 1995). The growing importance and use of outcome measures by different **stakeholders** has helped propel the field of community indicators significantly forward in the past decade and has generated a flurry of activities. Such activities largely adhere to the premise that performance, not process, counts. Activities also focus on achieving results rather than simply guaranteeing exposure to services (Corbett, 1997). This chapter focuses on the history, development, and current use of community indicators. Although much is happening around the globe, especially in the area of children's well-being indicators (Ben-Arieh & Goerge, 2001), we will concentrate on work in the United States. Examples of community indicator projects and suggested future directions for the movement will also be included.

History

The roots of community indicators are closely linked to the social indicator movement. **Social indicators** have been defined as "quantitative data that serve as indexes to socially important conditions of the society" (Biderman, 1966, p. 69). Although this definition may seem broad, it reflects the sheer depth of topics that can be illustrated through the use of indicators. Community-level social indicators, as some have called them (Gibbs & Brown, 2000), can, for example, be used to help gauge the progress of early childhood education (as measured by indicators such as the rate of children entering school ready to learn). Other examples for which community indicators can be used are to track the increasing prevalence of asthma (as measured by changes in the rate of children hospitalized with asthma) or to track fluctuations in the unemployment rate.

The history of public health is rife with health-related statistics that make up one of the major subdivisions of social indicators. *Vital statistics*, indicators of vital events such as births and deaths, have long guided public health efforts and policies to improve the health of the population. One of the first quantifications of patterns of diseases in a population occurred in Europe and predates such epidemiologic work here in the United States. John Graunt's 1662 work *The Nature and Political Observations Made upon the Bills of Mortality*, in which he analyzed the weekly reports of births and deaths in London, is typically identified as the basis of modern **epidemiology** (Hennekens & Buring, 1987). It was not, however, until 1839, when the physician William Farr set up a system for the routine compilation of the numbers and causes of death, that the now well known tradition of using vital statistics in evaluating the public's health became established (Hennekens & Buring, 1987). In the United States, data on morbidity and mortality, such as the hallmark public health indicator of the infant mortality rate, go back to the beginning of the twentieth century (Moore, 1999).

In fact, the gathering of statistics, which we typically now call data collection, has long been a priority in the United States. The nation's founders recognized the importance of obtaining regular data on the population when they wrote the U.S. Constitution with a provision for a decennial census (Article I, Section 2). Later, beginning in the late 1800s with the creation of the U.S. Bureau of Labor, labor statistics were among the first social statistics collected for official purposes, with an interest primarily in demonstrating the terrible conditions of workers (Cobb & Rixford, 1998). Religious groups and other social reformers led the development of social indicators in this country.

At the beginning of the twentieth century, the formation of the Children's Bureau (Hutchins, 1994), now the Maternal and Child Health Bureau, used indicators as a primary strategy to document the relationship of family earnings, maternal employment, and access to health care on the health and survival of children (Skocpol, 1992). However, it was not until 1933 that all states were included in the newly established birth registry that was created as one of the bureau's first priorities.

The term *social indicator* rose to popularity in the mid-1960s, during which time numerous proposals for the use of such indicators were advanced (Land & Spilerman, 1975). The mid-1960s was the most intense period of scholarly and policy interest in social indicators (Kingsley, 1999). Significant societal changes, such as the civil rights and women's movements, as well as the beginnings of the space program, helped set the stage for this interest. Proposals of the mid-1960s argued that social indicators could be used to evaluate particular public programs, establish a system of social accounts analogous to the national economic accounts, establish social goals, and set social policy (Land & Spilerman, 1975).

The first proposal to be endorsed by an official government panel came from the National Commission on Technology, Automation, and Economic Progress (Land & Spilerman, 1975). This commission was established by public law "to identify and assess the pace and impact of current and prospective technological change on production, employment, and community and human needs and to recommend actions which could be taken by private and public agencies with respect to technological change and its consequences" (p. 6). The commission conceived the creation of a system of social accounts as the means to indicate the social benefits and social costs of investment and services to reflect the true costs of a product (National Commission, 1966). The focus was on building a system of social accounts analogous to the traditional economic indicators of the time (such as the gross national product and unemployment) in an effort to improve the means of public decision making and provide a more balanced picture of the meaning of social and economic progress. For example, such a social indicator system would take into account broad social ills (such as crime) or unforeseen burdens that might result from technological advances such as automation (displacement of workers with a certain skill set). It would also take into account the negative by-products of a new production plant in a community (air pollution) in addition to documenting the more obvious economic benefits of new jobs.

In the same year that the commission's report was completed, one of the first contemporary books to present the idea of using indicators to do precisely what the commission describes, *Social Indicators*, was published (Bauer, 1966). In this volume, Raymond Bauer describes the National Aeronautics and Space Administration (NASA)–funded evaluation of the social impacts of the space program and delineates the components of an ideal information system to capture relevant information. Bauer describes this ideal as a "system of feedback in the society for detecting the full range of consequences of its actions, and for guiding future actions" (p. 20). He describes the three major components of the system as (1) regular trend series of social indicators, (2) special mechanisms for gathering data on new developments falling outside those regular trend series, and (3) some means of reporting this information with appropriate speed, in appropriate form, to the appropriate agency.

Some observers have suggested that the historical social indicators movement in the United States was a disappointment to its originators (Innes, 1990a) and that it failed to serve one vitally important function: to make indicators practical tools (Cobb & Rixford, 1998). Brown and Corbett (1998) have delineated five general purposes for which indicators are now commonly used:

1. *Description:* Indicators are used to describe the circumstances of a community. They provide information in such areas as health, economic situation, and social environment.

2. *Monitoring:* Indicators are used to track what is happening in a community over time.

3. *Setting goals:* Organizations and other groups use indicators to set goals for their programs and activities.

4. *Outcome-based accountability:* The presence of indicators provides people with the information needed to hold community organizations, the government, and other groups responsible for what occurs within their communities.

5. *Evaluation:* Indicators are used in program evaluation to determine a program's effectiveness.

Until very recently, indicator use had not begun to reach its full potential. Moreover, although indicators yielded important information, the link between the data that indicators provide and actual use of the data was absent, perhaps due to a top-down approach. The current social indicators movement, which is now more commonly termed the "community indicators movement" or even the "community-level social indicators movement," strives to rectify that failure by making the "democratization of information" of paramount importance. That is, stakeholders (such as community organizations, nongovernmental groups, and other leaders) now participate in community indicator initiatives from the development phase through implementation. The entire process emphasizes facilitating the direct practical use of data by city and community leaders (Kingsley, 1999). Community members themselves design, develop, and research community indicator systems (Norris & Atkisson, 1997). This more inclusive process helps ensure that the indicators can be used by the community and applied to relevant issues in their own neighborhoods.

Although calls for the increased use of data on social conditions were heard much earlier, the use of social indicators did not truly flourish until the 1990s (Gibbs & Brown, 2000). Kingsley (1999) cites the cost and work of constructing the computer-based information systems needed to develop and track indicators as the primary reason for the lack of progress from earlier eras. Scholars in every field of social science and professional practice now give explicit attention to indicators (Innes, 1990b). There is, however, a notable exception: although many professional disciplines have been using indicators for several decades, those involved in the field of child and family services lag far behind. Mark Friedman (2000) of the Fiscal Policy Studies Institute has said, "We are 100 years behind the business community, 70 years behind the labor movement, 50 years behind the public health services in creating timely, reliable comparable data on the well-being of children and families." Nevertheless, there is now great public and policymaker pressure to include community indicators in child and family service work.

Gibbs and Brown (1999) cite three major factors that have contributed to the tremendous recent growth in the use of community indicators as tools of governance and advocacy: (1) advances in computer technology such as accessibility to the Internet, (2) the devolution or the transfer of control from higher levels to lower levels of government, and (3) a renewed emphasis on service coordination and integration. Nearly two hundred cities have now adopted a community indicators process to track community conditions, inform policy choices, build consensus, and promote accountability (Besleme, Maser, & Silverstein, 1999). Demand for readily accessible and understandable community-specific data has been fueled, in part, by a more general awareness of outcomes or what is sometimes termed "results-based accountability." Such accountability-based public policy requires increasing amounts of data to provide more accurate measures of children's conditions as well as the outcomes various programs achieve (Ben-Arieh & Goerge, 2001).

Community indicator–based documentation of child health in the community at large can provide this needed actionable information for a broad range of child health stakeholders, including child health services researchers. As discussed by Paul Kurtin in Chapter One, those stakeholders may also include individuals and groups who now recognize that health care policy debates and contract negotiations need to shift from cost alone to a focus on quality and include purchasers, payers, regulators, and consumers of child health services.

The contemporary widespread interest in community-level indicators is documented in a September 2000 publication from the U.S. Department of Health and Human Services' Office of the Assistant Secretary for Planning and Evaluation (Gibbs & Brown, 2000), which describes the current state of the art as follows: "Local governments, private civic improvement organizations, community foundations and private community-based services organizations are beginning to build and use data sets to create local indicator systems that, in turn, have become fundamental tools for tracking and understanding community viability, health, and social functioning" (p. 1).

Although the collection of data is certainly not a new concept, its pragmatic adoption by such stakeholders, including community residents, is a key feature of the current community indicators movement. The democratization of information will not become a reality unless such groups are involved at all phases and levels. **Child health services research (CHSR)** can play an important role in advancing the movement by facilitating the effective use of data by all concerned.

The advancement of the community indicators agenda is closely linked with the general desire for improving community health or what is frequently referred to as the "healthier communities" movement (see Chapter Five, by Dennis and Simmes). It has been said that indicators are the road map to progressing toward healthier communities (Redefining Progress, 1998). For children's health, a community emphasis is appropriate because the majority of children are well and their health care needs are preventive and often provided at the community or household level (see Chapter Three, by Sobo).

Framework

Whereas the earlier social indicator work largely lacked an organizing conceptual framework and any consensus on single or aggregate indicators of community health (Slater, 1999), it is now believed that the selection of a theoretical framework is a prerequisite to indicator design. Contemporary community indicator projects quantify community health and well-being in terms of one of the three most prominent models in current use: health, quality of life, and sustainability (Besleme & Mullin, 1997). The traditional health-based, or *epidemiological,* approach typically measures the total amount of ill health in the community and uses that measurement to allocate resources for different diseases (Billings & Cowley, 1995). Adopting a "quality of life" approach focuses on factors such as housing, jobs, and public safety that may not fall under a traditional medical service delivery model (Norris & Atkisson, 1997). The third predominant framework, sustainability, has given the community indicators movement a boost via the increasing requirements for more effective monitoring of environmental conditions (Kingsley, 1999). A major body of work has been developed based on a grant awarded to Tufts University in 1992 by the U.S. Environmental Protection Agency to initially define and then develop indicators to measure progress toward achieving a "sustainable community" (Kline, 1997).[1]

The framework that is chosen naturally influences the composition of the project and any resulting product, coalition, or action that derives from it. However, some observers have argued that positing a completed framework up front puts an unrealistic strain on data production (Innes, 1990b) and thereby limits indicator coalition possibilities. Looking at the broader determinants of a community's health leads an indicator coalition to a much different outcome than taking a more narrow view of the community's health, such as adopting a strictly epidemiological viewpoint that relies heavily on morbidity and mortality data, as opposed to being concerned with the percentage of students taking the Scholastic Assessment Test (SAT) or the supply of affordable high-quality child care.

The Language Trap

In addition to arriving at a consensus as to which framework will drive a project, a community indicator coalition must agree on the terms it will use to describe its processes and outcomes. As simple as this may seem, achieving consensus on a framework and terminology is a significant issue, in our experience. Many others have called for building a common language to clear some of the fog that is apparent in this field (Ben-Arieh & Goerge, 2001). However, because this field is community-based, has no central literature (as academic fields do), and is multidisciplinary, one obstacle that indicator coalitions must overcome is what Mark Friedman (2000) has termed the "language trap."

In Figure 4.1, the term *indicator* is related to several important concepts, terms for which are often used interchangeably (such as **outcome** and **benchmark**). Further complications typically arise when several disciplines come together with different perspectives and definitions, thereby adding to the confusion of these terms and causing some indicator coalitions to become trapped in a game of semantics. One solution to alleviate the confusion is the development of consistent definitions within the movement. Because community indicators are used for comparing communities, benchmarking, identifying best practices, and ultimately making improvements within a community, a common vocabulary is fundamental. The following definitions hold the greatest currency today:

Accountability: Demonstrating value through outcomes (Seid, Sadler, Peddecord, & Kurtin, 1996)

Community health report card: Document that provides a snapshot of the community's health by presenting objective information about past trends and current realities through the use of indicators, or measurements of local trends (Fielding & Sutherland, 1998)

Community-level social indicator: A social indicator that can be collected, reported, and meaningfully interpreted for geopolitical units such as neighborhoods, towns, cities, metropolitan areas, or regions (Gibbs & Brown, 2000)

Health status: A description or measurement of the health of an individual or population at a particular point in time against identifiable standards, usually by reference to health indicators (World Health Organization, 1998)

Needs assessment: The process of identifying the problems and needs of a target population (Butler, 1994)

Performance measure: A measure of how well agency or program service delivery is working. Some examples include police response time, percentage of teen parents keeping clinic appointments, and child abuse investigations initiated within twenty-four hours of a report of abuse (Friedman, 2000)

The lack of a common vocabulary has been an issue with indicator coalitions, in our experience, and can impede early progress.

The Underwriters: The Role of Foundations and the Government

The evolution of the community indicators movement has been fostered, in large part, by the federal government and several major foundations that have sought to expand the knowledge base and

Figure 4.1. The Language Trap.

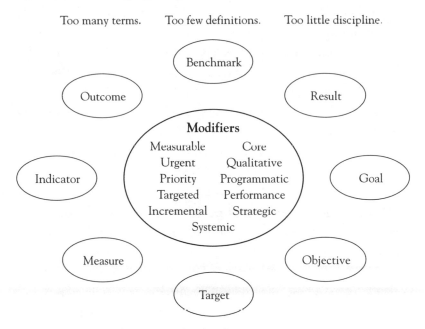

Too many terms.   Too few definitions.   Too little discipline.

Benchmark

Outcome

Result

Modifiers

Measurable   Core
Urgent   Qualitative
Indicator   Priority   Programmatic   Goal
Targeted   Performance
Incremental   Strategic
Systemic

Measure

Objective

Target

Source: From Friedman, 2000. Used with permission.

move the community indicators field forward. By making significant investments, these funding agencies have helped contribute to the evolution of community indicators and the resulting data-based advocacy. Local community foundations have helped institutionalize indicator efforts in their own neighborhoods, thereby increasing the likelihood of the democratization of information.

The Role of Foundations

In 1990, the Annie E. Casey Foundation started the Kids Count initiative to raise the nation's awareness and accountability about the condition of children and families and has since become the foundation's signature product (www.kidscountnetwork.net). Kids Count uses community indicators to measure the educational, social, economic, and physical well-being of children and families by state, by metropolitan area, and by specific topics such as teen pregnancy. The foundation began supporting state-level Kids Count projects

in 1991 and urged these various efforts to network and form partnerships. Highly successful projects like Kids Count have helped
disseminate information on the community indicators movement
and contributed to the increased appeal of creating indicator coalitions. There now are Kids Count projects in all fifty states, the District of Columbia, and the Virgin Islands. The annual Kids Count
nationwide report has spawned numerous additional reports such as
"City Kids Count."

Similarly, the Robert Wood Johnson Foundation's Child Health
Initiative, conceived in the late 1980s and initiated in 1991, funded
nine communities throughout the United States to improve the coordination and integration of health services for children with
greater than average health and social service needs (Halfon,
Newacheck, Hughes, & Brindis, 1998). Part of this initiative required that each community develop a health report to heighten
community awareness of children's health needs. In addition, some
developed models of community-based and school-based programs.
This initiative is significant in that it helped inform others beginning to work in this newly reenergized field. The role of foundations
is integral and must be appreciated. Foundations provide a general
structure within which to work, networking and peer learning opportunities, and operational support in addition to showcasing national models (Redefining Progress, 1998).

The Role of Government

In addition to foundations, the federal government has played, and
continues to play, an important role in children's health. Developing better monitoring of children's health in a community, including the use of **community health report cards**, is one of the eight
strategies proposed for implementing the national research agenda
on improving the quality of health care for children (Halfon, Schuster, Valentine, & McGlynn, 1998). To develop such improved monitoring, the following key steps were proposed: (1) use a core set of
indicators to facilitate benchmarking capabilities; (2) develop software and standard data collection procedures for local communities;

(3) enhance communities' technical capacity for data collection, analysis, and presentation; and (4) provide funding to support these activities and coordination at the national level. The proposed agenda was developed at a 1997 conference, sponsored by the Association for Health Services Research (AHSR), on developing a research agenda focused on improving the quality of care for children.

The federal government has funded several important initiatives aimed toward improving the collection and use of community indicators. In 1998, the U.S. Department of Health and Human Services' Office of the Assistant Secretary for Planning and Evaluation (ASPE)[2] awarded grants to thirteen states to promote their efforts to develop and monitor indicators of the health and well-being of children and to help institutionalize the use of indicators in policy-making. This coincided with welfare reform and other major policy changes (Reidy & Moorehouse, 2002) that have been predicted to have far-reaching consequences for children's health. In September 2000, the ASPE, in conjunction with the Research Triangle Institute and Child Trends, Inc., released *Community-Level Indicators for Understanding Health and Human Services Issues: A Compendium of Selected Indicator Systems and Resource Organizations* (Gibbs & Brown, 2000). This compendium provides many examples of outstanding community, regional, and statewide indicator systems as well as public and private resource organizations for community indicator practitioners. These organizations serve as useful starting points for newcomers to this rapidly evolving field.

Public health professionals have also been actively involved in developing indicators at the national level. A variety of national initiatives centered on health-specific community indicators proliferated in the 1990s. In 1991, the Centers for Disease Control and Prevention (CDC) released its consensus set of health status indicators for the general assessment of community health status (National Center for Health Statistics, 1991). This consensus set of eighteen specific indicators, which enjoys widespread use by state health departments (Zucconi & Carson, 1994), was developed to help communities gauge their general health status as well as track progress toward achieving the nation's official health objectives found in *Healthy People 2000* (U.S. Department of Health and Human Services, 1991). The scope of indicators in *Healthy People 2000*, originally called *The Objectives for the Nation's Health* in the late 1970s, is vast. *Healthy People 2000* was developed over the course of three years by a consortium of nearly three hundred national membership organizations and all fifty state health departments that solicited and analyzed comments and suggestions from people across the nation. Various regional and national hearings were held, including public review and comment. *Healthy People 2000* includes hundreds of indicators in more than twenty domains with specific targets, such as reducing the death rate for children by 15 percent to no more than 28 per 100,000 children aged one through fourteen and for infants by approximately 30 percent to no more than 7 per 1,000 live births. A companion document, *Healthy Communities 2000: Model Standards: Guidelines for Community Attainment of the Year 2000 National Health Objectives*, was released at the same time (American Public Health Association, 1991) and was designed for use by individual communities to put the *Healthy People 2000* objectives into achievable health targets of their own.

In support of these goals, the Health Resources and Services Administration (HRSA)[3] sponsors the Community Health Status Indicators (CHSI) project. This project was created in response to grassroots-level requests from local health officials for health data at the local level (www.communityhealth.hrsa.gov). These reports provide county-level indicator data in nine major categories and allow counties to compare themselves to the Healthy People targets as well as to "peer counties" that are similar in population size, density, age distribution, and poverty. Operating under the premise that community health improvement begins with an assessment of needs, quantification of vulnerable populations, and measurement of preventable disease, disability, and death, the CHSI focuses largely on federal data sources, such as the Environmental Protection Agency and the Census Bureau. Because the project adheres to the traditional epidemiological framework, the reports may be less useful to indicator coalitions interested in the broader aspects of community health. They do, however, provide valuable models for the development of indicators with higher local specificity. These numerous high-profile national efforts have helped set the tone for many groups working in the area of health-specific community indicators.

Development of Indicator Initiatives

Undoubtedly, community indicators are increasingly being used to document the health and well-being of children throughout the United States. Using well-measured and systematically collected indicators enables communities to monitor how well children are doing at one point in time, as well as over longer periods. However, developing relevant and sensitive community indicators, especially child and family well-being indicators, presents numerous conceptual, methodological, and political challenges (Coulton, 1995). Community indicator initiatives are frequently caught in the balancing act of accommodating the various stakeholders' perspectives on what is important to include while at the same time using valid and reliable data points.

The Federal Interagency Forum on Child and Family Statistics, an organization created to "foster coordination and collaboration in the collection and reporting of Federal data on children and families" (2001, p. i), developed guidelines to help direct communities through their indicator selection process. The Forum recommends that an indicator be easy to understand by an array of audiences, objectively based on research and reliable data, measured regularly, and representative of a large portion of the population rather than one particular group. CHSR investigators working with community indicators must bear these practical matters in mind.

Application of Community Indicators:
The Report Card Trend

Report cards, one of the more common applications of community indicator data, are used in many different fields. We are all familiar with report cards used to grade children's school achievement. In the health care industry, report cards have been used to present concise quality assessments to help consumers choose health plans and providers (Wicks & Meyer, 1999) and by public and private employers alike (such as the California Public Employees Retirement Systems and General Motors). Report cards have been used to compare quality between physician medical groups, as is done by the Pacific Business Group on Health, and to publish hospitals' performance (Wicks & Meyer, 1999). Research has found that consumers make limited use of such data for decision making; they may find it conflicting or difficult to understand, or they may be overwhelmed by the quantity of information presented (Hibbard, Peters, Slovic, Finucane, & Tusler, 2001). Environmental lobbies have used report cards as communication tools for public interest groups, as in determining the impact of ski resorts on the environment (Goodman, 2001). Therefore, it is not surprising that report cards have also made their way into the arena of children's health.

The development of community-level indicator projects and the emergence of community report cards (also known as "state of the child reports," "community status reports," "scorecards," or "community profiles") are directly related. Community-level indicators are the building blocks of community report cards, as they are comprised of data and information on conditions in a defined geopolitical area. Most often they are illustrated as charts and graphs, allowing people to see trends at a glance (Norris & Atkisson, 1997). One of the main benefits of community report cards is that they centralize information, providing a complete picture of a community's well-being. Child health stakeholders can use this snapshot in a variety of ways. For example, indicators and report cards are part of a growing trend to inform communities about children's needs so that services can be adjusted and improved (Halfon, Newacheck, et al., 1998). Report cards can also be used to raise awareness about specific issues within the community, educate the public about problems in the community, or provide the basis for programs and projects geared to aid community residents.

Pragmatics

Children Now, a California-based child policy and advocacy organization, has guided many community indicator coalitions through the development process via its step-by-step guide to producing such report cards (1998). This guide emphasizes that organizations creating a report card must first determine their goals and then develop an agenda for how it can be used to fuel action in their community. This requires that indicator coalitions know the target audience and consider how the report card will be useful to their community. Creating broad categories in which to group the indicators is also necessary to ensure a basis for choosing appropriate indicators and finding the corresponding data. This requires input and collaboration from a variety of organizations that are representative of the community as a whole. End users of the report card need to participate in the planning process to ensure that the indicators are useful not only to certain organizations within the community but also to the community as a whole (United Way of America, 1999).

Because report cards are comprehensive documents, the development process tends to be extensive and generally inclusive in successful cases. In fact, some observers have argued that the process is really the point and that using indicators is trivial compared what is gained during the development process (Innes, 1990b). Indeed, a resulting by-product of creating a local indicator coalition and selecting the indicators can be community building. (See Chapter Five, by Dennis and Simmes, for a thorough discussion of conducting community-based research.)

In addition to consensus-building activities, accurate and objective evaluation of the data is necessary. Evaluating potential data sources may be greatly aided by the inclusion of a neutral third party, such as a scientific advisory committee, that can lend credibility to the effort. State and national data are essential for benchmarking purposes; if local, state, and national comparison data are not available for an indicator, analysis will be somewhat limited. For example, in San Diego County, data were collected on low birthweight, and the rate for people grouped as Asian Americans and Pacific Islanders was 7 percent (San Diego County Health and Human Services Agency, 2001). The next step for community leaders, policymakers, and programs working on this issue is to compare that percentage to a percentage calculated on a larger scale (for example, regions of California, the state of California, or the entire United States) to determine if San Diego County is doing better, worse, or the same. This type of information can further guide program development, media campaigns, and funding requests for services that focus on decreasing racial disparities for low-birthweight births.

In addition to comparative data, it is helpful to include explanations of why the data should matter to the community in the first place. In our experience, keeping these considerations in mind during report card development increases its usefulness for the broadest range of child health stakeholders.

Report Card Projects: Some Examples

The CDC, under a cooperative agreement with the Association of Schools of Public Health, provided funding for the development of the 1998 *National Directory of Community Health Report Cards* (Fielding & Sutherland, 1998). This was the first directory of community health report cards and was developed on the basis of questionnaire responses from 250 public health officials and public and private organizations with an interest in community health improvement from around the country (Fielding, Sutherland, & Halfon, 1999). The *National Directory* catalogues more than fifty projects and provides a description of the community characteristics, report card characteristics, and outstanding features of each indicator project. We now take a closer look at two of the outstanding report card projects.

Jacksonville, Florida

Exemplary work has been done by communities like Jacksonville, Florida, one of the early adopters of the grassroots community indicators approach. The city's "Quality Indicators for Progress" report has been under continuous development since 1985 and is widely regarded as one of the most forward-thinking and effective tools for monitoring quality-of-life indicators reflective of community values and priorities (Norris & Atkisson, 1997). The Jacksonville Community Council is the driver and is credited with having the longest-standing community health report card project in the country.

San Diego, California

San Diego County's population is the second largest in California and the fourth largest in the United States. The 2.7 million people of the region represent diverse ethnoracial backgrounds, presenting many challenges to providers of public health and social services. Moreover, changes such as welfare reform, the movement of Medicaid to managed care, and the restructuring the county's health and human services agency further challenge the ability to improve outcomes for children and families. With these contextual factors in mind, the county's board of supervisors and the community at large wanted to know what impact these changes might have on the health and well-being of San Diego's children and families. In response, the San Diego County Child and Family Health and Well-Being Report Card was developed in 1998 under the leadership of the local health and human services agency, Children's Hospital San Diego, and the Alliance Healthcare Foundation (Simmes, Blaszcak, Kurtin, Bowen, & Ross, 2000).

Following the guidelines set forth by Children Now, stakeholders first determined the goal of the report card, which was to monitor the effects of the various changes on children and families in San Diego County. Next, the report card developers researched how the report card might be useful to the community. This entailed obtaining input from more than forty local community groups. Information gathered from the community resulted in the selection of twenty-nine indicators, grouped into five broad domains—economics, health, safety, access to services, and education. Once the indicators were selected, the data were gathered and evaluated for inclusion against a strict set of criteria.

As emphasized by Children Now and other organizations invested in the community report card effort, these documents not only present information about a community but are also used to fuel action and make changes within communities. The San Diego County Child and Family Health and Well-Being Report Card has been developed and produced on a yearly basis since 1999. The success of the project is due, in part, to the usefulness of the report card to local policymakers, community-based organizations, and child health service providers.

The "So What?" Question: What Is the Applied Usefulness of This Area of Research?

There are many specific examples, which will be discussed in the following sections, of how communities have used indicator data in real life settings. Data provided by indicators allow a community to act from a position of knowledge by providing a common information base and can foster the development of an outcomes-based culture of accountability. Knowledge gained from such a system of indicators ultimately has the potential to improve the programs and services that are delivered to children. Without documentation of the baseline status of a community through some type of monitoring system, it becomes difficult to measure progress, or lack thereof, from one point in time to another.

Community indicators are like the gauges on the dashboard of a moving car: their purpose is to alert the driver that something is going on. Just as any driver uses the fuel gauge to monitor the level of gas available, any concerned individual, policymaker, or service provider can use a community indicator to assess the general state of health and well-being of the community and help determine when intervention is needed. Research conducted by Redefining Progress (1998) distinguishes between **descriptive** and **prescriptive community indicators**. Descriptive community indicators allow us to name and quantify problems to help us understand where we are now, while prescriptive community indicators help identify root causes and the impact of existing assumptions on which potential policy decisions are based and can lead to actual change.

A population-based community health status assessment is just the first step in addressing the health-related needs of a given community. Once the data have been collected, stakeholders need to develop sustainable, meaningful improvement efforts (Felix & Burdine, 1995). Indicators are the least common denominator of such efforts, the starting point of a common information base. They are tools, not end products, providing basic descriptive information that can inform priority setting through the provision of data on specific health issues (Durch, Bailey, & Stoto, 1997). However, which specific factors predict which community indicator initiatives are or can be effectively linked to an actual community health "improvement" process remains an unanswered question at this point (Fielding et al., 1999). Ideally, community indicators do not just monitor progress; they help make it happen (Norris & Atkisson, 1997).

The chasm between documentation of a community's health, through the use of community indicators, and community health improvement can be vast. In *Children's Advocate*, a bimonthly advocacy newsmagazine, Franklin (2000) noted that while many groups are releasing community indicator reports that look impressive, whether the effort makes a difference remains unanswered. Notwithstanding the outcomes research that needs to be done to provide evidence of the link, the editors of the issue provided three specific examples of how report cards have been used for child advocacy projects: in launching local campaigns, influencing policy, and linking issues to data in order to secure funding. Responsibility for making indicators cross the chasm ultimately lies squarely on the shoulders of community indicator practitioners, including researchers new to the field of applied CHSR.

Tools of the Trade: Examples from the Trenches

Various stakeholder groups are applying indicators in a wide variety of areas. Advocacy organizations such as Children Now and the

Children's Defense Fund have used indicator data to raise awareness of infant mortality and draw attention to other issues, such as the plight of poor children. Local and state governments have sanctioned, and even legislated, the use of indicators for advancing specific child health agendas.

In 1991, the state of Oregon released its first "Oregon Benchmarks" report based on a twenty-year strategic vision for the state (Council of State Governments, 1997). The Oregon Benchmarks are a set of quantifiable indicators for the economy, communities, and the environment that was unanimously adopted by the Oregon legislature as state policy and that have been widely used by Oregon counties and communities (www.econ.state.or.us/opb). The Benchmarks articulate the state's goals as a set of measurable indicators, identify short- and long-term priorities, and establish targets.

In November 1998, California voters passed Proposition 10, the California Children and Families Act. This statewide ballot initiative increased the excise tax on tobacco products by 50 cents. It earmarked the resulting revenue to fund comprehensive, integrated systems to promote early childhood education development from the prenatal period to age five. Health and safety code section 130140(1)(C)(ii) of the act requires each county's Proposition 10 Commission's strategic plan to include a description of how measurable outcomes of funded programs will be determined using appropriate reliable indicators (www.ccfc.ca.gov). The statewide commission established a strong and clear agenda for early accountability and feedback via what it calls "short-term results," which are measured by various proposed indicators (such as the number of children with a primary care provider or the percentage of children with up-to-date immunizations at age two). In addition, individual counties need to establish an environment of results-based accountability, as outcomes are the primary criterion for continued funding of local projects (Illig, 1999).

Although the idea of monitoring outcomes through indicators is not a new idea, it is revolutionary to legislate their inclusion in an act of this significance for children's health. As part of the new focus on outcomes, or what Schorr (1997) describes as a revolution in our ability to know whether programs, policies, and tax dollars are achieving their intended purpose, **performance measures** are seen as an important aspect by the community-level indicators movement.

Technology

One way to facilitate the inclusion of indicator initiatives in community-specific projects is to incorporate information technology. For example, the use of indicators has been integrated with various computer software packages to monitor the performance of programs and services within a community. One example is the "Outcomes Toolkit" developed by the Healthcare Forum to aid community organizations in demonstrating their outcomes. Based on the growing demand for accountability, this user-friendly tool approaches planning and evaluation comprehensively (Healthcare Forum, 1998). Features include a community profile builder, a database of indicators, a report generator, useful Internet links, a "best practices" workbook, and references. All of these features are used together to develop goals, track progress, and present measurable results.

Geographic Information Systems

Geographic information systems (GISs) add a new dimension to community indicators by presenting a large amount of information visually. A GIS is "a computer system capable of assembling, storing, manipulating, and displaying geographically referenced information, i.e. data identified according to their locations" (U.S. Geological Survey, 2002). Moreover, a total GIS is typically regarded as including both operating personnel and the data that feed the system. For example, a GIS is used to take information from a database and present the data geographically on a computer-generated, multilayered map of a defined area (Redefining Progress, 1998). Data gathered on the number of clinics within a community, type of housing, location of freeways, and asthma hospitalizations can all be placed on one map. GIS maps illustrate the proximal linkages between these separate phenomena through a technique called layering. It also enables people without extensive data training to understand the multidimensional nature of circumstances in a community. Indeed, the power and mass appeal of information technology–based systems like GIS rely heavily on the notion that anyone can use them. Ultimately, maps can be used to influence public policy (Redefining Progress, 1998) and make recommendations within a given community for programs and services (see Figure 4.2).

What's Next?

Among the many challenges for the community indicators movement, including obtaining greater participation of government and business representatives in indicator coalitions (Redefining Progress, 1998), four major areas are ripe for development: (1) use and analysis of finer-grained data, (2) advancement of asset-based community indicators, (3) development of new indicators, and (4) transitioning projects from description to action and community health improvement.

The first area ready for development, and in many ways the easiest, is shrinking the unit of analysis. As CHSR investigators continue to live in an increasingly technological society, they will have access to an expansive body of information about the communities that they work with and study. Available data sets will provide them with information in increasingly smaller geographical units (such as by street intersection). Whereas some researchers in the field have traditionally focused their major work on issues of access to and use of health care services on a broader scale through the analysis of larger data sets, CHSR investigators are now perfectly poised to study community- and neighborhood-specific data points that make up these larger aggregated data sets. Interesting work has been done, for example, on the relationship between neighborhood

Figure 4.2. Children's Hospital and Health Center Pediatric
Hospitalizations in San Diego County in 2001, by ZIP Code.

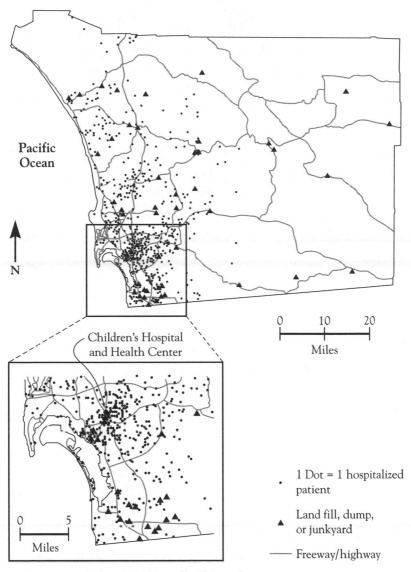

Pacific
Ocean

N

Children's Hospital
and Health Center

0   10   20
Miles

0   5
Miles

1 Dot = 1 hospitalized
patient

Land fill, dump,
or junkyard

Freeway/highway

Note: No causality should be inferred from this map.

socioeconomic characteristics and birthweight in different ethno-racial groups (Pearl, Braveman, & Abrams, 2001). Such data allow for more precise estimates and analyses regarding conditions of fundamental interest to the field of CHSR (such as hospitalization rates and injuries). Although the concept of examining health through the lens of geography is not novel, given John Snow's ground-breaking work on the geographically centered origins of a major cholera epidemic in London in the 1850s (Hennekens & Buring, 1987), computer technology increases the likelihood of this type of information's being widely accessible to all child health stakeholders, including applied CHSR investigators.

The second area of development is the creation of asset-based community indicator systems. The "democratization of information" movement strives to facilitate data use by stakeholders such as community and leadership groups (Kingsley, 1999). In recent years, several newsletters and listservs have been created, constituting an informal network for people involved in the community indicators field and supporting the democratization of information including best practices. The first issue of *The Child Indicator: The Child, Youth, and Family Indicators Newsletter* appeared in November 1999. This newsletter, published by Child Trends and funded by the Annie E. Casey Foundation, communicates the major developments within each sector of the child and youth indicators field to the larger community of interested users (such as community-based organizations, researchers, and data developers) on a regular basis (Brown & Van-divere, 1999). *Data Matters,* first published in 1999 by Georgetown University's National Technical Assistance Center for Children's Mental Health, features stories about promising practices concerning the evaluation of children's services and interagency management information systems. Moreover, the National Neighborhood Indicators Partnership started a listserv in 1999 in which indicator practitioners can post comments and questions regarding developing and using indicators, data sources, and helping community organizations understand and use data (www.urban.org/nnip/nnip_news.html).

As various stakeholders have become involved, the call for measuring positive aspects of children's lives, or assets, rather than only deficits, has grown increasingly strong. Recently, much work has been done on varying forms and thoughts of measuring positive aspects of children's lives to get beyond indicators of children's survival alone (Ben-Arieh & Goerge, 2001). Safe and clean streets, access to health care resources, employment opportunities, and youth-serving programs are a few examples of asset-based community indicators.

Despite high interest among stakeholders, the development of a true asset-based community indicator system is yet to come. A major barrier is the extensive paradigm shift needed among professionals who have been trained to measure deficits and count incidents of morbidity and mortality. For example, the medical model forces the focus to be on a specific symptom or medical problem rather than on a person's overall health and well-being (McKnight, 1999). In some respects, a negative focus can be beneficial when, for example, an emphasis on negative attributes enables the community to attract resources (Kretzmann & McKnight, 1993, cited in Sharpe, Greaney, Lee, & Royce, 2000). However, deficit-based thinking can also have a substantial negative impact on communities, especially those already labeled as disadvantaged through the reinforcement of stereotypes.

Though it may be tempting to simply invert a negative indicator in order to solve the problem (such as converting an infant mortality rate to an infant survival rate), this is a far cry from measuring the true assets of a community. A genuine asset-oriented community assessment "allows community members to identify, support, and mobilize existing community resources to create a shared vision of change, and encourages greater creativity when community members do address problems and obstacles" (Sharpe et al., 2000, p. 205). When assets are clearly identified, they may be built on and replicated. To increase the usability and visibility of indicators, community members must take action and develop indicators that are representative of their own community. In so doing, community members use their resources, skills, and other assets to directly benefit their community (McKnight, 1999).

The third area of development is the creation of new indicators. Continuously evolving indicators are important in the sustainability of community indicator initiatives. Schorr has said, "In efforts to select the right outcomes, no one should be under the illusion that any one set of outcomes or outcome measures will be perfect. They will have to be refined always, sometime renegotiated, and evolve continuously" (1997, p. 125). Several recommendations for new indicators can be found in *America's Children: Key National Indicators of Well-Being, 2001* (Federal Interagency Forum, 2001). In addition, there are areas that need further research and data collection. In the area of population and family characteristics, the key recommendation is to gather data on how children spend their time. Moreover, there is a lack of information related to children's economic security, including how their economic well-being has changed over time, the impact of long-term poverty, and the issue of homelessness. In addition to indicators related to early childhood development, health indicators regarding disability, mental health, and child abuse and neglect are also needed. Finally, in the area of behavior and social environment, the key recommendations are to gather data on indicators of positive behaviors, neighborhood environment, and youth violence.

The final, and in many ways most difficult, area of development is transitioning indicator projects from description to action and community health improvement. One way to ensure the development of new indicators, as well as improved data collection, is to actively solicit and use community input. Community members must determine their own needs and assets. In doing so, they can take a more active role in ensuring that the most useful and relevant information for their community is being collected and widely reported.

Adopting the concept of the democratization of information, the report card project in San Diego County is currently making the transition from documentation to action through the provision of data-related technical assistance to local community-based organizations. Although general feedback about the San Diego County Child and Family Health and Well-Being Report Card has been positive, the actual use of the document by community-based organizations was relatively unknown. In an effort to determine how the data in the report were being used to improve the health and well-being of communities in San Diego County, a technical assistance program was implemented. The goal of the technical assistance curriculum is to train community-based organizations in the collection, analysis, interpretation, and reporting of data to meet the increasing challenge of demonstrating organization and program outcomes. In addition, the technical assistance program aims to help participating organizations use report card data to evaluate and improve their services and ultimately the lives of the people they serve.

Conclusion: CHSR as a Bridge

We have argued that outcomes research directed at achieving accountability of the health care system and the development of community health information systems (such as community indicators) have been pursuing parallel but unconnected tracks for the past decade (Slater, 1999). The design of CHSR must take into account lessons learned from the failures of earlier decades, during which time the full potential of community indicators were never realized. Although the use of community indicators as a tool to document child health and well-being has made significant advancements in recent years, their application to improvement methodologies is not yet widely accepted. Community indicators are the yardsticks by which CHSR should not only measure but also direct improvements for the health of all children in a given community. CHSR investigators, particularly those working in an applied setting, can make significant strides toward bringing the two fields together and can become involved through existing indicator coalitions in their own communities, the creation of new ones, or providing the outcomes research base to promote their use.

Notes

1. For a discussion of theoretical frameworks previously proposed, see Innes (1990b).

2. Additional support was provided by the Administration for Children and Families and the David and Lucile Packard Foundation.

3. In conjunction with the Association of State and Territorial Health Officials and the National Association of County and City Health Officials, and the Public Health Foundation.

References

American Public Health Association. (1991). *Healthy communities 2000: Model standards: Guidelines for community attainment of the year 2000 national health objectives* (3rd ed.). Washington, DC: Author.

Bauer, R. (Ed.). (1966). *Social indicators*. Cambridge, MA: MIT Press.

Ben-Arieh, A., & Goerge, R. (2001). Beyond the numbers: How do we monitor the state of our children? *Children and Youth Services Review, 23*, 603–631.

Besleme, K., Maser, E., & Silverstein, J. (1999). *A community indicators case study: Addressing the quality of life in two communities*. Redefining Progress. Retrieved from http://www.rprogress.org/pubs/pubtable.html

Besleme, K., & Mullin, M. (1997). Community indicators and healthy communities. *National Civic Review, 86*, 43–53.

Biderman, A. (1966). Social indicators and goals. In R. Bauer (Ed.), *Social indicators* (pp. 68–153). Cambridge, MA: MIT Press.

Billings, J. R., & Cowley, S. (1995). Approaches to community needs assessment: A literature review. *Journal of Advanced Nursing, 22*, 721–730.

Brown, B., & Corbett, T. (1998). Social indicators and public policy in the age of devolution. Madison, WI: Institute for Research on Poverty.

Brown, B., & Vandivere, S. (1999). Welcome to the premier issue of *The Child Indicator*. *Child Indicator, 1*(1), 1.

Butler, J. (1994). *Principles of health education and health promotion*. Englewood, CO: Morton.

Children Now. (1998). *The report card guide: A step-by-step guide to producing a report card on the conditions of children in your community*. Retrieved from http://www.childrennow.org/reportguide.html

Cobb, C., & Rixford, C. (1998). *Lessons learned from the history of social indicators*. Redefining Progress. Retrieved from http://www.rprogress.org/pubs/pubtable.html

Corbett, T. (1997). Foreword. In R. Hauser, B. Brown, & W. Prosser (Eds.), *Indicators of children's well-being* (pp. xix–xxi). New York: Russell Sage Foundation.

Coulton, C. (1995). Using community-level indicators of children's well-being in comprehensive community initiatives. In J. Connell, A. Kubisch, L. Schorr, & C. Weiss (Eds.), *New approaches to evaluating community initiatives: Concepts, methods, and contexts* (pp. 173–200). Washington, DC: Aspen Institute.

Council of State Governments. (1997). *Managing for success: A profile of state government for the 21st century*. Lexington, KY: Council of State Governments.

Durch, J., Bailey, L., & Stoto, M. A. (1997). *Improving health in the community: A role for performance monitoring*. Washington, DC: National Academy Press.

Federal Interagency Forum on Child and Family Statistics. (2001). *America's children: Key national indicators of well-being, 2001*. Washington, DC: Government Printing Office.

Felix, M. R., & Burdine, J. N. (1995). Taking the pulse of the community. *Healthcare Executive, 10*(4), 8–11.

Fielding, J. E., & Sutherland, C. E. (1998). *National directory of community health report cards*. Chicago: Health Research and Educational Trust.

Fielding, J. E., Sutherland, C. E., & Halfon, N. (1999). Community health report cards. Results of a national survey. *American Journal of Preventive Medicine, 17*, 79–86.

Franklin, M. (2000, November-December). Making the grade: "Report card" advocacy. *Children's Advocate*, p. 3.

Friedman, M. (2000). *The results and performance accountability implementation guide*. Retrieved from http://www.raguide.org/complete_paper.htm

Gibbs, D., & Brown, B. (2000). *Community-level indicators for understanding health and human services issues: A compendium of selected indicator systems and resource organizations*. Office of the Assistant Secretary for Planning and Evaluation, U.S. Department of Health and Human Services. Retrieved from http://www.aspe.hhs.gov/progsys/Community/intro.html

Goodman, A. (2001, January). Report cards: Why they work. *Free-Range Thinking*. Retrieved from http://www.agoodmanonline.com/newsletter/2001_01.htm

Halfon, N., Newacheck, P., Hughes, D., & Brindis, C. (1998). Community health monitoring: Taking the pulse of America's children. *Maternal and Child Health Journal, 2*, 95–109.

Halfon, N., Schuster, M., Valentine, W., & McGlynn, E. A. (1998). Improving the quality of healthcare for children: Implementing the results of the AHSR research agenda conference. *Health Services Research, 33*, 955–976.

Healthcare Forum Foundation. (1998). *Outcomes toolkit information*. Retrieved from http://www.act-toolkit.com/toolkit_info.cfm?login=0

Hennekens, C., & Buring, J. (1987). *Epidemiology in medicine*. Boston: Little, Brown.

Hibbard, J., Peters, E., Slovic, P., Finucane, M., & Tusler, M. (2001). Making health care quality reports easier to use. *Journal on Quality Improvement, 27*, 591–604.

Hutchins, V. L. (1994). Maternal and Child Health Bureau: Roots. *Pediatrics, 94*, 695–699.

Illig, D. (1999). Thoughts on implementing Proposition 10: The California Children and Families First Act. *California Research Bureau Note, 6*(1), 1–23.

Innes, J. (1990a). Disappointments and legacies of social indicators. *Journal of Public Policy, 9*, 429–432.

Innes, J. (1990b). *Knowledge and public policy: The search for meaningful indicators* (2nd ed.). New Brunswick, NJ: Transaction.

Kingsley, T. (1999). *Building and operating neighborhood indicator systems: A guidebook*: Washington, DC: Urban Institute.

Kline, E. (1997). *Sustainable community: Topics and indicators*. Tufts University, Global Development and Environment Institute. Retrieved from http://www.ase.tufts.edu/gdae

Kretzman, J. P., & McKnight, J. L. (1993). *Building communities from the inside out: A path toward finding and mobilizing a community's assets*. Chicago: ACTA Publications.

Land, K., & Spilerman, S. (1975). Social indicator models: An overview. In K. Land & S. Spilerman (Eds.), *Social indicator models* (pp. 1–3). New York: Russell Sage Foundation.

McKnight, J. (1999). Two tools for well-being: Health systems and communities. *Journal of Perinatology, 19*(6, Pt. 2), S12–S15.

Moore, K. (1999, September 13). *Indicators of child and family well-being: The good, the bad and the ugly*. Presentation to the Office of Behavioral and Social Sciences Research, National Institutes of Health.

National Center for Health Statistics. (1991). Consensus set of health status indicators for the general assessment of community health status. *Morbidity and Mortality Weekly Report, 40*, 449–451.

National Commission on Technology, Automation and Economic Progress. (1966). *Technology and the American economy* (Vol. 1). Washington, DC: Government Printing Office.

Norris, T., & Atkisson, A. (1997). *The community indicators handbook: Measuring progress toward healthy and sustainable communities*. San Francisco: Redefining Progress.

Pearl, M., Braveman, P., & Abrams, B. (2001). The relationship of neighborhood socioeconomic characteristics to birthweight among 5 ethnic groups in California. *American Journal of Public Health, 91*, 1808–1814.

Redefining Progress. (1998, December 3–5). *Proceedings of the California Community Indicators Conference*. Paper presented at the California Community Indicators Conference, San Francisco.

Reidy, M., & Moorehouse, M. (2002). *Taking an indicator approach to monitoring school readiness: Reflections from the State Child Indicators Project: A working paper*. Unpublished manuscript.

San Diego County Health and Human Services Agency. (2001). *San Diego County child and family health and well-being report card, 2001*. San Diego, CA: Author.

Schorr, L. (1997). *Common purpose: Strengthening families and neighborhoods to rebuild America*. New York: Bantam Doubleday Dell.

Seid, M., Sadler, B. L., Peddecord, K. M., & Kurtin, P. S. (1996). *Accountability: Protecting the well-being of America's children and those who care for them*. Alexandria, VA: National Association of Children's Hospitals and Related Institutions.

Sharpe, P. A., Greaney, M. L., Lee, P. R., & Royce, S. W. (2000). Assets-oriented community assessment. *Public Health Reports, 115*, 205–211.

Simmes, D. R., Blaszcak, M. R., Kurtin, P. S., Bowen, N. L., & Ross, R. K. (2000). Creating a community report card: The San Diego experience. *American Journal of Public Health, 90*, 880–882.

Skocpol, T. (1992). *Protecting soldiers and mothers: The political origins of social policy in the United States*. Cambridge, MA: Belknap Press.

Slater, C. H. (1999). Outcomes research and community health information systems. *Journal of Medical Systems, 23*, 335–346.

U.S. Department of Health and Human Services. (1991). *Healthy people 2000: National health promotion and disease prevention objectives*. Washington, DC: Government Printing Office.

U.S. Geological Survey. (2002). *Geographic information systems: What is a GIS?* Retrieved from http://www.usgs.gov/research/gis/title.html

United Way of America. (1999). *Community status reports and targeted community interventions: Drawing a distinction*. Alexandria, VA: United Way of America.

Wicks, E., & Meyer, J. (1999). Making the report cards work: Two researchers reflect on the report card movement—its purpose, pitfalls, and prospects for improvement. *Health Affairs* (Millwood), *18*, 152–155.

World Health Organization. (1998). *Health promotion glossary*. Geneva: Author.

Zucconi, S. L., & Carson, C. A. (1994). CDC's consensus set of health status indicators: Monitoring and prioritization by state health departments. *American Journal of Public Health, 84*, 1644–1646.

5

Partnering with the Community

Implementation, Evaluation, and Impact

Kimberly Dennis, Diana R. Simmes

In the words of Donald Schön, "There is a high hard ground where practitioners can make effective use of research-based theory and technique, and there is a swampy lowland where situations are confusing 'messes' incapable of technical solution. The difficulty is that the problems of the high ground . . . are often relatively unimportant to clients or to the larger society, while in the swamp are the problems of greatest human concern" (1983, p. 42). That "swampy lowland," in contrast to the ivory towers of academia, includes the local communities in which children and families live their daily lives.

Increasingly, researchers are finding that they need to immerse themselves in the community—both literally and figuratively—to fully understand and address issues of child health and well-being. In other words, it is difficult to understand and study a community without going into it and asking residents about their lives and experiences there. As Ann Vander Stoep and colleagues so aptly put it, "By the same logic that it takes a village to raise a child, it also takes a village to name, study, and meet its challenges" (Vander Stoep, Williams, Jones, Green, & Trupin, 1999, p. 332).

Given that child health is so interconnected with economic, social, political, and other factors embedded in the community, **child health services research (CHSR)** professionals and health care providers alike must move beyond their focus on individual health—what E. Jose Proenca (1998) calls an "enrolled population" approach—to consider the dynamics of the communities in which they live. Further fueling this shift, notes Lisbeth Schorr (1997), is the limited effectiveness of traditional evaluation and research strategies when applied to complex and interactive interventions aimed at improving multiple child health and well-being outcomes.

A system of applied CHSR is thus emerging that is more responsive to intensely local problems. There is a growing cadre of researchers who are generating community-based research and finding solutions to local problems that traditional health services researchers and institutions have not provided. For instance, the Childhood Cancer Research Institute (CCRI) seeks to prevent childhood cancer by investigating the causes of the disease and educating the public on the findings. CCRI has worked closely with Native American communities, living for extended periods of time in their communities and sharing meals with community members. This has resulted, among other things, in CCRI's working with the Centers for Disease Control and Prevention (CDC) on innovations for incorporating community knowledge into the CDC's existing environmental and health research methods (Sclove, Scammell, & Holland, 1998).

To fully appreciate the health issues affecting children, CHSR investigators must have a deep understanding of the child's family and home environment (see Chapter Three, by Sobo). To fully comprehend the family and home environment, researchers need to grasp the dynamics of the community in which the child and family reside. This chapter is intended to help applied CHSR professionals better understand the community and incorporate it into their work. We discuss how researchers, particularly those trained in traditional methods, need to rethink their design strategies and expand their conventional mind-set. We first provide an overview of the changing world in which CHSR personnel are working to serve as context for why research grounded in the community is imperative.

The Changing World in Which Researchers Work

Five important developments have taken place in the past two decades that have affected and will continue to affect the nature of CHSR and evaluation. These developments provide useful insights into the world in which applied CHSR investigators are working and offer context for thinking about their research strategies, especially when working in the community. These developments are (1) a broader understanding of the nature of health and its determinants, (2) the changing nature of the health care system, (3) a shift in responsibility and accountability of programs for children and families to the local level, (4) increased collaboration among individuals and organizations at all levels to improve child health and well-being, and (5) a shift to an outcomes-based framework to improve the quality of health and other related services in public and private settings.

These developments are interconnected. For instance, adopting a more holistic view of health entails the realization of the need for greater collaboration to address the complexity inherent in health-related issues. The shift in responsibilities from the national to the state and local levels is linked to the development of local outcomes-based systems to measure success at the level where program control actually resides.

Broader Understanding of Health

To strengthen the health care system requires an understanding that there is more to health care than just the delivery of medical care. We will succeed in strengthening the health and well-being of children only if we comprehensively examine community safety, health, and economic interventions. CHSR investigators thus need to cast a wide net in considering what influences children's health and well-being. Researchers also need to incorporate a broad range of perspectives to identify both underlying causes and solutions to complex child health problems.

Changing Nature of the Health Care System

In most states, the health care system has undergone a structural shift from fee-for-service financing to managed care. The shift to managed care brought forth several key health policy issues, including monitoring the activity of managed care plans, organizing health care providers, and evaluating the quality of care delivered to patients (Institute for the Future, 2000). The need to address these issues has had an impact on the design and conduct of CHSR. For example, research endeavors are increasingly soliciting the input and involvement of families to design managed care programs that respond to their needs, as well as seeking to help consumers better access and navigate the managed care system. The Community Tracking Study, a major research project of the Center for Studying Health System Change, seeks to learn how the health system is changing in sixty communities across the United States and how these changes affect people (Center for Studying Health System Change, 1999).

Shift in Responsibility to the Local Level

Federal policies in the 1980s and 1990s shifted responsibility for solving public problems, such as moving families from welfare to work, from national to state and local levels. Such **devolution** entails more than just a simple transfer of authority. It encompasses a dramatic redistribution and renegotiation of responsibilities among various community organizations involved with children and their families, emphasizes the need to develop a community rather than state agency agenda, and calls for increased capacity for local governance (Center for the Study of Social Policy, 1995). In short, it calls for community-based solutions to address significant social challenges.

In the wake of this shift, local governance partnerships have emerged. Such partnerships involve a new decision-making process by which local communities take responsibility for designing and implementing community-supported plans of action to achieve desired results for children and families (Center for the Study of Social Policy, 1995; Farrow & Gardner, 1999). The result is a change in the way services are organized, delivered, and financed. Many different community organizations and agencies, rather than a single entity, now play a role in acting on problems. Consequently, CHSR professionals will need to work more closely and cooperatively with the communities in which they are working and the various local organizations responsible for designing and implementing programs to strengthen child health and well-being.

The Urban Institute's Assessing the New Federalism (ANF) project, which examines social policy changes in income security, employment, health, and social services areas, is a good example of how devolution has led to new research strategies. The Urban Institute's Stephen Bell (1999) explains, for example, that rather than relying on a single national research study to guide policy for the country as a whole, devolution has resulted in a need for research findings at the site or state level, where program authority and accountability now lie. He identified three key research challenges emerging from devolution: (1) many social policies changing at once, (2) a lack of basic information on program activities and costs, and (3) the shift from federal to state and foundation oversight of evaluation research. Bell also highlights several early lessons learned: broad-based analyses are hard, limits on research breadth and depth are essential, data needs cannot be compromised (even if that means narrowing the analysis agenda), and clear and timely presentation of results is more important than ever. He maintains, "The large number of policy questions the [ANF] program seeks to address—and the vast, diverse 'canvas' on which the answers are unfolding—necessitates the use of new, and potentially controversial, combinations of research and analysis tools" (p. 1).

Increased Collaboration

More than half a century ago, the World Health Organization (1948) defined health as "a complete state of physical, mental, and social well-being, and not merely absence of disease." This holistic definition of health has been widely adopted in the United States to emphasize the complex underpinnings of most health problems. Its comprehensive nature makes **collaboration** essential among various public and private entities seeking to improve child health.

As Jane Durch and colleagues note, "In communities, health is a product of many factors, and many segments of the community can contribute to and share responsibility for its protection and improvement" (Durch, Bailey, & Stoto, 1997, p. 1). Because so many different individuals and organizations affect a child's health status, collaboration is an indispensable way to achieve the improvements in health that individuals and communities care about.

Indeed, collaboration is at the heart of the Healthy Communities movement, which the World Health Organization set in motion in the 1980s. In 1989, the U.S. Department of Health and Human Services (HHS) tapped the National Civic League to launch the initiative in the United States. Now in its second decade, more than one thousand communities in the nation embrace the Healthy Communities collaborative philosophy. All strive for the same goal: "to achieve radical, measurable improvement in health status and long-term quality of life" (Norris & Pittman, 2000, p. 118). They seek to do so through local and regional collaborative efforts, recognizing that no one organization, sector, or program can effectively address the complexity of today's health and quality of life issues.

The American Hospital Association, too, has recognized the importance of collaboration and promotes the concept of Community Care Networks (CCNs), in which hospitals, physicians, other health providers, and social services agencies work closely together to improve care delivery and coordination. A community health focus, community accountability, seamless continuum of care, and management with limited resources are the four central features of CCNs (Proenca, Rosko, & Zinn, 2000; see also www.communitycare.org).

Collaboration as a standard way of doing business affects applied CHSR in at least two fundamental ways: not only will researchers need to expand their perspective to include and study the impact of collaboration on child health and well-being, but they will also increasingly need to become a more active partner in these larger collaborative efforts to ensure that their work is meaningful and relevant to the groups directly affected by a given problem. Community members are more likely to support and embrace a research effort if they know and trust the researchers. By being active and engaged collaborative members, researchers can develop trusting relationships and gain credibility. Schorr (1997) adds that as collaborative partners, researchers can focus more on issues of why and how and help people learn from their experiences to improve their programs and services.

Shift to an Outcomes-Based Framework

The outcomes movement originated in demands for accountability, shortcomings of quality assurance, a change in focus from structure and process to outcomes, and changes in health services research techniques. The movement coincided with growing acceptance of the importance of evidence-based medicine (see Chapter One, by Kurtin). As Sarah Hayward and colleagues surmise, "The impact of health care can no longer be measured by elements of structure or process; health outcomes are becoming the currency of health care exchange" (1996, p. 413).

The shift to outcomes-based accountability is gathering speed. Around the United States, health care service providers, governmental agencies, nonprofit organizations, community-based organizations, and others are moving away from a focus on tallying the number of children who walk in their doors ("inputs") and toward a vested interest in outcomes or results (the effect programs have on children's lives). U.S. society's expectations of health services are also changing. According to Schorr, "Most legislators want to know what works when they vote on laws and appropriations; parents want to know how well their children are being educated; foundations want to know about the impact of their support; and the staff of social programs want to know how effective they are.

Taxpayers, having given up on compassion, demand to know whether public funds are accomplishing what their proponents promise" (1997, p. 115).

The Healthy People initiative, a national health improvement strategy designed to help communities identify and set health priorities and measure their progress, is one product of the outcomes shift. The Healthy People objectives are used in a variety of ways, on several different levels. For example, Congress uses the objectives to measure the progress of various block grant programs, such as the Maternal and Child Health Block Grant. The National Committee on Quality Assurance (NCQA) incorporated Healthy People targets into HEDIS (Health Plan Employer Data and Information Set) 3.0 to help assess the performance of managed care plans in certain areas (such as immunizations). To date, nearly all fifty states have developed their own Healthy People plans, using the national objectives as a foundation on which to build and tailor their own specific agendas. In addition, local individuals, groups, and organizations integrate the objectives into community-based programs and other child and adult health-related activities (U.S. Department of Health and Human Services, 2000). *Healthy People 2010* is the third version of the Healthy People initiative, which was first launched in 1979. It seeks to improve on earlier versions by identifying a small number of key health and social issues—*leading health indicators*—that are designed to engage the general public as well as traditional public and private health organizations to take action on these priority health issues (Institute of Medicine, 1999).

As outcomes-based accountability becomes the standard way of doing business and the everyday lens through which people view programs and policies, Schorr (1997) argues that the researcher's role will change considerably. This change will be most apparent when researchers are examining interventions that not only cut across multiple disciplines and systems (such as health, education, child welfare, and community development) but also seek to have an impact on children, families, institutions, and entire communities. For instance, the community, rather than the researcher, will drive the process in selecting which outcomes will be used to judge a program's success. The result, according to Schorr, is the use of more meaningful and relevant outcomes, as opposed to measures derived from scales "constructed by researchers primarily for research purposes" (p. 138). She goes on to outline four characteristics of new research and evaluation approaches. They (1) are built on a strong theoretical and conceptual base, (2) emphasize shared interests of evaluators and program people, (3) employ multiple methods and perspectives, and (4) offer both rigor and relevance. (See Chapter Four, by Simmes, Lim, and Dennis, for a more detailed discussion of the outcomes movement.)

In this chapter, we focus primarily on what the effects of devolution and collaboration (developments 3 and 4) mean for CHSR investigators' approach to their work. The next section offers a more detailed look at the collaboration movement, as we believe this new way of doing business has far-reaching influences on the nature of CHSR.

The Collaboration Movement

In conducting applied CHSR, researchers are sure to encounter one or more collaborative community partnerships within a given community that bring together various people and organizations to address issues of child health and well-being. These partnerships, collectively and individually, play a role in creating community and systems change and improving child health. By better understanding the role of collaboratives, researchers have an opportunity to strengthen the science and practice of community health promotion (Roussos & Fawcett, 2000). For CHSR professionals to capitalize on this opportunity, they must understand what collaboration is, what drives it, and the special challenges it presents for researchers, especially those trained in traditional or academic research methods.

What Is Collaboration?

The term *collaboration* is often used loosely when people, organizations, and communities describe their efforts to strengthen the health and well-being of children, families, and communities. A key defining characteristic of collaboration is that it is action-oriented: "decisions are made, resources are shared, and activity brings about success and benefit" (Berkowitz, 2000, p. 67). Collaboration is more than simply coordinating or partnering on efforts, often in response to an immediate child health crisis. Rather, it is about creating an interdependent system where members have clearly defined roles and responsibilities, follow by-laws and procedures, complement and support one another's efforts, and share a sense of community. Collaboration is not an end goal in itself but a means to achieve the larger goal of providing more comprehensive and appropriate child health services (Hodges, Nesman, & Hernandez, 1999).

Collaboration is also a developmental process. Sid Gardner (2000) outlines four progressive stages of collaboration: (1) information exchange, (2) joint projects, (3) changing the rules, and (4) systems change. As a first step, groups must exchange information about what their agencies now do; for example, they must share data on which children and families they serve, the kinds of problems and challenges they face, and the types of programs and services they provide. As groups move forward in their collaborative efforts, the next major step is to undertake some form of joint project, often driven by an external funding opportunity for which collaboration is needed. At this juncture, groups understand and are convinced that they need to work together to address a shared problem; they have realized that they cannot achieve a goal solely on their own, within their own organizations. Unfortunately, this is typically where most collaboratives or coalitions get stuck. What allows a collaborative to move forward is the recognition that the current rules (for example, budgeting or the use of state and federal categorical funds) governing the collaborative's member agencies and organizations prevent the collaborative from achieving its particular goal or outcome. In stage 3, they actually do something about this. For example, various staff from health and human services agencies (such as health care providers, social workers, counselors, police, or probation officers) may be outstationed or co-located at a school site to provide more integrated and accessible services to children and youth. Or collaborating agencies may institute cross-disciplinary staff training to serve families who are involved in multiple systems, such as mothers on welfare who may also be dealing with child welfare, substance abuse, mental health, and domestic violence issues.

The fourth and ultimate stage of collaboration comes when the collaborative seeks to change the larger system in which it operates. The collaborative is able to weave together the elements of rule changes, new personnel, and new forms of accountability in a strategic package that represents real systems change. For example, the Healthy Start Support Services for Children and Families Act, passed in 1991 by the California State Legislature, funds local sites to develop collaborative partnerships between schools and local health and service agencies to deliver education and support services to children and their families more efficiently and more effectively. Evaluation of sixty-five Healthy Start sites showed such positive outcomes as better grades for students; improved attendance; schoolwide increases in standardized test scores in reading and math; increased parental involvement in school; decreases in reported need for child care, food, clothing, and emergency funds; better family access to health and dental care; and decreased emergency room use for illness or injury (California Department of Education, 2001).

Sharon Hodges and colleagues (1999) offer another perspective. They identify five stages of collaboration. The first involves individual action on behalf of children (by a single agency) but recognizes the need to move away from this internal agency focus. The second stage, one on one, occurs when an individual from one agency contacts an individual from another agency, typically to resolve a specific issue. They recognize, however, the potential for further collaboration to improve service delivery focus. The third stage is new service delivery, in which agency-centered thinking concerning service delivery shifts to a more collaborative approach and a formal collaboration structure is established. The fourth stage, professional collaboration, involves well-established collaboration at the agency, program, and service provider levels; it is characterized by group decision making, established guidelines and procedures, funding for collaborative service delivery, and a common vision or mission. At this stage, the collaborative recognizes the need to view children holistically and integrate families into the process. Indeed, in the final stage, true collaboration, families are full partners in the system of care. Additional results are broader community involvement in the collaborative, interdependence and shared responsibility among stakeholders, role clarity for families and service providers, and vision-driven solutions.

How Collaboration Has Evolved

A major impetus for increased collaboration around child health is the fact that in many communities, the current education, health, and social service systems are not achieving optimal results for children and families (Center for the Study of Social Policy, 1995). Lack of an integrated service delivery approach continues to be a major problem facing children in need; services tend to remain predominantly categorical and fragmented. Lawrence Green and colleagues explain that because an agency or organization typically serves a particular group, it has limited impact across the larger childhood population (Green, Daniel, & Novick, 2001). In addition, in an environment of constrained resources, policymakers are calling for interagency collaboration to decrease spending and improve outcomes. Managed care's focus on reducing duplication in services and increasing efficiency and accountability has further fu-

eled collaborative efforts. Finally, given that most children have little consistent contact with the health care system after the age of
three, partnerships between health, education, early intervention,
child development, and other systems serving children are essential
to improving overall child health and well-being.

Governmental changes in the administration, management, delivery, and funding of health and social services for children and
families have spurred various collaborative efforts. For example, in
1993, California passed Assembly Bill 1741 to establish the California Youth Pilot Project, a five-year program authorizing a few select pilot counties to blend various categorical funds and implement
new approaches to provide integrated, comprehensive services to
low-income, high-risk, multiple-need children and youth and their
families. The A.B. 1741 Collaboratives, as they are known, focus
on health and well-being, safety and security, and community and
organizational capacity building. The Collaboratives were recognized, in later legislation to extend the program (S.B. 1352), as a
promising method of increasing state support for local integration
of services to these children and their families. At the federal level,
a similar initiative, Boost4Kids (*Boost* stands for "Better Opportunities and Outcomes Starting Today"), was launched in 1999. At
selected Boost4Kids sites, local communities partner with state and
federal agencies in efforts to pool administrative savings from discretionary grant programs, streamline administration, and provide
greater flexibility to communities in administering grant funds. In
the area of children's mental health, the Center for Mental Health
Services and the Substance Abuse and Mental Health Services Administration (both within HHS) have administered a grant program
since 1993 to assist communities in building fully inclusive organized systems of care for children who experience serious emotional
problems and their families. The Comprehensive Community Mental Health Services for Children and Their Families program supports more than forty comprehensive systems of care, maintaining

that service delivery is "not the responsibility of a single agency, but should involve a collaborative network of child-serving agencies that includes mental health, child welfare, education, juvenile justice, and other appropriate services" (Hodges et al., 1999, p. 17).

Grantmaking institutions are also promoting collaboration through their funding requirements. Foundations of all shapes, sizes, and influence are embracing collaboration as a way to enhance their investments as well as to improve the outcomes of children, families, and communities. The Foundation Consortium, for example, is a collaboration of fifteen foundations whose mission is to improve the well-being of California's children, families, and communities. They use a "community approach"—schools, communities, and government work together to improve outcomes for children and their families—to promote collaboration and cooperation across organizations for more effective governance, service delivery, and community building. Rather than directly making grants, the consortium partners with others in the public and private sectors to lay the groundwork for change. The consortium's approach embraces key principles of family involvement, community partnership, and shared accountability (see www.foundationconsortium.org).

Despite advances, many funders struggle with operationalizing collaboration, as do the community-based individuals and organizations they support. Like these organizations, they have often used the word *collaboration* without fully appreciating its meaning. Moreover, they have had difficulty moving beyond the fragmented, categorical, piecemeal nature of funding that has dominated past funding practices (Gardner, 2000). Research has suggested that certain efforts, such as parent education and community health promotion, are not effective unless linked to a larger community collaborative effort, yet funding continues for these isolated programs (Gardner, 1996). Further, a particular program may offer a wide range of child health-related services in one central location (such as primary health care, developmental assessments, oral health screening and treatment, and mental health services) yet may be forced to rely on dozens of separate funding streams, each of which is earmarked for a very specific type and limited scope of service.

Benefits and Challenges of Collaboration

As Roz Lasker and colleagues note, "The connective power of collaboration has the potential to create a real health system in this country—one that focuses on health and well-being as well as the financing of medical care; one that actively involves people most affected by health problems in decisions and actions related to their health; and one that enables communities to take innovative and comprehensive actions to address the full range of environmental, economic, social, behavioral, and biological factors that influence health" (Lasker, Weiss, & Miller, 2000, p. 18). Although collaboration is not an easy fix, it does have significant benefits. First and foremost, it enhances an organization's or community's ability to address issues; to improve child, family, and community outcomes; and to influence public policy. Collaboration leads to information sharing among agencies and a greater understanding of how children's needs might be served by a variety of programs. Further, collaborative partners can acquire new skills and knowledge, may be better able to meet performance goals, and may increase their ability to secure additional funds to support the activities of the collaborative as well as individual partners. In addition, partners may enjoy the development of new and valuable relationships and heightened public recognition as a result of demonstrated improved outcomes, increased client satisfaction, increased savings due to the decrease in unnecessary duplication of services, and greater visibility for the issues at hand (Hodges et al., 1999; Lasker et al., 2000).

Despite the known benefits of collaboration, it is difficult to implement. Collaboration requires an optimal mix of partners, yet the very diversity of people and organizations that must come together to effectively address a problem often increases the difficulty of collaborating. For example, efforts to provide optimal care for children with asthma require that various health care providers, schools, child care providers, community-based organizations providing asthma education and awareness, and children and their families all work together. All may come from different disciplines or hold diverse perspectives that influence how they define and tackle the issue and which outcomes are important to achieve.

Even with the right mix of people, developing interagency collaboration is a time-consuming and process-intensive effort, often requiring multiyear planning and support. Partners, including researchers, must be willing to dedicate adequate time and resources and must balance these needs with their organization's primary activities. Reaching consensus on the collaborative's mission, goals, and priority issues can be a challenge, especially if partner agencies describe the target population in different ways and narrowly define their agency's role by discipline (such as health, education, or social work) rather than by services provided.

Other challenges to ensuring a successful partnership may include less independence in decision making, fragmented funding streams that do not support collaborative efforts, competing mandates for each member agency, lack of influence (real or perceived) in collaborative activities, and minimal credit for contributions, as well as organizational fragmentation, bureaucracy, and rapid turnover in leadership. Add to that barriers concerning data use and confidentiality, and it is no wonder that the word *collaboration* instills frustration for many practitioners, as well as researchers. These challenges notwithstanding, "the intrinsic value of coalition building is a deeply held conviction among practitioners, community organizers, researchers, and funding organizations" (Kreuter, Lezin, & Young, 2000, p. 50).

Does Collaboration Really Work?

Even though the popularity of and investment in collaboratives have grown, the amount of empirical evidence that exists on their effectiveness in improving community-level outcomes and changing health status remains limited (Berkowitz, 2000; Kreuter et al., 2000; Roussos & Fawcett, 2000). Sharon Hodges and colleagues conclude, "The literature indicates that collaborative endeavors can bring about improved and more appropriate services for children and their families, but continued research is needed to describe this process and its outcomes" (1999, p. 33). For instance, multidisciplinary teams are a frequent tool used by interagency collaboratives, yet their benefits "have not yet been documented by any collaborative in a way that has built a solid case for [their] replication and expansion" (Gardner, 2000, p. 12).

Stergios Roussos and Stephen Fawcett's review of more than thirty evaluation studies suggests that "collaborative partnerships can contribute to widespread change in a variety of health behaviors, but the magnitude of these effects may not be as great as intended" (2000, p. 376). They, too, call for further research, using an interdisciplinary approach, to better understand how collaborative efforts affect "the diverse, interconnected, and distant outcomes they seek" (p. 382). Further, Anne Kubisch and colleagues warn that if researchers focus on the discrete program pieces of a comprehensive collaborative, they are likely to miss the effects of this interaction. However, they acknowledge, "tracking and measuring 'synergy' is a problem that methodologists have yet to solve" (Kubisch, Weiss, Schorr, & Connell, 1995, p. 4).

Since the rise of community coalitions and collaboratives in the late 1980s and early 1990s, researchers and practitioners have been struggling to find evaluation strategies and methods that correspond well to the goals and designs of the initiatives (Connell & Kubisch 1998). Out of the literature emerge a number of challenges researchers are likely to encounter in trying to document the effectiveness of collaboration in strengthening the health and well-being of children. These include the dynamic nature of collaboratives, the magnitude of change they seek, the amount of time it takes to see results, the difficulty in measuring change, and other broader forces that may affect their success. The next section discusses the implications of these challenges and the general changing world in which researchers work.

What the New Landscape Means for CHSR Investigators

To improve child health services delivery, community-based health and social service agencies have had to evolve in response to funding changes, expanded or limited mandates, restructuring, new forms of local governance, and changes in priorities. CHSR investigators, too, must change their focus to develop more effective strategies for improving child health and well-being and learn how to incorporate the effects of increased collaboration and devolution into their research strategies. They must also become more involved in the very efforts they seek to understand. To advance our knowledge, traditional research methods will have to make room for alternative, innovative methods. We shall discuss seven key implications for what the new landscape means for the world of CHSR.

Research Should Be Applied and Lead to Sustainability

Applied research is better suited to meet a community's needs than traditional, academic, discipline-oriented research, as the latter is often driven by academic debates in the field rather than the concerns of the community. In applied research, the relationship between researchers and the community is different—program delivery shifts from an experimental context controlled by researchers to a naturalistic or real-world situation influenced by community organizations (Altman, 1995). Results from applied research can better enhance service delivery, inform the development of sound public policy, and help build a community's infrastructure. In other words, applied research can help create community capacity and facilitate sustainability.

Yet the ability to design and implement interventions that are useful to community systems after the formal phase of research ends is an inherent challenge to applied research endeavors. David Altman explains: "Most researchers view sustainability as a late phase in the research process, attended to once efficacy data are available. An alternative approach is to consider issues around sustainability as an essential component to all phases of the research project" (1995, p. 533). He goes on to identify five dynamic, interactive phases in the community research cycle that ultimately lead to sustainability:

1. The *research* phase, which is where projects, as well as relationships, often begin and end

2. The *transfer* phase, in which a project is transferred from researchers to community

3. The *transition* phase, in which community organizations adapt, replicate, and sometimes expand interventions

4. The *regeneration* phase, in which researchers and community members communicate to each other about insights, experiences, and results and possibly identify further research questions

5. The *empowerment* phase, in which a community assumes ownership, power, and control and is able to acquire needed resources to maintain the effort

Research Should Reflect the Shared Goals of Researchers and the Community

To ensure success and benefit for all involved, an explicit match between the mission and goals of the community and those of the researchers is needed. Identification of shared goals and objectives needs to happen up front. Yet researchers and practitioners do not necessarily have similar views regarding the research process. Professional and organizational constraints (such as political struggles, funders' constraints, and tensions of conflicting community organizations) often take precedence over research design considerations (Nyden & Wiewel, 1992; Perkins & Wandersman, 1990). In addition, in the face of very real budget constraints, "it will take real vision and creativity to nurture new initiatives" (Ansley & Gaventa, 1997, p. 53).

The Dilemma of Conflicting Priorities

The researcher's agenda is often influenced by funders' priorities; a dilemma occurs when researchers are funded to investigate an issue that the community does not see as a priority. For example, investing resources in reducing childhood lead burden may not be a top priority when affordable housing, food, clothing, community violence, and employment are more pressing community concerns (Jordan, Lee, & Shapiro, 2000).

It is often not just the priority area itself that is contested. The underlying philosophy driving the respective efforts of researchers and communities may be fundamentally different: theory development and data collection versus delivery of services. Community-based service providers often get caught up in the day-to-day realities of running an organization and face pressure to devote scarce resources to direct services, not research (Nyden & Wiewel, 1992). At times, the quest for data interferes with service delivery, and vice versa. For community organizations, the "time invested in a research partnership is time away from activities which may be more immediately and visibly associated with their goals and their survival" (Schulz, Israel, Selig, Bayer, & Griffin, 2000, p. 62).

Further, there may be differences in perspective, priorities, assumptions, values, beliefs, and language within the same organization as well as across participating organizations. Resolving such conflicting priorities is essential to achieve sustainability. But researchers must realize that the process of getting to common ground is inherently a political, as well as a scientific, one. Various collaborative partners may hold different views about what it will take to

produce the desired outcomes, and it is not uncommon for collaborative efforts to be launched without these various perspectives'
being articulated, much less reconciled (Connell & Kubisch, 1998).

The Challenge of Politics

Several obstacles may emerge during the researcher's and community's journey to get to common ground, one of which is resistance to change. Researchers must be aware that in some cases,
maintaining the status quo is the preferred course of community action, as it is less turbulent and more cost-effective than developing
new service delivery approaches (Altman, 1995). A related challenge is navigating the political and social dynamics within a community. Community members and providers from institutional
settings (such as, schools, clinics, and hospitals) may be more concerned about the potential political consequences of their work
than the community's best interests and thus place a higher value
on conforming to bureaucratic norms (Rotheram-Borus, Rebchook,
Kelly, Adams, & Neumann, 2000). In addition, research findings
can be politically sensitive, and researchers have to take into account competition among groups (especially in a managed care market) and different values among partners.

The Problem of Time

Another challenge to balancing the community's and researcher's needs is time. Traditional researchers tend to emphasize
the careful long-term study of issues. They seldom arrive at quick
conclusions, opting instead to continually test, refine, and revise,
reserving judgment until sufficient data are available. In contrast,
communities require quick decisions based on limited information.
They often fail to see the need for scientifically valid and reliable
data and instead opt to rely on common sense, anecdotal data, or
strategies that have worked in the past. "A central issue here is understanding and being sensitive to different time orientations and
working within them to achieve a mutually acceptable solution"

(Altman, 1995, p. 529). Time, though less of an obstacle in conducting applied research, can still pose problems. For example, short funding cycles may not provide sufficient time to develop and maintain the community trust needed for a project to succeed.

Designing and conducting CHSR is thus not a one-size-fits-all endeavor. "At each stage in the evaluation process, marked differences in perspective among team members emerge, demanding lengthy discussions and major compromises" (Vander Stoep et al., 1999, p. 336).

Research Should Encompass a More Comprehensive and More Integrated Approach

Health services researchers and practitioners alike are calling for increased attention to the complex issues that affect the health of children, particularly those living in marginalized communities. Widening the lens through which we view child health and its determinants is a useful starting point for researchers. However, we must also widen the lens through which we have typically viewed research to encompass how issues related to service delivery, budgets, and governance affect child health outcomes.

Embracing a more comprehensive approach also means that researchers must understand the cultural context of the communities in which they work and carry out their efforts in a culturally appropriate manner (see Chapter Three, by Sobo). For example, Michael Quinn Patton points out that for certain groups, such as Native Americans, who have strong oral traditions and whose cultures are very story-oriented, using flowchartlike diagrams to show relationships between strategies and outcomes can be insensitive and ineffective. A more appropriate approach, Patton says, might be the use of storyboards, where stories are arranged in a sequence of images (Coffman, 2002). The Substance Abuse and Mental Health Services Administration also stresses that family involvement and cultural diversity issues must be addressed and supported in the use of information. They recognize that ethnicity and culture are critical factors in developing and understanding any evaluation program and its findings. Ahoua Koné and colleagues found that hiring people of color was "an important step in increasing cultural competence of research teams and also as a means to provide training and opportunities for skill-building for members of communities of color" (2000, p. 247).

Research Must Move out of the Laboratory

Researchers need to "venture beyond the hallowed walls of research institutions to the frontlines of communities" (Altman, 1995, p. 534). But what do we mean by "community"? John McKnight speaks of the dilemma researchers face in the use of the term **community**. "At the very least, community usually means 'not in a hospital, clinic or doctor's office.' Community is the great 'out-thereness' beyond the doors of professional offices and other facilities. It is the social space beyond the edges of our professionally run systems" (2000, p. 13). Community typically encompasses a group of people who share a common interest such as living in the same geographical area, sharing a similar ethnic or cultural background, speaking the same language, experiencing the same history, or sharing the same profession (Koné et al., 2000; McKnight, 2000).

Getting out of the laboratory requires researchers to adapt to a constantly changing environment. They must take a different approach, master a different set of skills, and establish different types of relationships. For example, researchers will need to negotiate with various individuals and organizations about the research focus, design, and timelines (Nyden & Wiewel, 1992).

McKnight expands on this challenge: "The dilemma we face is that while we have great professional skills in managing and working within our systems, our skills are much less developed once we leave the system's space and cross the frontier into 'the community.' Indeed, one is impressed by the immediate confusion and frustration experienced by many professionals when they attempt to work in community space, for it often seems very complex, disordered, unstructured, and uncontrollable" (2000, p. 13).

In short, to navigate the world of applied research in the community, CHSR professionals will need to master the skills of community health development, partnership and team building, communication and listening, negotiation, conflict resolution, and working across traditional system boundaries (for example, between health care and education) as well as across differences of socioeconomic status, education, and ethnoracial and cultural backgrounds (Meyer, 2000; Schulz et al., 2000; Torres, 1998). They will also have to recognize that "solutions cannot be delivered exclusively by elites in institutions but must be approached and maintained as a collaborative enterprise with feedback loops to, between, and within [community-based organizations] and other stakeholders" (Levesque & Chopyak, 2001, p. 6).

Research Must Acknowledge a Web of Causation

Once researchers move out of the laboratory, they must also rethink their research approach. Community interventions often do not fit well with the narrow model of causation—linking single causes with single effects—that drives **randomized controlled trials (RCTs)**. Quite simply, "social policy changes do not have the protection that occurs in a controlled medical research environment" (Heymann, 2000, p. 372). Controlled experiments are also inclined to stress individual rather than social or environmental risk factors and to separate researchers and practitioners from the public at large as the "health experts." The emphasis on individual-level risk factors tends to obscure the impact of social and economic conditions—most visible in a growing health disparities gap (Israel, Schulz, Parker, & Becker, 1998). Judith Stephenson and John Imrie agree, noting that RCTs "may have little to contribute in terms of explaining how and why [complex social and economic] factors affect health and behavior" (1998, p. 612).

The Reality of Multiple, Evolving Settings

Relevant research models should refer to a web of causation and emphasize the context of care (Hayward et al., 1996). "Traditionally, research-based interventions are developed and tested in a limited number of research settings and with a limited number of populations . . . under a limited number of program and intervention parameters" (Rotheram-Borus et al., 2000, p. 59). In reality, community efforts may involve multisite initiatives in which all sites have the same charge but their individual approaches and program components will vary. Contrary to the traditional researcher's view that this reflects poor planning, such chameleonlike changes are a valid response to the complex reality of the service delivery world and the myriad needs of children and families. Such real-world dynamics, however, can make it difficult to establish stable baselines or comparative groups (Kubisch et al., 1995).

Other Forces at Work

CHSR personnel must also understand that community efforts do not take place in a vacuum. Circumstances and events—many of which a community collaborative has no control over—will have a direct bearing on the initiative's success. Roussos and Fawcett (2000) identify several factors that may influence a collaborative's ability to achieve desired health outcomes. They include the following:

1. Social and economic factors, such as age and gender, ethnicity, educational attainment and social status, concentrations of poverty, and income inequality

2. **Social capital** (a community's norms, networks, and store of social trust), which may be a factor in both facilitating the relationships needed for collaboration and affecting the desired outcomes

3. Partnership context, including the conditions that give rise to the partnership, the community's history of collaboration, and its political climate

4. Community control in agenda setting, reflected in who identifies the collaborative's primary goals and the desired indicators used to measure success in achieving those goals

In addition, Roussos and Fawcett note, "for any given community health concern, such as preventing injury or promoting early childhood development, a new collaborative partnership may be one of many initiatives within and outside the community working on that concern" (2000, p. 390). In essence, it is difficult to pinpoint a direct causal relationship between the collaborative's efforts and population-level health outcomes. In discussing the Urban Institute's research on devolution, Bell comments that "even isolating the combined effect of a state's entire policy package can be quite difficult given the many nonpolicy factors that influence participants' outcomes over time and across states" (1999, p. 11).

Research Should Be Methodologically Innovative

Nyden and Wiewel (1992) point out that leaders of community-based organizations want immediate positive results and are uneasy about researchers who have one foot in the ivy-covered academic world and talk of models of scientific inquiry. At the same time, however, these community leaders seek out the legitimacy (perceived or real) that the incorporation of scientific research brings. Thus, as Schorr argues, "it will not be easy to break with the dogma of experimental designs using random assignment as the only source of reliable knowledge" (1997, p. 146). However, Thomas Rundall and colleagues make it clear that "virtually all of the phenomena of interest to health services research . . . are embedded in a dynamic context that demands new approaches to inquiry" (Rundall, Devers, & Sofaer, 1999, p. 1091).

Randomized or true experimental designs are generally touted as the most rigorous of all designs and the strongest in isolating program effects and establishing a cause-and-effect relationship between a program and its outcomes. However, this type of design can be intrusive and difficult to carry out in applied child health services settings; community initiatives typically seek to benefit all children, making it impossible to randomly assign certain children to a treatment or control group (Hollister & Hill, 1995). Charles Bruner elaborates that randomized trials "are not an appropriate research technique if one of the key attributes of the service strategy is its inclusiveness and community-embeddedness. Randomized trials violate the premise that services be open and voluntary" (1994, p. 3). Further, traditional sampling methods such as random-digit dialing may not be feasible for hard-to-reach populations (Muhib et al., 2001).

As already noted, it is difficult to establish direct cause and effect in applied research. In conducting a participatory community-based survey for a community health intervention in Detroit, Amy Schulz and colleagues determined, "Without the power to control, or resources to monitor in enough detail, changes that might occur in a 'control' community, real questions arose about the extent to which such a study design would contribute to an understanding of the process or effects of the intervention. Instead resources were focused on documenting change within the intervention community" (1998, p. 21).

New Tools and Instruments May Be Needed

With a greater understanding of the dynamic nature of child health and increasingly complex interventions that involve numerous service providers, a host of delivery strategies, and variations in timing, intensity, and duration of services, the capability of traditional CHSR approaches and tools is severely tested. Applied researchers must be more flexible and willing to rework existing validated instruments to better reflect the needs and backgrounds of the children and families involved. Attribution of specific outcomes to specific interventions will be more difficult as increasing emphasis is put on communitywide strategies, client empowerment, and community development. Indeed, there are many situations in health care in which good quantitative data will never be available (Hayward et al., 1996).

Qualitative Data Can Help Fill In the Gaps

Catherine Pope and John Mays (1995) note that health care involves people, and people tend to be more complex than the subjects of the natural sciences. In researching childhood diseases like asthma or diabetes, CHSR professionals are likely to need answers to additional questions about patient behavior and the communities in which these children live. Quantitative methods may not be able to provide these much-needed answers. Indeed, "many health professionals begin to discover that their powerful tools and techniques seem weaker, less effective, and even inappropriate in the community" (McKnight, 2000, p. 13). However, a sea change is under way.

The research community is placing greater emphasis on the importance of and need to collect qualitative data to complement hard numbers and deepen our understanding of issues. Pope and Mays (1995) explain that qualitative studies help us answer questions such as "What is X, and how does X vary in different circumstances and why?" rather than simply "How many Xs are there?" (p. 43). The National Institutes of Health concludes: "When the goal is to understand the lived experience from the social actor's perspective within a specific context, qualitative methods are appropriate" (2001, p. 11).

Qualitative data may be collected through surveys, ethnographic interviews, cognitive interviews, case studies, focus groups, interpretive techniques such as phenomenological or narrative analyses, content analysis of relevant documents, and observational research. **Ethnography**, for instance, which is the long-term descriptive study of an individual culture or community, enables us to investigate such things as social networks, the process of community change, and institutional structure, all of which influence how a community functions (Horsch, 1997) and which in turn influence child health and well-being. This and related qualitative methods tend to emphasize interaction between the researcher and participant and require the researcher's acknowledgment that the participant is the best informant about his or her own experience. These methods rest on the assumption that experience is based on perceptions that differ from one individual to another and change over time and that knowledge accrues additional meaning in a given situation or life context.

Using qualitative methods to complement quantitative methods is valuable on many different fronts. For example, qualitative data can illuminate statistical results and address secondary questions that arise; help explain how various stakeholders view an issue and why; provide contextual information to explain differences in statistical findings across study groups; be used in the development of theories or conceptual frameworks; describe many kinds of complex settings and interactions; clarify differences in values, language, and meanings; give voice to individuals and groups who are rarely heard; and provide insights to inform the design of quantitative methods (Hoff & Witt, 2000; National Institutes of Health, 2001; Sofaer, 1999).

In short, as Shoshanna Sofaer argues, "researchers and funders cannot afford to ignore the potential contributions of qualitative methods in identifying important questions, in building capacity to conduct and replicate research, and in constructing useful theories" (1999, p. 1116).[1]

Balancing Scientific Rigor with Community Need

Barbara Israel and colleagues (1998) note that at the same time that community-based methods can increase the quality and relevance of the data, such strategies are continually plagued by questions of scientific validity, reliability, and objectivity. Researchers have expressed concern that community members do not have sufficient understanding of scientific methods to design valid research tools, to interview without bias, and to interpret the results of quantitative analyses. These issues are especially important to address in the field of child health research, where parents are surrogates of their children and researchers often rely on parent reports of a child's health and well-being.

Still others may question a researcher's objectivity if he or she is working closely with the community. They may wonder how a researcher can support the family's or community's change agenda without letting that agenda bias the research effort. Establishing appropriate feedback mechanisms and communication structures between the researcher and key stakeholders is one way that researchers can help clarify their role and relationship with the initiative being studied (Horsch, 1997).

Tension also exists between meeting the demands of scientific rigor and the needs and desires of multiple community stakeholders. For instance, in integrating data from multiple sources, potential conflicts may arise in deciding how to best integrate and prioritize the results. More specific problems include inadequate measures, limited availability and quality of data, lack of integrated data systems, and confidentiality. Further, concepts such as sampling, measurement, reliability, and validity may have different meanings and be applied differently in a qualitative versus quantitative context (National Institutes of Health, 2001).

The issue of what scientific standards can and should be used to assess the quality of research grounded in the community is an ongoing tension. Yet Brown argues, "Having a more complex appreciation of the realities of life and dynamics of change within a distressed neighborhood should add a richness and force to evaluators' assessments rather than either undermine their ability to make judgments and/or contribute to a paralysis of action" (1995, p. 214; see also Mays & Pope, 1995).

Research Must Recognize the Complex Nature of Change

Communities are not static; they are complex, dynamic, flexible systems that evolve over time and are responsive to local conditions, needs, and day-to-day events. It follows, then, that community collaborative efforts to improve child health and well-being are dynamic ventures whose goals are constantly changing. These efforts and their outcomes are difficult to evaluate in part because their designs evolve over time. Further, as they evolve, they undertake multiple interventions whose goals are constantly changing (Kreuter et al., 2000; Kubisch et al., 1995). As an initiative unfolds, its look and feel may scarcely resemble the original design. As James Connell and Anne Kubisch note, "A common answer to the question, 'What do you expect to be doing in the fifth year of the initiative?' is 'Ask us in the fourth year, and we'll tell you'" (1998, p. 28).

Change Takes Time

Two additional measurement challenges arise from the fact that community collaboratives typically seek to create large-scale change, and such change takes time. In seeking large-scale change, collaborative efforts must address a wide range of factors (social, economic, and political) affecting health and well-being on the individual, family, and community levels. These efforts often work across sectors and employ a dizzying array of activities, making it difficult, for example, to figure out what exactly should be measured and how and what level of change is considered significant. Michelle Alberti Gambone explains that "thresholds that would determine meaningful improvement are unknown or unspecified. There may be 'tipping points' that must be reached before significant change can be expected in certain areas" (1998, p. 155).

Visible changes in both community and child health and well-being may not be evident for several years. For instance, early childhood development efforts (for children up to three years old) are intended to help children enter school ready to learn (at age five or six), with the ultimate goal of having productive adult working lives. This example highlights the importance of collecting baseline data and tracking changes over time, as well as the need for long-term follow-up (or longitudinal) studies of children that assess the various influences on a child's health and well-being. Short-term studies often do not allow enough time to detect differences in population-level outcomes.

Do Appropriate Data Exist to Measure Change?

In collaboratives that cut across sectors and seek to address a host of related but distinct issues, the use of **indicators** (measures for which data are available that help quantify the achievement of a desired outcome) can help ensure that the efforts of all partners are having their intended effects. The challenge lies in choosing appropriate indicators for the multiple outcomes of interest: communitywide; cross-systems (such as outcomes shared by health and education); within a single system (such as health care), at the agency or organization level (within a children's hospital, for example), at the program level (for a pediatric asthma disease management program, for instance), and at the individual level. The selection of outcomes and indicators must also be balanced across the interests, contributions, and available resources of the various community partners. Thus in examining large-scale and far-reaching systems of care, researchers must be able to interpret and communicate results influenced by multiple perspectives (Woodbridge & Huang, 2000).

Typically, comprehensive community collaboratives seek improvements in areas where there may be few agreed-on definitions and indicators. For instance, different researchers may operationalize and then measure the concept of "community empowerment" quite differently. Even for many agreed-on child health and well-being concerns, such as long-term poverty, homelessness, mental health, neighborhood environment, school readiness, and disability, accurate and sensitive indicators are lacking or still being developed (Federal Interagency Forum on Child and Family Statistics, 2001). And where suitable indicators have been defined, data may be hard to come by due to differing protocols and data storage systems, issues around data ownership, confidentiality requirements, insufficient documentation, and limited data resources and time (see Chapter Four, by Simmes, Lim, and Dennis).

These difficulties are equally relevant for both long-term and short-term (or interim) indicators. Connell and Kubisch (1998) note that scientific and experiential knowledge about links between early, interim, and long-term outcomes is not well developed in many of the key areas in which collaboratives operate. Further, they caution that specifying intermediate outcomes and how they may lead to long-term change can be a politically charged process, especially if those outcomes might imply major resource allocation or power shifts. Bruner (1994) also cautions that any improvements made by individual children or families as a result of a new service or program strategy may be linked only indirectly to desired communitywide child and family outcomes. Carol Rodat and colleagues conclude, "Regardless of the type of indicators selected, it is important that they be closely linked to the community expectations of what the project or intervention is intended to produce" (Rodat, Bader, & Veatch, 1994, p. 16).

Though it may indeed be difficult to specify short- and long-term indicators that adequately measure conditions of well-being for children, families, and communities that cut across agencies, process measures can at least help indicate if a reform is moving in the right direction. Process measures that assess what is done and how it is done (such as number of clients served, types of services provided, or whether services were provided in a timely manner) can help determine how a particular agency's efforts and operations are contributing to the desired results for the larger child population or community. For a community whose desired long-term outcome is that all children are in a safe environment, looking at how long it takes to respond to child abuse complaints may be one useful process measure to track.

The New Paradigm: A Community-Based Research Approach

CHSR investigators clearly have their work cut out for them in designing and conducting research that will produce informative, meaningful, and actionable results to improve child health and well-being. This section provides a brief overview of what we consider a logical response: a community-based research approach.

Why Bring the Community into CHSR?

A **community-based research** approach rests on the underlying belief that the population's health needs will be better understood and improved in a research environment in which local needs are identified and local decision makers are made aware of current research findings and who is doing the research (Anderson, Cosby, Swan, Moore, & Broekhoven, 1999). Community participation helps ensure that the research truly reflects the community's immediate needs and that the program design is actually feasible in a given community setting (Center for AIDS Prevention Studies, 2001). In addition, as Charles Bruner and Veronica Kot state, community members "may be particularly skilled at uncovering information that is qualitative and asset-based rather than quantitative" and deficit-oriented (1999, p. 3).

Although citizens have historically been entrusted as research participants, very little research has been conducted by, with, or for citizens or their communities; it has been typically on behalf of private business, the military, the federal government, or the scientific and academic community (Sclove et al., 1998). Schön explains that after World War II, the U.S. government "began an unparalleled increase in the rate of spending for research," which resulted in a proliferation of research institutions that all sought to generate new scientific knowledge that could be used to "create wealth, achieve national goals, improve human life, and solve social problems" (1983, p. 38). Resulting research agendas set at the national level tended to support more academic and intellectual interests rather than local community concerns.

Historically, communities served as little more than laboratories for demonstration projects and the testing of ideas (Axel-Lute, 2000). Communities were not typically informed about the risks or results of research and rarely derived any direct benefit from it. Further, the research may have led to important policy decisions that were not in the community's best interest and in which residents had no input (Cheadle, 1996; Jordan et al., 2000). In short, communities, rather than being equal partners, were more the object of research and treated as "little more than data points" (Cordes, 1998, p. A37). For example, the Tuskegee Syphilis Study, which took place in Alabama from 1932 to 1972, is widely cited as an example of "medical research gone wrong," according to the CDC. Researchers did not view study participants as part of their community, did not fully inform them of the study's true purpose, and did not give them adequate treatment for their disease (Centers for Disease Control and Prevention, 2001). As a result of this history, many communities, particularly those with large ethnic minority populations, have strong negative feelings about research.

Human subject research protections emerged, in part, from the mistakes of Tuskegee and other studies. Although such protections are necessary and important, especially in traditional research settings, investigators conducting community-based research are concerned about how such policies might affect their efforts. For example, establishing a trusting relationship with a given community— especially one that has been exploited in the past—may already be a challenge; implementing consent forms may prove to be an added barrier. Currently, there is no clear-cut criterion that allows researchers to determine when innovative efforts intended to benefit a community move from collaboration or relationship building to more formal research.

Traditionally, the role of researchers has been to "do to" or to paternalistically seek to "do for" the community (for example, acting as evaluator or program developer) and to focus on quantifying individual health risks. The assumption has been that "certain people are incapable of articulating their own needs" (Vander Stoep et al., 1999, p. 332).

But the environment is changing. In the wake of devolution, increased collaboration, and outcomes-based accountability, researchers are recognizing the importance of giving something back to the community being studied "instead of just taking the data and running" (Perkins & Wandersman, 1990, p. 41). Researchers are paying more attention to how social policy, which is informed and shaped by their research, affects resource allocation, and they are becoming increasingly focused on developing and evaluating alternative service delivery systems (Altman, 1995).

Perhaps most important, researchers are adopting a "do with" philosophy, playing the role of collaborator, codiscoverer, trainer, facilitator, or scientific adviser. They are helping initiatives clarify and outline their goals so that their progress in improving child health and well-being can be tracked over time (Brown, 1995). "Embracing a *doing with* philosophy will assist both researchers and community groups in achieving consensus on the vision, goals, objectives, and methods underlying the research program" (Altman, 1995, p. 530; emphasis in original). This more engaged role is due in part to the increased support and necessity for local, community-based solutions to global issues (such as youth violence or access to health care). Communities are eager to learn about and use research to address their problems. They are looking to researchers to provide information that can help them improve organizational performance; build their capacity to self-assess and monitor progress; determine whether the initiative has achieved its goals; hold initiative partners accountable to the funder, community, or other stakeholders; or enhance their ability to get additional funding (Brown, 1995). For most researchers, this kind of approach requires a paradigm shift.

The Youth Action Project, a collaborative research project between a community-based health center and a university-based researcher that sought to evaluate HIV prevention programs for street youth engaging in HIV risk behavior, involved youth as both collaborators and research participants. Youth collaborators were extensively trained on a variety of research topics and involved in all aspects of the research. They helped develop questionnaires, surveyed outreach sites, translated measures into street language, and provided feedback on whether survey questions were too invasive or personal. Gary Harper and Lisa Carver concluded, "Without the synergistic energy and abilities of the team approach, it is doubtful that these high-risk youth would have been accessed, surveyed, and served" (1999, p. 259).

Richard Sclove and colleagues (1998) identify three common ways that community-based research projects are initiated:

1. A community group proposes a research project to a preexisting community research center or researchers who have a track record of community-based research.

2. A community-based research project is proposed and conducted by an already established community partnership that includes experts and community members (again highlighting the need for researchers to become active members of community collaboratives).

3. In the absence of a preexisting infrastructure that supports such research initiatives, a community group or organization embarks on a community-based research project on its own.

A Brief History of Community-Based Research in the United States

In the 1940s, social scientist Kurt Lewin introduced the idea of "action research" (Meyer, 2000; Minkler, 2000). By the late 1970s, community-based research (CBR) work was under way throughout the world as researchers sought to study causes and find solutions to health, literacy, welfare, economic, and other problems. The 1980s brought formal presentations at international and academic conferences and a significant body of literature demonstrating the importance of involving residents in research for community assessments and other aspects of health planning (Torres, 1998).

An increased focus on a community-based approach grew from community development and adult education work in communities where domination and oppression were key underpinnings of social and health problems and attempts were being made to address issues through permanent political or social change (Green et al., 1997). CBR was used in areas including, but not limited to, community organizing, agricultural extension education, environmental health, and community development (Schulz et al., 2000). As Peter Levesque and Jill Chopyak (2001) conclude, community-based, problem-focused research may help effectively address problems of inequities across regions and communities.

Community-based research currently accounts for a small fraction of the total government, industry, and foundation investment on research but is beginning to capture increased attention of funders. At the federal level, one of biggest pushes for CBR comes from the National Institute of Environmental Health Sciences (NIEHS), which requires researchers to work with local groups and community leaders to help design and carry out studies. The Environmental Justice: Partnerships for Communication Program is a cornerstone of NIEHS's Translational Research Program. This program links members of low-income and minority communities who are directly affected by adverse environmental conditions with researchers and health care providers and ensures that the research addresses community issues in such a way that "communities, environmental health scientists, and health care providers all contribute their resident expertise using participatory methodologies" ("Environmental Justice," 2001). Environmental health issues addressed by the program include mercury contamination in children associated with ritualistic use in Afro-Caribbean and Hispanic populations and pediatric asthma in urban African American children.

Other federal agencies and major institutions, including the CDC, the White House Office of Science and Technology Policy, the Department of Education, the Environmental Protection Agency (EPA), HHS, the Department of Housing and Urban Development (HUD), and the World Bank, are also supporting community-based research to plan and develop programs, assess problems, and set research priorities (Ansley & Gaventa, 1997; Cordes, 1998; Levesque & Chopyak, 2001). In addition, several private foundations, including the W. K. Kellogg Foundation, the C. S. Mott Foundation, the David and Lucile Packard Foundation, and the Carnegie Corporation, are funding collaborative research projects (Levesque & Chopyak, 2001).

Though not universally embraced, community-based research approaches are being accepted as a legitimate research alternative. Mainstream academic journals have begun to publish special issues on community-based research and to address questions about how to weigh the quality and validity of projects that use a participatory approach (Ansley & Gaventa, 1997).

Overview of Community-Based Research

Community-based research is grounded in the belief that partnerships between researchers and communities can contribute both to the development of knowledge and to the ability of communities to address their problems. A community-based approach facilitates collaborative partnerships and encourages all partners to participate as equal members in all phases of the research, including identifying the problem and formulating the research questions, selecting the research methods or instruments, analyzing or interpreting the results, applying the results, and disseminating the results. The underlying premise is that the community has particular insights about the problem and solutions (Green et al., 1997). Involving various constituencies as partners early in the process is a precondition to successful sustainability. Such an approach is meant to improve research quality while also promoting community self-determination and well-being. Most definitions of community-based research emphasize the integration of research, education, and action. The researcher's authority is diffused by incorporating the community's expert knowledge, enhancing the quality and applicability of the research. In addition, as Harper and Carver write about their research on HIV education programs for youth, information about the unique life experiences and circumstances that affect a population's health may be lacking: "Bringing youth into the research arena as full collaborators may hold one of the missing links to improving the impact of prevention efforts for adolescents" (1999, p. 251).

Community-based research offers a means to reduce the gaps among theory, research, and practice that have been problematic in the field. Because CBR emphasizes integrating knowledge into strategies to effect community and social change and ensure the provision of needed services, this approach is particularly aimed toward working with marginalized communities, whose members experience limited access to resources and decision-making processes (Israel et al., 1998). As Schulz and colleagues note, "Community-based research that is grounded in community concerns and linked with reflection and action can begin to address underlying social and political inequalities that contribute to differentials in health status" (1998, p. 22).

Myriad terms describe community-based research, as the field has evolved during the past two decades from various disciplines, each of which uses its own vocabulary. Depending on who is talking (a sociologist, anthropologist, geographer, and so on) and what his or her goals are, CBR might be called participatory research, action research, cooperative inquiry, feminist research, empowerment evaluation, conscientizing research, policy-oriented action research, dialectical research, collaborative inquiry, emancipatory research, participatory action learning research, or something else entirely (Green et al., 1997; Israel et al., 1998). Though the nuances of these approaches may differ, all share the underlying principles of commitment to the researcher-community exchange and commitment to using results to inform action for change. Placing the good of the community first guides the CBR decision-making process. For example, in one urban neighborhood seeking to combat lead exposure in children, residents and researchers worked together to design the project and arrive at a mutually acceptable methodology. The community set the agenda for future research directions, while researchers educated residents about the lead burden and scientific methods. Residents contributed knowledge about their community, such as ethnic traditions or public policies, which in turn informed participant recruitment and retention strategies. In addition, community members were hired as project staff and worked with researchers to disseminate the results. In working with community members, researchers were able to change city policy and ensure that lead-safe transitional housing was available to families affected by lead burden (Jordan et al., 2000).

Sclove (1997) tells the story of children in Woburn, Massachusetts, who were contracting leukemia at alarming rates and also experiencing an unusually high incidence of urinary tract infections and respiratory disease. The families were the first to identify a geographical pattern to the prevalence and began gathering data about sick children. They enlisted the help of several scientists at the Harvard School of Public Health and John Snow, Inc., who conducted additional research both with and on behalf of the affected families. Their research ultimately established a link between the existence of a cluster of leukemia cases and industrial carcinogens leaked into the water supply. The resulting civil suit against the corporation led to an $8 million settlement and was the major impetus for federal Superfund legislation to clean up our country's worst toxic waste sites.

Defining Characteristics of CBR

Several characteristics distinguish a community-based approach from other research strategies (Cheadle, 1996; Green et al., 1997; Israel et al., 1998; Schulz et al., 2000; Vander Stoep et al., 1999). In addition to the active engagement of interested partners in virtually all aspects of the research, defining characteristics include the underlying goal of sustainability, the aim of community empowerment, a focus on problem resolution and action, the use of both traditional and innovative research methods, a cyclical and iterative process, and the acceptance of a broad definition of health and its determinants. These distinguishing characteristics parallel the key issues raised throughout this chapter.

A Broader Definition of Health and Its Determinants

Community-based research emphasizes a child's and family's mental, physical, and social well-being. It accounts for biomedical, social, economic, cultural, historical, and political factors as determinants of health and disease. It emphasizes the local relevance of health problems and examines the social, economic, and cultural conditions that influence health status and the ways in which these affect lifestyle, behavior, and community decision making. For example, in one community health collaborative located in an area with major toxic pollution and substandard housing, lead was the leading cause of death for children. The lead did not come from waste sites or paint chips; rather, it came from handguns. "Successfully addressing a problem like this involves much more than epidemiology. . . . [It] requires a community as well as scientific approach" (Brunner, 2001, p. 2).

Underlying Goal of Sustainability

Productive partnerships between researchers and community members optimally last beyond the life of the project. Altman (1995) describes *sustainability* as the long-term maintenance of the effects of collaboration between researchers and community leaders. Sustainability includes interventions that are maintained, organizations that modify their actions as a result of participating in research, and individuals who, through the research process, gain knowledge and skills that are used in other life domains.

Though Altman says that sustaining interventions is critical because it is the interventions that ultimately bring value to a community and help it improve the population's health, he argues that sustainability is more than the continuation of interventions. Ideally, he says, collective action and purpose lead to community ownership of problem definition, intervention goals and objectives, resources to resolve the problems, and solutions.

Empowerment of Community Members

In CBR, researchers acknowledge and attempt to address social inequalities by sharing information, decision-making power, resources, and support. The community's strongest financial and human resources are pooled in a way that does not create an imbalance in power and responsibility among researchers and community participants. CBR explicitly recognizes and seeks to support or expand social structures and processes that contribute to the ability of community members to work together to improve health. Further, while researchers gain knowledge from the community, community members acquire skills in how to conduct research, empowering them to initiate their own research projects that address self-identified needs.

Focus on Problem Resolution and Action

CBR begins with community members encountering and identifying a practical problem and moves to seeking solutions to address the problem and its underlying causes. The information gathered informs actions, and new understandings emerge as participants reflect on actions taken. There is a commitment to integrating results with community change efforts, with the intent that all involved partners will benefit.

To facilitate action and empowerment, findings and knowledge gained must be disseminated to all partners in ways that will be useful for community action. Ongoing feedback of data and the use of results to inform action is key. Researchers consult with community members prior to the release of findings and, as appropriate, are asked to collaborate as coauthors. Residents help analyze and interpret data by meeting regularly with researchers to discuss findings and provide input on the dissemination of results.

A Combination of Traditional and Innovative Techniques

Community-based research is a process that may entail any number of research methods. Choosing the methods that fit the question at hand and are appropriate in light of a community's cultural, economic, and political issues is key. The usual standards of science regarding generalizability take a back seat to the community's expressed needs. As previously discussed, community interventions do not fit well with the narrow model of causation that drives randomized, experimental designs in which results can be generalized to other settings.

A Cyclical and Iterative Process

In CBR, data are verified through an iterative process and must be refined according to the particular needs, language, and cultural context to which they apply. This cyclical and iterative process entails partnership development and maintenance, community assessment, problem definition, development of methodology, data collection and analysis, interpretation of data, determination of action and policy implications, dissemination of results, action taking, and establishment of mechanisms for sustainability.

Conclusion

Calls for increased attention to the issues affecting child health and well-being have been voiced in major reports and translated into funding initiatives and policy statements by several private foundations and federal and international organizations (Israel et al., 1998). The Children's Health Act of 2000, for example, "expands, intensifies, and coordinates research, prevention, and treatment activities for diseases and conditions having a disproportionate or significant impact on children, including autism, diabetes, asthma, hearing loss, epilepsy, traumatic brain injuries, infant mortality, lead poisoning, and oral health."

Though great strides have been made, there is still more work to be done. To effectively address the determinants of child health will require a more comprehensive and integrated approach to research and practice, including the expanded use of both qualitative and quantitative methods and new, innovative research tools that can capture the social, economic, and political dimensions of child health and well-being. Applied CHSR investigators must also embrace greater community involvement and broader participation in determining what research questions are asked, as well as show increased sensitivity to and competence in working within diverse cultures. This will require CHSR professionals to immerse themselves in the community, build different types of relationships with the community, and develop additional skills. All involved will need to stretch beyond their comfort zones; be willing to compromise, listen and try to understand one another's perspectives; and embrace a sense of adventure to explore uncharted territory (Vander Stoep et al., 1999).

Community-based research is neither simple nor easy. Indeed, working collaboratively with the community "does not offer protection from chaos, but rather doubles the chances of encountering it" (Center for AIDS Prevention Studies, 2001). Yet collaboration is necessary if applied CHSR investigators are serious about improving and strengthening child health and well-being. Meaningful research will require CHSR professionals to develop a deep understanding of the communities in which children and their families live and to apply that knowledge to ask and answer the tough questions that will ultimately advance child health service delivery. In the end, CBR "offers a fresh approach to local capacity building in applied research" (Riley, Jossy, Nkinsi, & Buhi, 2001, p. 1551).

Note

1. For a more in-depth discussion on the nature of qualitative methods in health services research, information on specific techniques, and guidance on how to improve qualitative health services research, see "Qualitative Methods in Health Services Research: A Special Supplement to *Health Services Research*" (1999, vol. 34, no. 5); see also Bernard (1995) and de Munck and Sobo (1998).

References

Altman, D. G. (1995). Sustaining interventions in community systems: On the relationship between researchers and communities. *Health Psychology, 14,* 526–536.

Anderson, M., Cosby, J., Swan, B., Moore, H., & Broekhoven, M. (1999). The use of research in local health service agencies. *Social Science and Medicine, 49,* 1007–1019.

Ansley, F., & Gaventa, J. (1997). Researching for democracy and democratizing research. *Change, 29*(1), 46–53.

Axel-Lute, M. (2000). Town and gown: Making research serve communities' needs. National Housing Institute Shelterforce Online. Retrieved from http://www.loka.org/town&gown.htm

Bell, S. H. (1999). *New federalism and research: Rearranging old methods to study new social policies in the states.* Washington, DC: Urban Institute.

Berkowitz, B. (2000). Collaboration for health improvement: Models for state, community, and academic partnerships. *Journal of Public Health Management Practice, 6,* 67–72.

Bernard, H. R. (1995). *Research methods in anthropology: Qualitative and quantitative approaches* (2nd ed.). Walnut Creek, CA: Alta Mira Press.

Brown, P. (1995). The role of evaluator in comprehensive community initiatives. In J. P. Connell, A. C. Kubisch, L. B. Schorr, & C. Weiss (Eds.), *New approaches to evaluating community initiatives: Vol. 1: Concepts, methods, and contexts* (pp. 201–225). Washington, DC: Aspen Institute.

Bruner, C. (1994). *Toward improved outcomes for children and families: A framework for measuring the potential of comprehensive service strategies.* Des Moines, IA: Child and Family Policy Center.

Bruner, C., & Kot, V. (1999). *Resident experts: Supporting neighborhood organizations and individuals in collecting and using information.* Des Moines, IA: Child and Family Policy Center.

Brunner, W. (2001). Community-based public health: A model for local success. *Community-Based Public Health Policy and Practice, 1,* 2–3.

California Department of Education. (2001). *Fact sheet: Healthy Start Support Services for Children Act.* Retrieved from http://www.cde.ca.gov/healthystart/hsfactsheet.pdf

Center for AIDS Prevention Studies. (2001). *Working together: A guide to collaborative research in HIV prevention.* San Francisco: University of California, AIDS Research Institute.

Center for Studying Health System Change. (1999). *An update on the Community Tracking study: A focus on the changing health system.* Retrieved from http://www.hschange.com

Center for the Study of Social Policy. (1995). *Changing governance to achieve better results for children and families.* Retrieved from http://www.cssp.org/kd12.htm

Centers for Disease Control and Prevention. (2001). *The Tuskegee Syphilis Study: A hard lesson learned.* Retrieved from http://www.cdc.gov/nchstp/od/tuskegee/time.htm

Cheadle, A. (1996, September). The community research partnership: Trying to build better relations between community groups and researchers in Seattle. *Networker, 1*(6). Retrieved from http://www.sehn.org/Volume_1-6_2.html

Coffman, J. (2002). A conversation with Michael Quinn Patton. *Evaluation Exchange, 8*(1), 10–11.

Connell, J. P., & Kubisch, A. C. (1998). Applying a theory of change approach to the evaluation of comprehensive community initiatives: Progress, prospects, and problems. In K. Fulbright-Anderson, A. C. Kubisch & J. P. Connell (Eds.), *New approaches to evaluating community initiatives: Vol. 2. Theory, measurement, and analysis* (pp. 15–44). Washington, DC: Aspen Institute.

Cordes, C. (1998, September 18). Community-based projects help scholars build public support. *Chronicle of Higher Education,* pp. A37–A39.

de Munck, V. C., & Sobo, E. J. (Eds.). (1998). *Using methods in the field: A practical introduction and casebook.* Walnut Creek, CA: Alta Mira Press.

Durch, J. S., Bailey, L. A., & Stoto, M. A. (1997). *Improving health in the community: A role for performance monitoring.* Washington, DC: National Academy Press.

Environmental justice: Partnerships for communication. (2001). *Environmental Health Perspectives, 109,* A545. Retrieved from http://ehpnet1.niehs.nih.gov/docs/2001/109-11/extram-speaking.html

Farrow, F., & Gardner, S. (1999). *Citizens making decisions: Local governance making change.* Sacramento, CA: Foundation Consortium.

Federal Interagency Forum on Child and Family Statistics. (2001). *America's children: Key national indicators of well-being, 2001.* Washington, DC: Government Printing Office.

Gambone, M. A. (1998). Challenges of measurement in community change initiatives. In K. Fulbright-Anderson, A. C. Kubisch & J. P. Connell (Eds.),

New approaches to evaluating community initiatives: Vol. 2. Theory, measurement, and analysis (pp. 149–163). Washington, DC: Aspen Institute.

Gardner, S. (1996). *Moving toward outcomes: An overview of the state of the art and key lessons for agencies.* Fullerton: California State University, Center for Collaboration for Children.

Gardner, S. (2000). *Changing the rules? County collaboratives' roles in improving outcomes for children and families.* Fullerton: California State University, Center for Collaboration for Children.

Green, L., Daniel, M., & Novick, L. (2001). Partnerships and coalitions for community-based research. *Public Health Reports, 116*(Suppl. 1), 20–31.

Green, L. W., George, M. A., Daniel, M., Frankish, C. J., Herbert, C. P., Bowie, W. R., & O'Neill, M. (1997). Background on participatory research. In D. Murphy, M. L. Scammell, & R. E. Sclove (Eds.), *Doing community-based research: A reader* (pp. 53–66). Amherst, MA: Loka Institute.

Harper, G. W., & Carver, L. J. (1999). "Out-of-the-mainstream" youth as partners in collaborative research: Exploring the benefits and challenges. *Health Education and Behavior, 26,* 250–265.

Hayward, S., Ciliska, D., Di Censo, A., Thomas, H., Underwood, E. J., & Rafael, A. (1996). Evaluation research in public health: Barriers to production and dissemination of outcomes data. *Canadian Journal of Public Health, 87,* 413–417.

Heymann, S. J. (2000). Health and social policy. In L. F. Berkman & I. Kawachi (Eds.), *Social epidemiology* (pp. 368–381). New York: Oxford University Press.

Hodges, S., Nesman, T., & Hernandez, M. (1999). Promising practices: Building collaboration in systems of care. *Systems of care: Promising practices in children's mental health, 1998 Series* (Vol. 6). Washington, DC: Center for Effective Collaboration and Practice, American Institutes for Research.

Hoff, T. J., & Witt, L. C. (2000). Exploring the use of qualitative methods in published health services and management research. *Medical Care Research and Review, 57,* 139–160.

Hollister, R. G., & Hill, J. (1995). Problems in the evaluation of community-wide initiatives. In J. P. Connell, A. C. Kubisch, L. B. Schorr, & C. Weiss (Eds.), *New approaches to evaluating community initiatives: Vol. 1. Concepts, methods, and contexts* (pp. 127–172). Washington, DC: Aspen Institute.

Horsch, K. (1997). Interview with Mercer Sullivan. *Evaluation Exchange, 3*(3–4), 5–6.

Institute for the Future. (2000). *Health and health care, 2010: The forecast, the challenge.* San Francisco: Jossey-Bass.

Institute of Medicine. (1999). *Leading health indicators for Healthy People 2010.* Washington, DC: National Academy Press.

Israel, B. A., Schulz, A. J., Parker, E. A., & Becker, A. B. (1998). Review of community-based research. *Annual Review of Public Health, 19,* 173–202.

Jordan, C., Lee, P., & Shapiro, E. (2000). Measuring developmental outcomes of lead exposure in an urban neighborhood: The challenges of community-based research. *Journal of Exposure, Analysis, and Environmental Epidemiology, 10,* 732–742.

Koné, A., Sullivan, M., Senturia, K. D., Chrisman, N. J., Ciske, S. J., & Krieger, J. W. (2000). Improving collaboration between researchers and communities. *Public Health Reports, 115,* 243–248.

Kreuter, M. W., Lezin, N. A., & Young, L. A. (2000). Evaluating community based collaborative mechanisms: Implications for practitioners. *Health Promotion Practice, 1,* 49–63.

Kubisch, A. C., Weiss, C. H., Schorr, L. B., & Connell, J. P. (1995). Introduction. In J. P. Connell, A. C. Kubisch, L. B. Schorr, & C. H. Weiss (Eds.), *New approaches to evaluating community initiatives: Vol. 1. Concepts, methods, and contexts* (pp. 1–21). Washington, DC: Aspen Institute.

Lasker, R. D., Weiss, E. S., & Miller, R. (2000). *Promoting collaborations that improve health.* New York: New York Academy of Medicine, Division of Public Health, Center for the Advancement of Collaborative Strategies in Health.

Levesque, P. N., & Chopyak, J. M. (2001, April). *Managing multi-sector research projects: Developing models for effective movement from problem identification to problem solving.* Paper presented at the Fifth International Research Symposium on Public Management, Barcelona, Spain.

Mays, N., & Pope, C. (1995). Qualitative research: Rigour and qualitative research. *British Medical Journal, 311,* 109–112.

McKnight, J. L. (2000). Rationale for a community approach to health improvement. In T. A. Bruce & S. U. McKane (Eds.), *A partnership model* (pp. 13–18). Washington, DC: American Public Health Association.

Meyer, J. (2000). Qualitative research in health care: Using qualitative methods in health related action research. *British Medical Journal, 320,* 178–181.

Minkler, M. (2000). Using participatory action research to build healthy communities. *Public Health Reports, 115,* 191–197.

Muhib, F. B., Lin, L. S., Stueve, A., Miller, R. L., Ford, W. L., Johnson, W. D., & Smith, P. J. (2001). A venue-based method for sampling hard-to-reach populations. *Public Health Reports, 116*(Suppl. 1), 216–222.

National Institutes of Health (2001). *Qualitative methods in health research:*

Opportunities and considerations for application and review. NIH Publication No. 02-5046. Bethesda, MD: Author.

Norris, T., & Pittman, M. (2000). The Healthy Communities movement and the Coalition for Healthier Cities and Communities. *Public Health Reports, 115,* 118–124.

Nyden, P., & Wiewel, W. (1992). Collaborative research: Harnessing the tensions between researcher and practitioner. *American Sociologist, 24,* 43–55.

Perkins, D., & Wandersman, A. (1990). "You'll have to work to overcome our suspicions": The benefits and pitfalls of research with community organizations. *Social Policy, 21,* 32–41.

Pope, C., & Mays, N. (1995). Reaching the parts other methods cannot reach: An introduction to qualitative methods in health and health services research. *British Medical Journal, 311,* 42–45.

Proenca, E. J. (1998). Community orientation in health services organizations: The concept and its implementation. *Health Care Management Review, 23*(2), 28–38.

Proenca, E. J., Rosko, M. D., & Zinn, J. S. (2000). Community orientation in hospitals: An institutional and resource dependence perspective. *Health Services Research, 35,* 1011–1035.

Riley, P. L., Jossy, R., Nkinsi, L. & Buhi, L. (2001). The CARE-CDC Health Initiative: A model for global participatory research. *American Journal of Public Health, 91,* 1549–1552.

Rodat, C. C., Bader, B. S., & Veatch, R. (1994). Measuring and improving community health. *Quality Letter for Healthcare Leaders, 6*(5), 2–21.

Rotheram-Borus, M. J., Rebchook, G., Kelly, J., Adams, J., & Neumann, M. S. (2000). Bridging research and practice: Community-researcher partnerships for replicating effective interventions. *AIDS Education and Prevention, 12*(Suppl. A), 49–61.

Roussos, S. T., & Fawcett, S. B. (2000). A review of collaborative partnerships as a strategy for improving community health. *Annual Review of Public Health, 21,* 369–402.

Rundall, T., Devers, K., & Sofaer, S. (1999). Introduction: Overview of the special supplement issue. *Health Services Research, 34*(Suppl.), 1091–1099.

Schön, D. A. (1983). *The reflective practitioner: How professionals think in action.* New York: Basic Books.

Schorr, L. B. (1997). *Common purpose: Strengthening families and neighborhoods to rebuild America.* New York: Anchor/Doubleday.

Schulz, A. J., Israel, B. A., Selig, S. M., Bayer, I. S., & Griffin, C. (2000). The research perspective: Development and implementation of principles for community-based research in public health. In T. A. Bruce & S. U. McKane (Eds.), *A partnership model* (pp. 53–69). Washington, DC: American Public Health Association.

Schulz, A. J., Parker, E. A., Israel, B. A., Becker, A. B., Maciak, B. J., & Hollis, R. (1998). Conducting a participatory community-based survey: Collecting and interpreting data for a community intervention on Detroit's East Side. *Journal of Public Health Management and Practice, 4*(2), 10–24.

Sclove, R. E. (1997). "Everyone contributes": Participation in technology research, development, and design. In D. Murphy, M. L. Scammell, & R. E. Sclove (Eds.), *Doing community-based research: A reader* (pp. 15–30). Amherst, MA: Loka Institute.

Sclove, R. E., Scammell, M. L., & Holland, B. (1998). *Community-based research in the United States: An introductory reconnaissance, including 12 organizational case studies and comparison with the Dutch Science Shops and the Mainstream American Research System.* Amherst, MA: Loka Institute.

Sofaer, S. (1999). Qualitative methods: What are they and why use them? *Health Services Research, 34,* 1102–1118.

Stephenson, J., & Imrie, J. (1998). Why do we need randomized controlled trials to assess behavioural interventions? *British Medical Journal, 316,* 611–613.

Torres, M. I. (1998). Assessing health in an urban neighborhood: Community process, data results, and implications for practice. *Journal of Community Health, 23,* 211–226.

U.S. Department of Health and Human Services. (2000). *Healthy people 2010: Healthy people in healthy communities.* Washington, DC: Government Printing Office.

Vander Stoep, A., Williams, M., Jones, R., Green, L., & Trupin, E. (1999). Families as full research partners: What's in it for us? *Journal of Behavioral Health Services and Research, 26,* 329–344.

Woodbridge, M. W., & Huang, L. N. (2000). Using evaluation data to manage, improve, market, and sustain children's services. *Systems of care: Promising practices in children's mental health* (2000 Series, Vol. 2). Washington, DC: Center for Effective Collaboration and Practice, American Institutes for Research.

World Health Organization. (1948). *Constitution of the World Health Organization.* Geneva: Author.

Part III

. . . .

Child Health in Conventional
Health Care Settings

Improving Organizational Performance

Part III

Child Health in Community Health Care Settings

6

Health-Related Quality of Life

Tara Smith Knight, Tasha M. Burwinkle,

James W. Varni

During the past twenty years, researchers, physicians, and other health care professionals have recognized the importance of evaluating health outcomes and measuring the quality of care offered to patients in health care settings. In the treatment and management of chronic illness, there is widespread agreement on the importance of understanding and improving quality of life in addition to promoting quantity, or duration, of life. The purpose of this chapter is to define **health-related quality of life (HRQL)**, discuss the measurement of HRQL and its applications within pediatric populations, examine the benefits and limitations of using survey instruments, and outline future directions in HRQL assessment.

Defining Health-Related Quality of Life

Numerous definitions of HRQL have been presented in the literature, leading to broad disagreement among researchers as to what constitutes HRQL. As a result, a solid, conceptual definition on which researchers can agree has yet to be widely accepted (Gladis, Gosch, Dishuck, & Crits-Cristoph, 1999; Leplege & Hunt, 1997). HRQL is often used interchangeably with terms such as *quality of life*, *health status*, or *functional status*. **Health status** and **functional status** typically refer to one's ability to perform the physical, mental, and social activities of daily life relative to age level (Spilker,

1996; Walker & Greene, 1991). In adults, for example, functional status might refer to the ability to dress oneself, drive a car, or balance a checkbook; in children, it might refer to the ability to engage in active play, run a short distance, or complete homework. Instruments that measure health status or functional status typically contain items dedicated solely to the measurement of physical functioning variables (Eiser, 1997; Stein & Jessop, 1990; Walker & Greene, 1991).

The term **quality of life (QOL)** is a broader construct that typically encompasses many aspects of an individual's life, including housing, environment, work, and school (Seid, Varni, & Jacobs, 2000). QOL has been defined as individuals' perceptions of their position in life in the context of the culture and value systems in which they live and in relation to their goals, expectations, standards, and concerns (World Health Organization Quality of Life Group, 1995). The term *quality of life*, however, can appear in the literature as if interchangeable with *health status, functional status, physical functioning, perceived health status, subjective health, health perceptions, symptoms,* or *functional disability* (Guyatt, Feeny, & Patrick, 1993; Hunt, 1997). As a result, some debate exists regarding how quality of life can be validly measured because it has different meanings for different individuals.

Researchers have agreed, however, that "health-related quality of life" is a more comprehensive concept (Guyatt et al., 1993). HRQL refers to those domains of an individual's health that can be influenced by the health care system (Seid et al., 2000) and can thus be conceptualized as a patient's perceptions of the impact of disease and treatment on functioning in a variety of dimensions, including physical and mental health functioning, social and role functioning, disease and treatment-related symptoms, and general perceptions of well-being (Gotay, Korn, McCabe, Moore, & Cheson, 1992; Jenney, Kane, & Lurie, 1995; Varni, Seid, & Kurtin, 1999; Varni, Seid, & Rode, 1999; Ware & Sherbourne, 1992). These dimensions were initially delineated by the World Health Organization (1948), which defined health as "a state of complete, physical, mental, and social well-being and not merely the absence of disease or infirmity." Instruments that measure HRQL tend to include items that assess not only physical functioning but also social and cognitive functioning, physical symptoms of disease, and other experiences related to chronic illness (Aaronson, 1998; Seid et al., 2000; Wilson & Cleary, 1995).

Uses of HRQL Instruments

Because HRQL instruments assess a broad range of concepts, they have multiple uses in the health care setting. They can be especially helpful to physicians, medical and outcomes research professionals, and other health care personnel for the evaluation of patients in a hospital or clinic setting. HRQL instruments are effective in assessing individuals, groups, and populations. For individuals, they can be used to measure a patient's progress over time, to compare the patient to others with a similar diagnosis or to healthy patients, to evaluate medical treatments, or to assess a patient's cognitive functioning or psychological symptoms. They can also be used to increase physician awareness and understanding of the significance of an individual patient's symptoms that might not be communicated during an appointment due to time constraints or patient reluctance to discuss problems (Their, 1992). For example, a child may be embarrassed or reluctant to tell his doctor that he is being teased at school due to his condition but may be more comfortable responding to such a question in a survey format.

HRQL instruments are useful not only in the assessment of individuals but also for assessing and comparing outcomes between patient groups (Deyo & Carter, 1992). For example, health care professionals can evaluate HRQL within an illness subgroup (diabetes, cancer, or asthma, for instance) to gain an understanding of the impact of a particular illness, to assess the efficacy of medical treatments or interventions, or to compare the functioning or symptoms of patients with different diagnoses. For example, a study using the Pediatric Quality of Life Inventory (PedsQL) in pediatric oncology demonstrated that children with cancer who were on treatment scored lower on all domains than children off treatment, particularly in the psychosocial domain (Varni, Burwinkle, Katz, Meeske, & Dickinson, 2002a). This information can be used to develop and implement interventions targeted at improving the psychological well-being of children with cancer who are undergoing treatment. HRQL assessment can also be helpful in clinical trials by identifying areas within an illness subgroup that are affected or improved by newly developed pharmacological agents. Furthermore, groups of patients can be compared to a group of healthy children, who serve as a benchmark from which to draw conclusions about the influence of a chronic health condition on overall functioning.

Finally, HRQL instruments can be used to measure the health and functioning of a population. In this way, they can help in evaluating the effectiveness of health care services, aid in identifying subgroups of children who are at risk for health or mental health problems, help determine the burden of a particular disease or disability, and guide efforts aimed at prevention and intervention. In addition, use of HRQL measures may assist in the evaluation of the health care needs of a community, and results can be used to influence public policy decisions, such as guiding the development of strategic health care plans, promoting policies and legislation related to community health, and aiding in the allocation of health care resources.

Benefits of HRQL Instruments

There are several benefits to using HRQL instruments in **applied child health services research (CHSR)**. First, HRQL instruments can identify physical, social, and emotional functioning deficits in individual patients (Lansky, Butler, & Waller, 1992) that physicians might otherwise overlook. Physicians consistently underestimate or fail to recognize functional and emotional disabilities reported by patients (Calkins et al., 1991; Golden, 1992; Nelson & Berwick, 1989; Wilson & Kaplan, 1995). This may be because they are concerned about alleviating reported physical symptoms such as pain, placing a lower priority on disability or functional limitations; they also have limited time to take patient histories and may experience communication difficulties with their patients. In this way, physicians can use HRQL instruments to identify areas that need attention or intervention. For example, in the rheumatology clinic at Children's Hospital San Diego, the clinic physician was able to use the PedsQL to inform clinical intervention. In cases where the physician's intervention was influenced by examining the child's PedsQL scores, the patient's scores in subsequent visits significantly increased by approximately 10 points (Varni et al., 2002b).

Second, HRQL instruments can provide the physician with valuable information in a short amount of time (Faden & Leplege, 1992; Their, 1992), indicating more precisely areas of concern for the patient. This is especially helpful in a clinic setting, where time constraints for examination and evaluation by the physician are prevalent.

A third benefit of HRQL instruments is that they can facilitate physician-patient communication (Lansky et al., 1992; Nelson & Berwick, 1989). For a number of reasons, a patient may be unable or reluctant to share meaningful information with a physician. Young children, for example, may not have the language skills necessary to communicate their symptoms accurately, or they may be fearful of talking to the physician. For these situations, scores on HRQL instruments, especially those that are sensitive to children's language development, can indicate problem areas that need to be further explored or problems in areas that are unrelated to the patient's chief complaint but could affect functioning.

HRQL instruments have several additional benefits. Data can help physicians inform patients that a certain treatment will have beneficial effects (Lansky et al., 1992), physicians can establish a baseline health status for all patients (Deyo & Carter, 1992), and assessments can provide information that can help improve patients' quality of life over time (Wasson et al., 1992). For example, if a patient's scores indicate that he or she is having physical functioning difficulties, a comprehensive treatment protocol can be introduced to address those areas of particular concern, thereby improving the patient's HRQL. In addition, if a patient's scores highlight problems in a domain outside of the physician's expertise, such as an emotional or behavioral problem, the physician can refer the patient to the appropriate professional.

Despite the obvious benefits of using HRQL instruments in clinic settings, several challenges have limited their use. Frederick Wolfe and colleagues (1988) state that HRQL instruments may not be consistently used in clinic settings because they might be too expensive or time-consuming to administer and may interfere with clinic operation. In addition, the information they provide might be difficult for the physician to interpret and may already be available through conventional testing methods. Reasons such as these turn up throughout the literature (Deyo & Carter, 1992; Greenfield & Nelson, 1992; Their, 1992; Wasson et al., 1992). Moreover, additional factors in the clinic setting, such as staff unavailability for data collection, the lack of skills to conduct careful data collection, little patience for data analysis, and a lack of confidence in the efficacy of questionnaires, might impede success with such instruments (Lansky et al., 1992; Nelson & Berwick, 1989). Nevertheless, in settings where health status measures have been employed with adults, researchers have found that most physicians report such measures as useful; in fact, between 25 and 45 percent of physicians say they altered their treatment based on HRQL assessments and that patients generally considered the instruments helpful in communicating their symptoms to the physician (Nelson, Landgraf, & Hays, 1990; Rubenstein et al., 1989; Wolfe & Pincus, 1991).

For the benefits of HRQL assessment to be realized in medical settings and within the field of CHSR, researchers must address these challenges and explore ways to improve the use of HRQL instruments. They must look for and develop instruments that are brief, are easy to score, and provide practical, relevant information to health care personnel. They should also seek measures that can be self-administered, when possible, to reduce the burden on clinic or office staff.

Issues in HRQL Assessment

The development and use of HRQL instruments for both children and adults has highlighted some important issues to be considered in HRQL assessment. For example, should an HRQL measure be broad enough to use in many populations, or should it be developed for specific disease symptoms? Should a child report his or her own HRQL, or is a **proxy** rater (for example, a parent or the physician) a more reliable source of information? These kinds of issues are discussed here.

Generic or Disease-Specific HRQL?

Two different approaches to measuring HRQL have been discussed in the literature. The first approach uses nonspecific or **generic measures** of physical, psychological, and social functioning, regardless of disease or treatment. Physical functioning (the ability to perform daily activities) is of considerable importance to children with illnesses that can result in severe physical limitations (such as cerebral palsy or juvenile rheumatoid arthritis). In these cases, assessment of physical functioning is particularly relevant, as it likely has a great impact on overall HRQL.

A child with a chronic health condition is affected not only by the potential loss of physical functioning but also possible difficulties in psychological functioning (Bouman, Koot, Van Gils, & Verhulst, 1999), typically represented by cognitive, mood, and behavior components. Children with chronic illness have been shown to have a higher incidence of a **comorbid** psychiatric disorder than healthy children (Cadman, Boyle, Szatmari, & Offord, 1987; Lavigne & Faier-Routman, 1992), which can have a negative impact on a child's HRQL. In fact, some studies have shown an increased risk for internalizing problems such as anxiety and depression at diagnosis or at some time after diagnosis in children with chronic illnesses such as rheumatic disease (Wallander, Varni, Babani, Banis, & Wilcox, 1989), diabetes (Grey, Lipman, Cameron, & Thurber, 1995), asthma (Padur et al., 1995), and sickle cell disease (Yang, Cepeda, Price, Shah, & Mankud, 1994). It is therefore important to assess psychological functioning in children with a chronic illness.

The social functioning domain typically addresses issues related to family functioning and support as well as peer relationships. Children with chronic health conditions may, for example, experience difficulties talking about their illness with their friends or teachers. They may also experience teasing or questions from peers with regard to their illness. In addition, family relationships may become strained as family members attempt to cope with the child's diagnosis and subsequent illness-related activities, such as going to the hospital for treatment or taking medications at home. Because family and peer relationships can have an impact on a child's psychosocial adjustment and social support (Wood, 1995), it is increasingly important to measure this domain in pediatric chronic illness populations.

In addition to physical, psychological, and social functioning, it is important to measure a child's functioning in the school environment. Adult HRQL instruments typically include items about role functioning, such as job- or work-related tasks; however, a child's role is typically conceptualized as going to school. Having a chronic health condition can affect one's memory, concentration, and attention (Brown, Sawyer, Antoniou, Toogood, & Rice, 1999; Noll et al., 2001; Northam et al., 2001; Wray, Long, Radley-Smith, & Yacoub, 2001), which can have a negative effect on school performance. Furthermore, children with chronic health conditions have been shown to miss more school days than healthy children (Charlton et al., 1991; Fowler, Johnson, Welshimer, Atkinson, & Loda, 1987; Newacheck & Halfon, 2000; Newacheck, McManus, & Fox, 1991; Rapoff, Purviance, & Lindsley, 1988; Sturge, Garralda, Boissin, Dore, & Woo, 1997). For these reasons, it is important to measure school functioning in children with chronic health conditions.

There are several benefits to using generic measures of HRQL in pediatric medical settings. Generic measures permit standard comparisons between ill and healthy children, between acutely and chronically ill populations, and across different illness groups. A single measure can be used in any population irrespective of the condition, making such measures particularly helpful in making health policy decisions, such as the allocation of resources related to health, education, or social services (Eiser, 1997; Ware, 1996). Generic measures also have the versatility of being applied in many different types of large-scale studies, and often have better-documented **psychometric properties** (the degree to which the instrument is reliable and valid).

The second approach to measuring HRQL employs **disease-specific measures**. These are intended to assess symptoms of disease, treatment effects, and other relevant HRQL issues not sufficiently covered in the generic core measure. They generally contain a symptom checklist in addition to questions about illness and treatment-related issues that characterize a specific disease. Given that approximately 18 percent of children in the United States have a chronic health condition (see Tables 2.3 and 2.4 in Chapter Two), it is increasingly important to evaluate the impact of these conditions. Numerous instruments exist for illnesses such as pediatric asthma (Christie, French, Sowden, & West, 1993; Townsend et al., 1991), diabetes (Ingersoll & Marrero, 1990), and cancer (Goodwin, Boggs, & Graham-Pole, 1994; Varni et al., 2002a). Disease-specific measures are presumed to be more sensitive to changes in disease states and consequently may be more useful than generic measures to compare different treatments of the same disease (Richards & Hemstreet, 1994). They are also useful to health care providers because the information provided may inform treatment goals and assist in the evaluation of new therapies. Disease-specific measures, however, are limited in their usefulness for comparison across different patient populations and with healthy population norms for benchmarking purposes.

Although generic and disease-specific measures assess different aspects of disease, a consensus is emerging that both general and disease-specific HRQL instruments should be administered together in order to gain comprehensive information about a patient's health status (Aaronson, 1991; Jacobson, de Groot, & Samson, 1994; Lohr, 1989). Ideas regarding integrating both generic core HRQL scales and disease-specific modules for children were influenced by the European Organization for Research and Treatment of Cancer (EORTC) study group. This study group has developed a **modular assessment** approach to investigate a variety of different adult cancers and has reported adequate **reliability** and **validity** of these measures (Sprangers, Cull, Bjordal, Groenvold, & Aaronson, 1993). The modular assessment strategy involves the administration of both a generic instrument to healthy patients and patients with acute or chronic illnesses and disease-specific modules designed for use in identified illness populations. Although the EORTC study group did not employ this strategy in pediatrics, the benefit of doing so is that it facilitates the measurement of disease and treatment-related symptoms in ill children and aids in the comparison of diverse groups of patients (Varni, Seid, & Kurtin, 1999).

Self-Report or Proxy Report?

In contrast to adult measures, which typically involve only a self-report, pediatric HRQL survey instruments may involve either a proxy report form (on which a parent or other proxy reports on the child's HRQL) or a self-report form (on which the child reports on his or her own HRQL), or a combination of the two. There is considerable debate about whether a child's self-report provides an accurate picture of a child's health and well-being. Given that HRQL derives from a person's own perception of the impact of disease and treatment (Schipper, Clinch, & Owleny, 1996), it makes sense to ask children about their health. Studies have suggested that patient self-reports may provide important information regarding HRQL that parents or other proxies cannot (Guyatt, Juniper, Griffith, Feeny, & Ferrie, 1997). Therefore, reliable and valid pediatric self-report instruments are needed to ensure that the child's perceptions are measured accurately (Gill & Feinstein, 1994; Varni, Katz, Cole-grove, & Dolgin, 1995). To this end, some authors advocate for pediatric patient self-reporting while others point to the benefit of proxy reports to evaluate the child's HRQL (Seid et al., 2000), especially because parents are the ones likely to introduce their child to a health care system based on their own perceptions of their child's health. However, proxy reports have been reported by some as a questionable method of assessment, due in part to the existence of imperfect concordance between patient and proxy responses on HRQL instruments (Seid et al., 2000).

This imperfect concordance, often termed **cross-informant variance** (Varni et al., 1995), has been documented between the reports of child or adolescent, parent, teacher, and health care professional in the assessment of physically healthy children (Achenbach, McConaughy, & Howell, 1987), as well as in the HRQL assessment of children with asthma (Guyatt et al., 1997), cystic fibrosis (Czyzewski, Mariotto, Bartholomew, Le Compte, & Sockrider, 1994), chronic headache (Langeveld et al., 1996), limb deficiencies (Varni & Setoguchi, 1992), and cancer (Varni et al., 1995). One reason for this discord may be that children may differ from adults in their understanding of health, the causes of illness, and their beliefs about how medications work (Eiser, 1997).

In addition, research has demonstrated that the psychological well-being and personal views of the child's primary caregivers may influence the assessment of child functioning and HRQL. Parental responses to questionnaires evaluating a child's health and well-being are largely influenced by the parent's psychological well-being and personal views. For example, a depressed parent may describe her child as less psychologically stable than a nondepressed parent evaluating the same child (Thompson, Gustafson, Hamlett, & Spock, 1992). Studies have noted that depressed mothers tend to overstate their children's behavior problems (Chilcoat & Breslau, 1997; Najman et al., 2000), thereby raising doubts regarding the validity of reports by persons who are mentally impaired or emotionally distressed. (For additional information about the influence of the home environment and the community on a child's health and well-being, see Chapter Three, by Sobo, and Chapter Five, by Dennis and Simmes).

A reliable and valid parent proxy report of HRQL in addition to a pediatric patient self-report is important in at least two ways. First, children are rarely in the position to refer themselves for treatment, and it is the parent's perceptions of the child's HRQL that influence the likelihood that care will be sought (Seid et al., 2000). Thus the parent's perception of HRQL, while not necessarily an accurate reflection of the patient's experience, is instrumentally important in seeking treatment for the child. Second, the use of a proxy rater to estimate patient HRQL may be necessary when the patient is either unable or unwilling to complete the HRQL measure (Seid et al., 2000). Given these considerations, the evaluation of HRQL with combined **parallel forms** (that is, forms with congruent items and domains) for pediatric patient self-report and parent proxy-report appears to be the best approach (Varni, Seid, & Kurtin, 1999).

Factors That Influence HRQL

Many factors can influence a child's health-related quality of life and hence a child's self-report. Adherence to medications and treatment, sociodemographic factors, family function, social support, pain, and other symptoms of disease are just some of the variables that can affect HRQL. Such factors should be considered when designing and interpreting measures to assess HRQL.

Adherence

The lack of **adherence** to medications and treatment regimens can be a major issue in pediatric medicine. There are a number of reasons why a child may not take medication, including negative side effects, unpleasant taste, forgetfulness, unclear instructions, or demanding dose regimens (Matsui, 2000). Such failure to adhere can compromise functional status and HRQL for both patients and their families (Varni, Jacobs, & Seid, 2000). For example, children who do not take their asthma medications can experience more wheezing and variability in pulmonary function that can limit their daily activities (Cluss, Epstein, Galvis, Fireman, & Friday, 1984). Furthermore, nonadherent patients with chronic diseases may be hospitalized or stay home for brief but repeated periods of time, adversely affecting their academic and social functioning (Rapoff et al., 1988). The prevalence of nonadherence, given the complexities and duration of most pediatric chronic health conditions, can have direct effects on the management of patient symptoms (Varni et al., 2000). It is important for researchers and other health care professionals to account for adherence failures, which can affect a patient's overall HRQL.

Sociodemographic Variables

Sociodemographic variables have been demonstrated to have a significant impact on child health (Aligne, Auinger, Byrd, & Weitzman, 2000; Inglis, 1991; Weissman, Stern, Fielding, & Epstein, 1991) and are essential to understanding and explaining individual and population differences. For example, studies in the United States have found parent education level to be a predictor of child health (Zill, 1996), and maternal reports of child health status appear to be affected by sociodemographic variables such as marital status (Bullers, 1994). Studies of family structure have suggested that mean HRQL scores for children in married families were significantly higher than for children living in single-parent families in a number of domains, including mental, physical, and psychosocial summary scores (Schor, 1995).

Worldwide, poverty has been unequivocally related to poor health and well-being (Calman, 1997). Impoverished patients, receiving health care in the public sector, are particularly vulnerable to barriers to care (see Chapter Seven, by Seid, Sobo, Zivkovic, Nelson, and Far). Barriers to health care, both real and perceived, include transportation, paucity of family and community support, and lack of health insurance (Andrulis, 1998; Mansour, Lanphear, & De Witt, 2000). The literature also suggests that children's access to and use of health care services is influenced to a great extent by parental variables including level of education, employment, and marital status (Landgraf & Abetz, 1998). Lack of access to health care is associated with poor health outcomes due to inadequate disease management, which has obvious implications for HRQL.

Family Functioning

The family is typically the most central influence in a child's life. The quality of family relationships can have a profound impact on HRQL in children. Family functioning, defined by Kantor and Neal (1985) as "the actions and interactions of the family members within the family system and across its boundaries" (p. 15), has emerged as an influencing factor in child health. In recent years, studies have documented a link between family adversity and increased risks of problems in children (Lewis & Khaw, 1982; Patterson, McCubbin, & Warwick, 1990). Recent studies have suggested that positive family relationships are related to metabolic control in children with diabetes (Hanson, De Guire, Schinkel, & Kolterman, 1995) and treatment compliance in adolescents with endstage renal failure (Kurtin, Landgraf, & Abetz, 1994). In a study examining pediatric bone marrow transplantation, improvements in quality of life six months posttransplant were most strongly associated with measures of family cohesion assessed pretransplant (Barrera, Boyd-Pringle, Sumbler, & Saunders, 2000). These findings suggest the role of family cohesiveness as a buffer to potential detrimental effects of disease.

Social Support

Social support has been identified as an important factor in predicting HRQL, the lack of which is associated with less than optimal health outcomes in a variety of disease states as well as in studies measuring general population health (House, Robbins, & Metzner, 1982; Pedro, 2001). Social support is a multidimensional construct and has been conceptualized in a number of different ways, with some studies emphasizing structural aspects of support (such as marital status, network extensiveness, and network stability), while others focus on the function of emotional or practical support in social relationships.

Positive social relationships are thought to enhance the quality of life of individuals and serve as protective factors from traumatic life events (Woodgate, 1999). Studies involving cancer patients suggest that social support has a positive influence on the adjustment to disease and impact on health outcomes (Waxler-Morrison, Hislop, Mears, & Kan, 1991). Although studies exploring the relationship between social support and HRQL in children are limited, studies with adult populations have found that individuals with larger social support networks report better overall quality of life (Dobkin et al., 1998; Gielen, McDonnell, Wu, O'Campo, & Faden, 2001). Of the studies that investigate the effects of social support on pediatric HRQL, many focus on the support network of the family, not the child. In a study of asthmatic children, child emotional and behavioral dysfunction was best predicted by the family's network of social support outside the immediate family, as well as general measures of family functioning including conflict, expressiveness, and cohesion (Bender et al., 2000). In the case of chronic illness, families that are challenged by factors such as weak social networks or lack of resources may perceive a child's illness as hugely disruptive, whereas a family characterized by stability and support may report little impact on the family. As mentioned before, the child is deeply embedded in and reliant on his or her family (see Chapter Three, by Sobo). Therefore, negative perceptions by the family (specifically, that the child's illness is burdensome) can have a profound impact on a child's perceptions of his or her role in the adversity of the family. This can have detrimental effects on a child's psychological well-being.

Although the majority of research supports the notion that less social support is related to negative health outcomes (such as a lower quality of life and higher rates of depression), it is important to recognize that larger and more cohesive networks are not always associated with positive outcomes. People in difficult social relationships may experience "social strain," defined as interpersonal interactions that lead to stress rather than improved well-being (Lunsky & Benson, 2001). For example, individuals with large family networks may feel extreme pressure when faced with a personal decision that is not consistent with the family's objectives, which then introduces a type of stress that can be as detrimental as the lack of a social network.

Pain

Pain can also affect a child's HRQL. James Varni (1983) delineated four types of pediatric pain: (1) pain associated with chronic diseases (arthritis, hemophilia, sickle cell disease, cancer, and so on), (2) pain associated with observable physical injuries or traumas (such as burns, lacerations, or fractures), (3) pain not associated with a well-defined or specific chronic disease or identifiable physical injury (such as migraine and tension headaches or recurrent abdominal pain syndrome), and (4) pain associated with medical and dental procedures (lumbar punctures, bone marrow aspirations, surgery, injections, extractions, and the like). Three different levels of pain have also been differentiated in the literature: acute pain, chronic pain, and recurrent pain (Varni, Walco, & Katz, 1989).

Pediatric acute pain has been defined as an **adaptive warning signal**, directing attention to an injured part or disease condition, and is associated with an anxiety reaction. Pediatric chronic pain has been defined as pain that lasts over a period of time and is not associated with an anxiety reaction; rather, it is associated with reactive features such as a lack of developmentally appropriate behaviors, depressed mood, and inactivity or restriction in the normal activities of daily living. Recurrent pain, by contrast, is conceptualized as pain that is sustained over a period of time but is not constant. Recurrent pain is prevalent in children with illnesses such as hemophilia, in which the child experiences recurrent acute pain during bleeding episodes (Varni et al., 1989).

Pediatric pain, whether it is acute, chronic, or recurrent, can impede a child's ability to perform daily activities, participate in sports activities or exercise, or enjoy group or individual activities. Pain has a direct effect on a child's health-related quality of life, especially in the physical functioning and emotional functioning domains, and efforts to reduce pain will have a positive impact on a child's HRQL.

Health-Related Quality of Life in Pediatric Populations

In recent years, HRQL assessment research has been more commonly applied to adult populations, and numerous measures for adults are currently used widely in clinical and effectiveness studies (Seid et al., 2000). In pediatrics, however, few practical, reliable, and valid measures are available. One reason for this discrepancy is that determining age-appropriate norms is complex and requires the development and use of outcome measures that focus on each critical phase of development (infancy, early childhood, and so on). Furthermore, pediatric instruments must be sensitive to a child's cognitive and language development (see Chapter Two, by Gidwani,

Sobo, Seid, and Kurtin) and are therefore more difficult to design. Furthermore, researchers assessing HRQL in children face an additional challenge in disentangling the effects of an intervention from effects due to the variations in typical development (Schor, 1995).

Pediatric HRQL Instruments

Despite the potential challenges to the design of pediatric HRQL measures, some researchers have developed useful measures with acceptable measurement properties. The Child Health Questionnaire, the Child Health and Illness Profile, the Functional Status Measure, and the Pediatric Quality of Life Inventory are perhaps the most widely used of the available pediatric HRQL instruments.

Child Health Questionnaire

The Child Health Questionnaire (CHQ) has been developed specifically to measure HRQL in children. It has a child report form and a parent report form, which are similar but not parallel. The CHQ contains several items relating to domains of physical health, mental health, and role functioning and is available in English, Spanish, French, and other languages (Landgraf, Abetz, & Ware, 1996). **Internal consistency reliability** for the instrument is acceptable, with **alpha coefficients** ranging from .62 to .97; validity statistics and normative data, however, are available only for the parent report form.

Although initial statistics indicate promise for the CHQ, the length of the instrument (eighty-seven items) may be problematic, especially for children. In fact, most respondents answer only 60 to 70 percent of the items (Landgraf et al., 1996), resulting in incomplete data that may affect the instrument's measurement properties. The length of the instrument can also be a barrier to its use in the clinic setting, where time to complete questionnaires is limited. Another limitation to the CHQ is that while the parent report is available for children aged five to eighteen, the child self-report form is only available for children aged ten to eighteen. Despite these limitations, the CHQ attempts to provide a comprehensive measurement of pediatric HRQL and has been widely used in health care settings.

Child Health and Illness Profile

The Child Health and Illness Profile (CHIP) assesses six domains of functioning and includes items concerning physical and psychological functioning, self-esteem and body image, achievement, and resilience (Starfield et al., 1993). The CHIP has demonstrated good **construct validity** and internal consistency reliability, with alpha coefficients ranging from .79 to .92. The CHIP contains 175 items and takes approximately forty-five minutes to complete.

Although the number of items in multiple domains makes the CHIP a comprehensive measure of pediatric HRQL, the length of the instrument is a limitation, especially for health care settings in which time for questionnaire completion is limited. Other limitations of the CHIP are that it was developed for use in adolescent populations (ages eleven to seventeen) and consists only of a child self-report. It is therefore not useful for assessing the HRQL of younger children and does not take into account a parent's perception of the child's HRQL.

Functional Status Measure

The Functional Status Measure (FSII-R) is an instrument that measures behavioral aspects of functioning. It is available as an interviewer-administered parent report instrument for children up to age sixteen and can be completed as a forty-three-item long form or a fourteen-item short form. Both forms have demonstrated good internal consistency reliability, with alphas ranging from .83 to .94 (Stein & Jessop, 1990), have shown acceptable construct validity, and are available in English and Spanish.

The drawbacks of the FSII-R short and long forms are that there is no child self-report available, it is more expensive to administer because it requires an interviewer, and the items are strictly behavioral. For example, they do not assess disease and treatment-related symptoms.

Pediatric Quality of Life Inventory

The Pediatric Quality of Life Inventory (PedsQL) is among the most practical measures of health-related quality of life in children and adolescents. The core instrument is brief, containing twenty-three items covering four domains (physical, emotional, social, and school functioning), supplemented by a series of disease-specific modules, available for cancer, diabetes, asthma, and rheumatic conditions. Additional modules are currently under development for cerebral palsy, brain tumors, medically fragile conditions, cardiac conditions, and other chronic diseases. The PedsQL has been translated into Spanish, German, Dutch, Arabic, Norwegian, Russian, and Tagalog, and additional translations are in progress.

A patient self-report of the PedsQL is available for children aged five to eighteen. Young children (aged five to seven) are aided by a research assistant who reads the items to the child, and older children (aged eight to eighteen) self-administer the instrument. In addition to a child self-report, a parent proxy-report for children aged two to eighteen is available. Recent findings have shown that the PedsQL 4.0 Generic Core and the PedsQL disease-specific modules are reliable measures of quality of life in all age groups, for both the self-report and parent-report forms, with alphas ranging from .83 to .90. The PedsQL 4.0 Generic Core and the PedsQL disease-specific modules have also demonstrated good validity, in part because they distinguish between children with various chronic health conditions and healthy children (Varni, Seid, & Kurtin, 2001). In addition, the PedsQL is responsive to change longitudinally (that is, it can assess changes in the HRQL of individual patients or patient groups over time) and has been shown to have a direct impact on clinical decision making (Varni et al., 2002c).

The PedsQL addresses many of the limitations found in similar pediatric HRQL instruments because it is brief, available as both a child report and a parallel parent report, can be administered to children as young as five years old, and assesses multiple domains of functioning. These qualities make the PedsQL an ideal instrument for use in a busy health care setting.

Illustrations of the PedsQL in Pediatric Rheumatology and Oncology

The PedsQL 4.0 Generic Core Scales and disease-specific modules for pediatric rheumatology and cancer were recently field-tested in outpatient clinics at Children's Hospital and Health Center in San Diego. Each of these studies will be discussed.

Rheumatology Clinic

Participants were children aged five to eighteen years ($n = 231$) and parents of children aged two to eighteen years ($n = 245; 272$ participants accrued overall). The four PedsQL 4.0 Generic Core Scales and five PedsQL 3.0 Rheumatology Module Scales (Pain, Daily Activities, Treatment, Worry, Communication) were administered during clinic visits. The sample included 81 (29.8 percent) children with juvenile rheumatoid arthritis—32 (11.8 percent) pauciarticular, 35 (12.9 percent) polyarticular, 14 (5.1 percent) systemic; 22 (8.1 percent) with systemic lupus erythematosis; 35 (12.9 percent) with juvenile fibromyalgia; 29 (10.7 percent) with spondyloarthritis; and 105 (38.5 percent) with other rheumatic diseases.

Internal consistency reliability for the PedsQL 4.0 Generic Core and the PedsQL Rheumatology Module scales were acceptable for group comparisons, with alphas ranging from .71 to .93 for both child and parent reports. Validity was demonstrated using the known-groups method, in that the PedsQL distinguished among healthy children and children with different rheumatic diseases. The responsiveness of the PedsQL was demonstrated through individual patient change over time (visit 1 to visit 6) as a result of clinical intervention. These results demonstrate the reliability, validity, and responsiveness of the PedsQL 4.0 Generic Core Scales and PedsQL 3.0 Rheumatology Module.

Oncology Clinic

Participants were children aged five to eighteen years ($n = 220$) and parents of children aged two to eighteen years ($n = 337$; 339 participants accrued overall). The four PedsQL 4.0 Generic Core Scales (Acute Version), eight PedsQL 3.0 Cancer Module (Acute Version) Scales (Pain and Hurt, Nausea, Procedural Anxiety, Treatment Anxiety, Worry, Cognitive Problems, Perceived Physical Appearance, and Communication), and three PedsQL Multidimensional Fatigue Scales (General Fatigue, Sleep/Rest Fatigue, and Cognitive Fatigue) were administered during clinic visits. Each of the instruments was administered with a seven-day **recall interval**, instead of the standard thirty-day recall interval.

The sample included children with acute lymphocytic leukemia (50.4 percent), brain tumor (7.1 percent), non-Hodgkin's lymphoma (5.9 percent), Hodgkin's lymphoma (3.2 percent), Wilm's tumor (5.6 percent), and other cancers (27.8 percent). Patients were classified into one of three treatment groups: newly diagnosed on treatment, off treatment for less than twelve months, and off treatment for more than twelve months (long-term survivor).

Internal consistency reliability for the PedsQL 4.0 Generic Core and the PedsQL Multidimensional Fatigue scales approached or exceeded the minimum alpha standard of .70 recommended for group comparisons (Nunnaly & Bernstein, 1994) for both child and parent reports. Internal consistency reliability for the PedsQL 3.0 Cancer Module (Acute Version) parent and proxy report also met or exceeded the minimum reliability standard of .70; the child self-report alphas, however, were more variable. All of the adolescent (ages thirteen to eighteen) self-report scales met or exceeded the standard of .70. Six of the eight child (ages eight to twelve) self-report scales met or exceeded the standard of .70. Two of the young child (ages five to seven) self-report scales met or exceeded the standard.

Validity was demonstrated using the known-groups method, in that the PedsQL 4.0 Generic Core Scales significantly distinguished among healthy children and children with different types of cancer. For the child self-report, the PedsQL 4.0 Generic Core Scales Total Score demonstrated significant differences between the healthy population group and children with cancer undergoing treatment. For the parent or proxy report, the PedsQL Generic Core Scales Total Score demonstrated significant differences between the healthy population group and children with cancer on treatment and off treatment.

In addition, the PedsQL Multidimensional Fatigue Scale subscales and Total Scale Score demonstrated statistically significant differences between the healthy population group and children with cancer as a group. For the child self-report, the PedsQL Multidimensional Fatigue Scale Total Score demonstrated significant differences between the healthy population group and children with cancer undergoing treatment. For the parent or proxy report, the PedsQL Multidimensional Fatigue Scale Total Score demonstrated significant differences between the healthy population group and children with cancer on treatment and off treatment.

For the PedsQL Cancer Module (Acute Version) Scales, the analyses among children with cancer revealed that for the child self-report, the group differences were observed on the Nausea, Treatment Anxiety, and Worry Scales between children on treatment versus off treatment greater than twelve months. For the parent or proxy report, group differences were observed on the Pain, Nausea, Procedural Anxiety, Treatment Anxiety, and Worry Scales between children on treatment versus off treatment. These results demonstrate the reliability and validity of the PedsQL 4.0 Generic Core Scales, the PedsQL Cancer Module (Acute Version), and the PedsQL Multidimensional Fatigue Scale.

Conclusions and Future Directions

Although a clear definition of HRQL is somewhat elusive, it is generally agreed that HRQL is a multidimensional construct that includes physical, social, emotional, and role functioning in addition to symptoms of disease and treatment. A number of instruments for measuring pediatric HRQL are currently available, but limitations such as length, lack of parallel parent and child reports, and problematic measurement properties remain to be addressed for some of these instruments. As a result, CHSR investigators should strive to design instruments that are brief, easy to administer, and cognitively appropriate for different age groups, that include multiple respondents, and that address methodological issues. In addition, research efforts should attempt to incorporate computer-assisted technology in the assessment of pediatric HRQL, allowing for ease and accuracy of child responses, as well as real-time capabilities for scoring and interpretation. This is especially important, as HRQL instruments have multiple uses in pediatric health care settings and have been shown to be beneficial in assessing individuals and patient groups.

Although great strides have been made in the development of pediatric HRQL measures in the past decade, several challenges remain to be addressed. First, there are few longitudinal studies to demonstrate the responsiveness of pediatric HRQL instruments over time. Second, the cross-cultural validity of many pediatric HRQL instruments has yet to be determined. Third, few researchers have investigated the influence of psychosocial, spiritual, and socio-demographic factors that influence HRQL in pediatric populations. Fourth, there have been few studies examining HRQL in non-clinical pediatric populations. Finally, large-scale HRQL population studies are lacking in the pediatric literature. Future efforts by CHSR investigators can address these challenges in an effort to support the value and application of HRQL assessment in pediatric populations.

References

Aaronson, N. K. (1991). Methodologic issues in assessing the quality of life of cancer patients. *Cancer, 67*(3 Suppl.), 844–850.

Aaronson, N. K. (1998). Assessing the quality of life of patients with cancer: East meets West. *European Journal of Cancer, 34*, 767–769.

Achenbach, T. M., McConaughy, S. H., & Howell, C. T. (1987). Child/adolescent behavioral and emotional problems: Implications of cross-informant correlations for situational specificity. *Psychological Bulletin, 101*, 213–232.

Aligne, C. A., Auinger, P., Byrd, R. S., & Weitzman, M. (2000). Risk factors for pediatric asthma: Contributions of poverty, race, and urban residence. *American Journal of Respiratory and Critical Care Medicine, 162*, 873–877.

Andrulis, D. (1998). Access to care is the centerpiece in elimination of socioeconomic disparities in health. *Annals of Internal Medicine, 129*, 412–416.

Barrera, M., Boyd-Pringle, L. A., Sumbler, K., & Saunders, F. (2000). Quality of life and behavioral adjustment after pediatric bone marrow transplantation. *Bone Marrow Transplantation, 26*, 427–435.

Bender, B., Annett, R. D., Ikle, D., Du Hammel, T. R., Rand, C., & Strunk, R. (2000). Relationship between disease and psychological adaptation in children in the Childhood Asthma Management Program and their families. *Archives of Pediatrics and Adolescent Medicine, 154*, 706–713.

Bouman, N. H., Koot, H. M., Van Gils, A., & Verhulst, F. C. (1999). Development of a health-related quality of life instrument for children: The quality of life questionnaire for children. *Psychology and Health, 14*, 829–846.

Brown, R. T., Sawyer, M. G., Antoniou, G., Toogood, I., & Rice, M. (1999). Longitudinal follow-up of the intellectual and academic functioning of children receiving central nervous system–prophylactic chemotherapy for leukemia: A four-year final report. *Journal of Developmental Behavioral Pediatrics, 20*, 373–377.

Bullers, S. (1994). Women's roles and health: The mediating effect of perceived control. *Women's Health, 22*(2), 11–30.

Cadman, D., Boyle, M., Szatmari, P., & Offord, D. R. (1987). Chronic illness, disability, and mental and social well-being: Findings of the Ontario Child Health Study. *Pediatrics, 79*, 805–813.

Calkins, D. R., Rubenstein, L. V., Cleary, P. D., Davies, A. R., Jette, A. M., Fink, A., et al. (1991). Failure of physicians to recognize functional disability in ambulatory patients. *Annals of Internal Medicine, 114*, 451–454.

Calman, K. C. (1997). Equity, poverty, and health for all. *British Medical Journal, 314*, 1187–1191.

Charlton, A., Larcombe, I. J., Meller, S. T., Morris Jones, P. H., Mott, M. G., Potton, M. W., et al. (1991). Absence from school related to cancer and other chronic conditions. *Archives of Disease in Childhood, 66,* 1217–1222.

Chilcoat, H. D., & Breslau, N. (1997). Does psychiatric history bias mothers' reports? An application of a new analytic approach. *Journal of the American Academy of Child and Adolescent Psychiatry, 36,* 971–979.

Christie, M. J., French, D., Sowden, A., & West, A. (1993). Development of child-centered disease-specific questionnaires for living with asthma. *Psychosomatic Medicine, 55,* 541–548.

Cluss, P. A., Epstein, L. H., Galvis, S. A., Fireman, P., & Friday, G. (1984). Effect of compliance for chronic asthmatic children. *Journal of Consulting and Clinical Psychology, 52,* 909–910.

Czyzewski, D. I., Mariotto, M. J., Bartholomew, L. K., Le Compte, S. H., & Sockrider, M. M. (1994). Measurement of quality of well-being in a child and adolescent cystic fibrosis population. *Medical Care, 32,* 965–972.

Deyo, R. A., & Carter, W. B. (1992). Strategies for improving and expanding the application of health status measures in clinical settings: A researcher-developer viewpoint. *Medical Care, 30*(5 Suppl.), MS176–MS186.

Dobkin, P. L., Fortin, P. R., Joseph, L., Esdaile, J. M., Danoff, D. S., & Clarke, A. E. (1998). Psychosocial contributors to mental and physical health in patients with systemic lupus erythematosus. *Arthritis Care Research, 11,* 23–31.

Eiser, C. (1997). Children's quality of life measures. *Archives of Disease in Childhood, 77,* 350–354.

Faden, R., & Leplege, A. (1992). Assessing quality of life: Moral implications for clinical practice. *Medical Care, 30*(5 Suppl.), MS166–MS175.

Fowler, M. G., Johnson, M. P., Welshimer, K. J., Atkinson, S. S., & Loda, F. A. (1987). Factors related to school absence among children with cardiac conditions. *American Journal of Diseases in Childhood, 141,* 1317–1320.

Gielen, A. C., McDonnell, K. A., Wu, A. W., O'Campo, P., & Faden, R. (2001). Quality of life among women living with HIV: The importance of violence, social support, and self-care behaviors. *Social Science Medicine, 52,* 315–322.

Gill, T. M., & Feinstein, A. R. (1994). A critical appraisal of the quality of quality of life measurements. *Journal of the American Medical Association, 272,* 619–626.

Gladis, M. M., Gosch, E. A., Dishuck, N. M., & Crits-Cristoph, P. (1999). Quality of life: Expanding the scope of clinical significance. *Journal of Consulting and Clinical Psychology, 67,* 320–331.

Golden, W. E. (1992). Health status measurement: Implementation strategies. *Medical Care, 30*(5 Suppl.), MS187–MS195.

Goodwin, D., Boggs, S. R., & Graham-Pole, J. (1994). Development and validation of the Pediatric Oncology Quality of Life Scale. *Psychological Assessment, 6,* 321–328.

Gotay, C. C., Korn, E. L., McCabe, M. S., Moore, T. D., & Cheson, B. D. (1992). Quality of life assessment in cancer treatment protocols: Research issues in protocol development. *Journal of the National Cancer Institute, 84,* 575–579.

Greenfield, S., & Nelson, E. C. (1992). Recent developments and future issues in the use of health status assessment measures in clinical settings. *Medical Care, 30*(5 Suppl.), MS23–MS41.

Grey, M., Lipman, T. H., Cameron, M. E., & Thurber, F. W. (1995). Psychosocial status of children with diabetes in the first 2 years after diagnosis. *Diabetes Care, 18,* 1330–1336.

Guyatt, G. H., Feeny, D. H., & Patrick, D. L. (1993). Measuring health-related quality of life: Basic science review. *Annals of Internal Medicine, 70,* 225–230.

Guyatt, G. H., Juniper, E. F., Griffith, L. E., Feeny, D. H., & Ferrie, P. J. (1997). Children and adult perceptions of childhood asthma. *Pediatrics, 99,* 165–168.

Hanson, C. L., De Guire, M. J., Schinkel, A. M., & Kolterman, O. G. (1995). Empirical validation for a family-centered model of care. *Diabetes Care, 18,* 1347–1356.

House, J. S., Robbins, C., & Metzner, H. L. (1982). The association of social relationships and activities with mortality: Prospective evidence from the Tecumseh Community Health Study. *American Journal of Epidemiology, 116,* 123–140.

Hunt, S. M. (1997). The problem of quality of life. *Quality of Life Research, 6,* 205–212.

Ingersoll, G. M., & Marrero, D. G. (1990). A modified quality of life measure for youths: Psychometric properties. *Diabetes Educator, 17,* 114–120.

Inglis, A. D. (1991). United States maternal and child health services: Part 2. A comparison with Western Europe and strategies for change. *Neonatal Network, 10,* 7–13.

Jacobson, A. M., de Groot, M., & Samson, J. A. (1994). The evaluation of two measures of quality of life in patients with type I and type II diabetes. *Diabetes Care, 17,* 267–274.

Jenney, M.E.M., Kane, R. L., & Lurie, N. (1995). Developing a measure of health outcomes in survivors of childhood cancer: A review of the issues. *Medical and Pediatric Oncology, 24,* 145–153.

Kantor, D., & Neal, J. H. (1985). Integrative shifts for the theory and practice of family systems therapy. *Family Process, 24,* 13–30.

Kurtin, P. S., Landgraf, J. M., & Abetz, L. (1994). Patient-based health status measurements in pediatric dialysis: Expanding the assessment of outcome. *American Journal of Kidney Diseases, 24,* 376–382.

Landgraf, J., & Abetz, L. (1998). Influences of socio-demographics on parental reports of children's physical and psychosocial well-being: Early experiences with the Child Health Questionnaire. In D. Drotar (Ed.), *Measuring health-related quality of life in children and adolescents* (pp. 105–126). Mahwah, NJ: Erlbaum.

Landgraf, J., Abetz, L., & Ware, J. E., Jr. (1996). *Child Health Questionnaire: A user's manual.* Boston: Health Institute, New England Medical Center.

Langeveld, J. H., Koot, H. M., Loonen, M.C.B., Hazebroek-Kampschreur, A.A.J.M., & Passchier, J. (1996). A quality of life instrument for adolescents with chronic headache. *Cephalalgia, 16,* 183–196.

Lansky, D., Butler, J.V.B., & Waller, F. T. (1992). Using health status measures in the hospital setting: From acute care to "outcomes management." *Medical Care, 30*(5 Suppl.), MS57–MS73.

Lavigne, J. V., & Faier-Routman, J. (1992). Psychological adjustment to pediatric physical disorders: A meta-analytic review. *Journal of Pediatric Psychology, 17,* 133–157.

Leplege, A., & Hunt, S. (1997). The problem of quality of life in medicine. *Journal of the American Medical Association, 278,* 47–50.

Lewis, B. L., & Khaw, K. T. (1982). Family functioning as a mediating variable affecting psychosocial adjustment of children with cystic fibrosis. *Journal of Pediatrics, 101,* 636–640.

Lohr, K. N. (1989). Advances in health status assessment: Overview of the conference. *Medical Care, 27*(3 Suppl.), S1–S11.

Lunsky, Y., & Benson, B. A. (2001). Association between perceived social support and strain, and positive and negative outcome for adults with mild intellectual disability. *Journal of Intellectual Disability Research, 45,* 106–114.

Mansour, M. E., Lanphear, B. P., & De Witt, T. G. (2000). Barriers to asthma care in urban children: Parent perspectives. *Pediatrics, 106,* 512–519.

Matsui, D. M. (2000). Children's adherence to medication treatment. In D. Drotar (Ed.), *Promoting adherence to medical treatment in chronic childhood illness: Concepts, methods, and interventions* (pp. 135–152). Mahwah, NJ: Erlbaum.

Najman, J. M., Williams, G. M., Nikles, J., Spence, S., Bor, W., O'Callaghan, M., et al. (2000). Mothers' mental illness and child behavior problems: Cause-effect association or observation bias? *Journal of the American Academy of Child and Adolescent Psychiatry, 39,* 592–602.

Nelson, E. C., & Berwick, D. M. (1989). The measurement of health status in clinical practice. *Medical Care, 27*(3 Suppl.), S77–S90.

Nelson, E. C., Landgraf, J. M., & Hays, R. D. (1990). The functional status of patients: How can it be measured in physician's offices? *Medical Care, 28,* 1111–1126.

Newacheck, P. W., & Halfon, N. (2000). Prevalence, impact, and trends in childhood disability due to asthma. *Archives of Pediatric Adolescent Medicine, 154,* 287–293.

Newacheck, P. W., McManus, M. A., & Fox, H. B. (1991). Prevalence and impact of chronic illness among adolescents. *American Journal of Diseases in Childhood, 145,* 1367–1373.

Noll, R. B., Stith, L., Gartstein, M. A., Ris, M. D., Grueneich, R., Vannatta, K., & Kalinyak, K. (2001). Neuropsychological functioning of youths with sickle cell disease: Comparisons with non–chronically ill peers. *Journal of Pediatric Psychology, 26,* 69–78.

Northam, E. A., Anderson, P. J., Jacobs, R., Hughes, M., Warne, G. L., & Werther, G. A. (2001). Neuropsychological profiles of children with type I diabetes 6 years after disease onset. *Diabetes Care, 24,* 1541–1546.

Nunnaly, J. C., & Bernstein, I. R. (1994). *Psychometric theory.* New York: McGraw-Hill.

Padur, J. S., Rapoff, M. A., Houston, B. K., Barnard, M., Danovsky, M., Olson, N. Y., et al. (1995). Psychosocial adjustment and the role of functional status for children with asthma. *Journal of Asthma, 32,* 345–353.

Patterson, J. M., McCubbin, H. I., & Warwick, W. J. (1990). The impact of family functioning on health changes in children with cystic fibrosis. *Social Science and Medicine, 31,* 159–164.

Pedro, L. (2001). Quality of life for long-term survivors of cancer: Influencing variables. *Cancer Nursing, 241,* 1–11.

Rapoff, M. A., Purviance, M. R., & Lindsley, C. B. (1988). Educational and behavioral strategies for improving medication compliance in juvenile rheumatoid arthritis. *Archives of Physical Medicine and Rehabilitation, 69,* 439–441.

Richards, J. M., & Hemstreet, M. P. (1994). Measures of life quality, role performance, and functional status in asthma research. *American Journal of Respiratory and Critical Care Medicine, 149*(2 Suppl.), S31–S39.

Rubenstein, L. V., Calkins, D. R., Young, R. T., Cleary, P. D., Fink, A., Kosecoff, J., et al. (1989). Improving patient function: A randomized trial of functional disability screening. *Annals of Internal Medicine, 111,* 836–842.

Schipper, H., Clinch, J. J., & Owleny, L. M. (1996). Quality of life studies: Definitions and conceptual issues. In B. Spilker (Ed.), *Quality of life and pharmacoeconomics in clinical trials* (2nd ed., pp 11–23). Philadelphia: Lippincott Williams & Wilkins.

Schor, E. L. (1995). The influence of families on child health: Family behaviors and child outcomes. *Pediatric Clinics of North America, 42,* 89–102.

Seid, M., Varni, J. W., & Jacobs, J. (2000). Pediatric health-related quality of life measurement technology: Intersections between science, managed care, and clinical care. *Journal of Clinical Psychology in Medical Settings, 7,* 17–27.

Spilker, B. (Ed.). (1996). *Quality of life and pharmacoeconomics in clinical trials* (2nd ed.). Philadelphia: Lippincott Williams & Wilkins.

Sprangers, M.A.G., Cull, A., Bjordal, K., Groenvold, M., & Aaronson, N. K. (1993). The European Organization for Research and Treatment of Cancer approach to quality of life assessment: Guidelines for developing questionnaire modules. *Quality of Life Research, 2,* 287–295.

Starfield, B., Bergner, M., Ensminger, M. E., Riley, A. W., Ryan, S. A., Green, B. F., et al. (1993). Adolescent health status measurement: Development of the Child Health and Illness Profile. *Pediatrics, 91,* 430–435.

Stein, R.E.K., & Jessop, D. J. (1990). Functional Status II-R: A measure of child health status. *Medical Care, 28,* 1041–1055.

Sturge, C., Garralda, M. E., Boissin, M., Dore, C. J., & Woo, P. (1997). School attendance and juvenile chronic arthritis. *British Journal of Rheumatology, 36,* 1218–1223.

Their, S. O. (1992). Forces motivating the use of health status assessment measures in clinical settings and related clinical research. *Medical Care, 30*(5 Suppl.), MS15–MS22.

Thompson, R. J., Jr., Gustafson, K. E., Hamlett, K. W., & Spock, A. (1992). Psychological adjustment of children with cystic fibrosis: The role of child cognitive processes and maternal adjustment. *Journal of Pediatric Psychology, 17,* 741–755.

Townsend, M., Feeny, D. H., Guyatt, G. H., Furlong, W. J., Seip, A. E., & Dolovich, J. (1991). An evaluation of the burden of illness for pediatric asthma patients and their parents. *Annals of Allergy, 67,* 403–408.

Varni, J. W. (1983). *Clinical behavioral pediatrics: An interdisciplinary biobehavioral approach.* New York: Pergamon Press.

Varni, J. W., Burwinkle, T. M., Katz, E. R., Meeske, K., & Dickinson, P. (2002a). The PedsQL in pediatric cancer: Reliability and validity of the Pediatric Quality of Life Inventory Generic Core Scales, Multidimensional Fatigue Scale, and Cancer Module. *Cancer, 94,* 2090–2106.

Varni, J. W., Jacobs, J. R., & Seid, M. (2000). Adherence to treatment as a predictor of health-related quality of life: An integrative conceptual model. In D. Drotar (Ed.), *Promoting adherence to medical treatment in childhood chronic illness: Concepts, methods, and interventions* (pp. 287–305). Mahwah, NJ: Erlbaum.

Varni, J. W., Katz, E. R., Colegrove, R., & Dolgin, M. (1995). Adjustment of children with newly diagnosed cancer: Cross-informant variance. *Journal of Psychosocial Oncology, 13,* 23–38.

Varni, J. W., Seid, M., & Kurtin, P. S. (1999). Pediatric health-related quality of life measurement technology: A guide for health care decision makers. *Journal of Clinical Outcomes Management, 6,* 33–40.

Varni, J. W., Seid, M., & Kurtin, P. S. (2001). The PedsQL 4.0: Reliability and validity of the Pediatric Quality of Life Inventory Version 4.0 Generic Core Scales in healthy and patient populations. *Medical Care, 39,* 800–812.

Varni, J. W., Seid, M., Knight, T. S., Burwinkle, T. M., Szer, I., & Brown, J. (2002b). The PedsQL in pediatric rheumatology: Reliability, validity, and responsiveness of the Pediatric Quality of Life Inventory Generic Core Scales and Rheumatology module. *Arthritis and Rheumatism, 46,* 714–725.

Varni, J. W., Seid, M., Knight, T. S., Uzark, K., Szer, I., & Kurtin, P. S. (2002c). The PedsQL Generic Core Scales: Sensitivity, responsiveness, and impact on clinical decision making. *Journal of Behavioral Medicine, 25,* 175–193.

Varni, J. W., Seid, M., & Rode, C. (1999). The PedsQL: Measurement model for the Pediatric Quality of Life Inventory. *Medical Care, 27,* 126–139.

Varni, J. W., & Setoguchi, Y. (1992). Screening for behavioral and emotional problems in children and adolescents with congenital or acquired limb deficiencies. *American Journal of Diseases of Children, 146,* 103–107.

Varni, J. W., Walco, G. A., & Katz, E. R. (1989). Assessment and management of chronic and recurrent pain in children with chronic diseases. *Pediatrician, 16,* 56–63.

Walker, L. S., & Greene, J. W. (1991). The Functional Disability Inventory: Measuring a neglected dimension of child health status. *Journal of Pediatric Psychology, 16,* 39–58.

Wallander, J. L., Varni, J. W., Babani, L., Banis, H. T., & Wilcox, K. T. (1989). Family resources as resistance factors for psychological and maladjustment in chronically ill and handicapped children. *Journal of Pediatric Psychology*, *14*, 157–173.

Ware, J. E., Jr. (1996). The SF-36 health survey. In B. Spilker (Ed.), *Quality of life and pharmacoeconomics in clinical trials* (2nd ed., pp. 337–345). Philadelphia: Lippincott Williams & Wilkins.

Ware, J. E., Jr., & Sherbourne, C. D. (1992). The MOS 36-item short form-health survey (SF-36): I. Conceptual framework and item selection. *Medical Care*, *30*, 473–483.

Wasson, J., Keller, A., Rubenstein, L., Hays, R., Nelson, E., & Johnson, D. (1992). Benefits and obstacles of health status assessment in ambulatory settings: The clinician's point of view. *Medical Care*, *30*(5 Suppl.), MS42–MS49.

Waxler-Morrison, N., Hislop, T. G., Mears, B., & Kan, L. (1991). Effects of social relationships on survival for women with breast cancer: A prospective study. *Social Science Medicine*, *33*, 177–183.

Weissman, J. S., Stern, R., Fielding, S. L., & Epstein, A. M. (1991). Delayed access to health care: Risk factors, reasons, and consequences. *Annals of Internal Medicine*, *114*, 325–331.

Wilson, I. B., & Cleary, P. D. (1995). Linking clinical variables with health-related quality of life: A conceptual model of patient outcomes. *Journal of the American Medical Association*, *273*, 59–65.

Wilson, I. B., & Kaplan, S. (1995). Clinical practice and patients' health status: How are the two related? *Medical Care*, *33*(1), AS209–AS214.

Wolfe, F., Kleinheksel, S. M., Cathey, M. A., Hawley, D. J., Spitz, P. W., & Fries, J. F. (1988). The clinical value of the Stanford Health Assessment questionnaire functional disability index in patients with rheumatoid arthritis. *Journal of Rheumatology*, *15*, 1480–1488.

Wolfe, F., & Pincus, T. (1991). Standard self-report questionnaires in routine clinical and research practice: An opportunity for patients and rheumatologists. *Journal of Rheumatology*, *18*, 643–644.

Wood, B. L. (1995). A developmental biopsychosocial approach to the treatment of chronic illness in children and adolescents. In R. H. Mikesell, D.-D. Lusterman, & S. H. McDaniel (Eds.), *Integrating family therapy: Handbook of family psychology and systems theory* (pp. 437–457). Washington, DC: American Psychological Association.

Woodgate, R. L. (1999). Social support in children with cancer: A review of the literature. *Journal of Pediatric Oncology Nursing*, *16*, 201–213.

World Health Organization. (1948). *Constitution of the World Health Organization*. Geneva: Author.

World Health Organization Quality of Life Group (1995). The World Health
    Organization quality of life (WHOQOL) assessment: Position paper from
    the World Health Organization. *Social Science Medicine, 41,* 1403–1409.
Wray, J., Long, T., Radley-Smith, R., & Yacoub, M. (2001). Returning to school
    after heart or heart-lung transplantation: How well do children adjust?
    Transplantation, 72, 100–106.
Yang, Y. M., Cepeda, M., Price, C., Shah, A., & Mankud, V. (1994). Depression
    in children and adolescents with sickle-cell disease. *Archives of Pediatric
    and Adolescent Medicine, 148,* 457–460.
Zill, N. (1996). Parental schooling and children's health. *Public Health Report,
    111,* 34–43.

7

Conceptual Models of Quality of Care and Health-Related Quality of Life for Vulnerable Children

Michael Seid, Elisa J. Sobo, Mirjana Zivkovic, Melissa Nelson, and Maryam Davodi Far

A pplied child health services researchers aim to generate knowledge that will improve the health care delivered to children. Consequently, an understanding of the system that delivers health care is essential. One way to understand systems, including the health care system, is to use conceptual models. Like all scientists, applied child health services researchers can use conceptual models as useful tools in the quest for knowledge. This chapter illustrates one such model for understanding vulnerable children's access to, use of, experiences with, and outcomes of the health care system. Beginning with a discussion of conceptual models, including what they are and what they can be used for, we describe a working model of quality of care and **health-related quality of life (HRQL)** for vulnerable children. This model draws from some of the major constructs and conceptual models in health services research to elucidate the links between quality of care and HRQL for vulnerable children.

Conceptual Models

A **conceptual model** is a set of informed assumptions that scientists make about their focus of study, including definitions of the variables under study, a description of the relationships among the variables, and delineation of the limits of the phenomena of interest.

Applied child health services researchers are like other scientists in that they try to make sense of complex phenomena, such as the state of a child's health, a mother's trust in her pediatrician's expertise, a physician's judgment about a caregiver's competence in caring for a discharged child, or an adolescent's preferences regarding management of a chronic disease. These **hypothetical constructs** are measured by observable indicators, which are in turn operationalized by specific measurements (see Figure 7.1). An explicit statement of how a researcher intends to measure a hypothetical construct is called an **operational definition**. For example, access to health care services (hypothetical construct) could be operationalized by the number of physician visits within the past year (observable indicator), as documented in a patient's chart (specific measurement). Similarly, health-related quality of life (hypothetical construct) could be operationalized by responses on a particular questionnaire (observable indicator) made up of specific items (specific measurement).

Conceptual models describe the relationships among variables. Scientists and philosophers of science call this set of relationships a *nomological network*. Consider a conceptual model of access to ser-

Figure 7.1. The Relationships Among Hypothetical Constructs, Observable Indicators, and Specific Measurements.

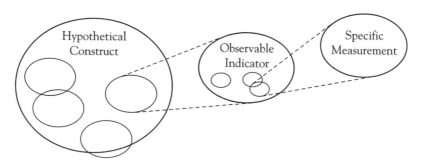

vices and HRQL. The first question is whether these two variables are related. If the variables are thought to be related, the conceptual model can attempt to define the nature of this relationship. Several types of relationships are possible between variables in a conceptual model. Two variables may be directly related (A causes B), and the researcher must specify which variable is the cause and which is the effect. The two variables may be related recursively (A causes B, which causes a change in A, which again affects B), or the two variables may be related indirectly through the influence of a third variable (A causes X, which then causes B). For example, in the model relating access to HRQL, a direct relationship might be hypothesized in stating that access to services is thought to affect HRQL (if a child goes to the doctor, she will feel better). Of course, it may be that the relationship works in the opposite direction—that HRQL affects access to services (if a child feels sick, her mother will take her to the doctor). A recursive relationship might be hypothesized if the researcher thought that HRQL affects access, which in turn affects HRQL (a child feels sick, her mother takes her to the doctor, and she feels better, so she doesn't have to go back to the doctor). An indirect relationship might be hypothesized if the researcher thought that access and HRQL were related by means of a third variable, such as quality of the care provided (a child goes to the doctor, the doctor provides high-quality care, and it is the quality of care, not just an appointment with a doctor, that improves HRQL).

Conceptual models also describe the limits of the inquiry. It is impossible to develop a model that accounts for every variable and relationship involved in a given phenomenon, including the bias imposed by one's theoretical orientation. By describing the variables of interest and their relationships, the researcher is describing the limits of what variables are deemed sufficiently relevant to warrant attention. In our example relating access to HRQL, much may depend on other variables not specified in the model, such as age, insurance status, chronic health condition, season of the year, or region of the country. While a good model encompasses much of what is known about a phenomenon, it is equally important to define what the model does not address. Researchers must take care to define the limits of the models they use.

What can conceptual models be used for? Conceptual models are tools for generating hypotheses and guiding research design. In our example, the position of access and HRQL in the conceptual model specifies a hypothesis: access is related to HRQL. The model also gives rise to competing hypotheses about the nature of the relationship: (1) access to services affects HRQL, (2) HRQL affects access to services, (3) access and HRQL are recursively interrelated, or (4) access and HRQL are related through some third variable. Specification of this model can therefore guide the research design. If the researcher is interested in testing whether access is related to HRQL, gathering data at one point in time using a cross-sectional design would be appropriate. However, if the researcher wanted to test the nature of the relationship, a more sophisticated design might be necessary. Testing whether one variable causes another, for example, requires a longitudinal design, gathering data at more than one point in time. Testing the effects of a third variable requires including that measurement in the research design.

Quality of Care and HRQL for Vulnerable Children

We now turn to an example of a conceptual model that may be useful for applied child health services researchers. This model attempts to increase understanding of vulnerable children's access to, use of, and experiences with the U.S. health system and resultant outcomes. We first describe a rationale for the model and then turn to the model itself, describing the hypothetical constructs involved and their supposed relationships.

Rationale for the Model

The Institute of Medicine, a branch of the National Academy of Sciences and the preeminent national advisory body on health care and health policy, has advocated that U.S. health care providers and stakeholders "should adopt as their explicit purpose to continually reduce the burden of illness, injury, and disability, and to improve the health and functioning of the people of the United States" (2001, p. 6). This statement implies that one important way to examine the U.S. health system is in the results it achieves in terms of the health of individuals and populations. If we are to focus on results, applied child health services researchers should have a set of informed assumptions about how the system works to produce those results.

Which Results of the Health System Are Important?

Researchers need to have an idea of which results are important and how to measure them. For applied child health services researchers, this means understanding and measuring child health. However, the conceptualization and measurement of child health per se is by no means universal (Szilagyi & Schor, 1998). *Health* may be defined by some as the absence of disease but is increasingly seen as a broad construct consisting of physical, psychological, and social well-being and role functioning (World Health Organization, 1948). Child health is seen as a multidimensional state, conceptualized as a continuum (Szilagyi & Schor, 1998). Szilagyi and Schor review four categories of individual health status indicators: (1) biological and physiological indicators, (2) symptoms, (3) functional status, and (4) perceived well-being.

Measuring the health of groups of children is challenging. There is no physiological marker for good health, and although public health indicators such as infant mortality are useful, mortality falls short as a child health measure because most health conditions of childhood are not fatal. The measurement of symptoms, or *morbidity*, is also lacking because there are a very large number of low-prevalence pediatric health conditions (see Chapter Two, by Gidwani, Sobo, Seid, and Kurtin); this makes it difficult to aggregate across health conditions and across healthy and ill children.

For children, one way to operationalize health and functioning is via HRQL, a multidimensional construct that includes primary domains of physical and mental health functioning and social and role functioning (Gotay, Korn, McCabe, Moore, & Cheson, 1992; Ware & Sherbourne, 1992). Thus the conceptualization of HRQL follows from the World Health Organization's 1948 definition of health as not only the absence of disease and infirmity but also the presence of physical, mental, and social well-being. Researchers have made great strides in conceptualizing and measuring HRQL for children (Landgraf, Abetz, & Ware, 1996; Starfield et al., 1995; Stein & Jessop, 1990; Varni, Seid, & Kurtin, 1999, 2001; Varni, Seid, & Rode, 1999). HRQL is increasingly recognized as an important outcome, and some observers contend that it is the *most* important outcome in child health services research (Forrest, Simpson, & Clancy, 1997; McGlynn, Halfon, & Leibowitz, 1995). For these reasons, the outcome of interest of the conceptual model discussed here is HRQL.

Why Do We Need a Separate Model for Children?

Children are not miniature adults. There are systematic differences between children and adults that strongly suggest the necessity of child-focused models for health services. The systematic differences have been summarized as the "four Ds" (Forrest et al., 1997): **developmental change**, **dependence**, **differential epidemiology**, and **demographics**. A fifth D, *disparities*, has also been proposed (see Chapter Two, by Gidwani, Sobo, Seid, and Kurtin). Children develop at a rapid pace, and their development in one domain affects development in others. Children are dependent on families, schools, and other social and political institutions for their welfare in general and for access to health care. Most children are healthy, and in contrast to adult epidemiology, where a few high-prevalence conditions account for most morbidity and mortality, pediatric epidemiology is characterized by a relatively large number of low-prevalence conditions. Demographically, children are disproportionately poor, of color, and uninsured, and **health disparities** among these groups of children are a major concern. (These concepts are discussed more fully in Chapter Two, by Gidwani, Sobo, Seid, and Kurtin.)

Why Vulnerable Children?

Compared to adults, children are more likely to be poor and of minority status, factors that have been conclusively associated with poorer health. Consequently, the conceptual model discussed here focuses on vulnerable children.

Vulnerability to poor health outcomes can be defined as an individual's risk for poor physical, psychological, and social health (Aday, 1993). In a general sense, vulnerability is a susceptibility to negative events or, for purposes of health care, refers to populations that are at higher risk of having health problems or are more susceptible than others to adverse health outcomes (Sebastian & Bushy, 1999). Aday's widely used model of vulnerability encompasses social status (age, sex, ethnicity), human capital (socioeconomic status, language ability), and social capital (family, community) factors that affect the risk of poor health outcomes (Aday, 1993). Though risk for poor health outcomes exists to some degree for every individual, certain groups are at increased risk for poor health outcomes because of a convergence of demographic characteristics, individual assets, and social assets. An implication of this "differential vulnerability hypothesis" (p. 5) is that vulnerability is not a personal deficiency but the result of the interaction among several factors, some of which are beyond the individual's control.

Socioeconomic status (SES) is one aspect of vulnerability often associated with health. Researchers have tended to conceptualize SES as an attribute of an individual, household, or community consisting of different dimensions. These dimensions generally include educational attainment, income, wealth, and occupational status and are viewed as objectively measurable, distinctive dimensions of social stratification (Williams, 1990). Although there are issues yet to be resolved in the conceptualization and measurement of SES, Krieger, Williams, and Moss (1997) have argued that the conceptualization and measurement of SES should match the research question at hand. For children, SES should be measured at the household level, as children are dependent on their families and other institutions for access to health services (Halfon, Inkelas, & Wood, 1995).

The link between SES and health has long been recognized, and there is little argument that the two are related in the United States (Feinstein, 1993; Gould, Davey, & LeRoy, 1989; Pappas, Hadden, Kozak, & Fisher, 1997; Pappas, Queen, Hadden, & Fisher, 1993; U.S. Department of Health and Human Services, 2000). As Starfield found in her review of the research linking poverty and child health, "Poor children are more likely to become ill, and when they do become ill they get sicker and die at higher rates than do nonpoor children" (1992, p. 17).

Another aspect of vulnerability is ethnicity, closely correlated with SES in the United States. However, many researchers (Schulman, Rubenstein, Chesley, & Eisenberg, 1995, among others) argue that these variables are best considered as distinct and related. That is, although demographic factors have traditionally been thought of as causal variables that determine physiological vulnerability, these variables are social constructs, the social dimensions of which influence health, as the American Academy of Pediatrics' Committee on Pediatric Research has emphasized (2000). Ethnicity is not a biological determinant of health, nor should it be used as a **proxy** for socioeconomic status (Schulman et al., 1995). It is best conceptualized as a marker for social processes that might affect health (American Academy of Pediatrics, 2000) (for further discussion, see Chapter Two, by Gidwani, Sobo, Seid, and Kurtin, and Chapter Three, by Sobo).

Because minority children are more likely to be poor (Institute on Race and Poverty, 1995), much of the research on SES and health also considers ethnicity. Income and ethnicity (sometimes conceptualized as race, but see Chapters Two and Three) affect the use of services (Gittelsohn, Halpern, & Sanchez, 1991) and health outcomes, including mortality (Gittelsohn et al., 1991; Howard, Anderson, Russell, Howard, & Burke, 2000), asthma hospitalizations (Goodman, Stukel, & Chang, 1998), and low-birthweight deliveries (Gould & LeRoy, 1988). Inner-city infants in New York State had a higher rate of admission for mandatory and discretionary hospitalizations, reflecting a higher illness burden and poorer access to preventive care (McConnochie, Roghmann, & Liptak, 1997). National survey data have shown that Latino children, those whose parents have little education, and those who live in families without an employed parent are at disproportionately high risk of being uninsured, lacking access to care, and being in fair or poor health (Weinick, Weigers, & Cohen, 1998). Overall, the health status of minority children is worse than that of non-Hispanic whites (Flores, Bauchner, Feinstein, & Nguyen, 1999; Mayberry, Mili, & Ofili, 2000).

What Do We Mean by Health Care Quality for Children?

Quality of care can be defined as the degree to which health services for individuals and populations increase the likelihood of desired health outcomes and are consistent with current professional knowledge (Institute of Medicine, 1996). More recently, the Institute of Medicine (2001) has proposed that the health system should deliver care that is safe, effective, patient-centered, timely, efficient, and equitable. High-quality care occurs when the person has the opportunity to obtain needed care, the care is appropriate and skillfully provided, the care is delivered in a humane manner consistent with patient (or parent) preferences, and the best possible outcomes are achieved (McGlynn, 1997).

Donabedian's model of health services, discussed by Gidwani, Sobo, Seid, and Kurtin in Chapter Two, provides a basic paradigm for assessing and improving the quality of care and is one of the most widely used models in research on health care quality (Donabedian, 1966, 1988). This eloquently simple model, which views care as a production system, entails the components (hypothetical constructs) of structure, process, and the resultant outcomes. **Structure** refers to who is delivering services, where services are delivered, and who is receiving services. **Process** is what is done and how it is done. Processes of care embody both the technical competence of the provider and the interpersonal or humanistic aspects of the patient-provider relationship (Lohr, 1988). A health delivery system is made up of multiple complex processes. **Outcomes** are the health results of the interaction between providers and patients (Vivier, Bernier, & Starfield, 1994) or a change, either positive or negative, in the health status of the individual, group, or population as a result of previous or concurrent care (Donabedian, 1966).

Partly because of the four Ds discussed earlier, measuring quality of care for children and for adults requires different approaches. In adults, measures of quality of care are often based on assessing health care quality for adult populations served by defined health delivery systems, usually health plans (McGlynn & Asch, 1998; Siu et al., 1992). Because of the emphasis on diagnosis and intervention in adult health services, the first step in these methods of quality assessment is usually choosing clinical areas to measure (McGlynn & Asch, 1998). As the epidemiology of adult health conditions is such that there are a relatively small number of highly prevalent conditions, quality measurement tends to focus on defined conditions (Siu et al., 1992).

Measuring quality of care for children requires a different approach (Kuhlthau et al., 1998). Because many children are uninsured (demographics) and because children receive health interventions from many systems including schools and community organizations (dependence), focusing on a defined population served by a defined health delivery system overlooks many children and many health interventions. An emphasis on prevention and health development (development), as well as diagnosis and intervention, requires that the focus be broader than only clinical interventions. The epidemiology of child health conditions is such that there are a large number of low-prevalence conditions (differential epidemiology), and quality measurement should not be based on particular conditions because "monitoring any single condition (as is typical in many current plans) provides an inadequate view of the overall quality and outcomes of care for children with chronic conditions"

(p. 43). Rather than developing measures that address care for a single condition, researchers have called for an exploration of ways of aggregating across services for several conditions (McGlynn et al., 1995).

Experts in pediatric quality-of-care measurement (Kuhlthau et al., 1998; Mangione-Smith & McGlynn, 1998; McGlynn et al., 1995) have advocated for a **noncategorical approach** to quality measurement, one that does not rely on classification by condition. The noncategorical approach has been used to describe children with special health care needs (CSHCN). Applied to CSHCN, this approach stipulates that although biologically diverse, pediatric chronic health conditions have in common the features of significant duration and potential long-term impact on the daily lives of children and their families (Perrin et al., 1993; Stein & Jessop, 1982; Varni, 1983; Wallander, Varni, Babani, Banis, & Wilcox, 1988). Consequently, descriptions of pediatric chronic health conditions are based not on specific diagnoses but on the degree of burden caused by the illness. The noncategorical approach obviates some of the problems in quality measurement stemming from the four Ds and has the advantage of potentially leading to efficient indicators, that is, indicators that can be used to measure quality of care for the broadest possible range of children.

One way to implement a noncategorical approach to measuring quality of care is to focus on noncategorical outcomes of care. Forrest and colleagues (1997) have called for child health services research to "incorporate assessments of children's health-related quality of life as the principal outcome for health services studies" (p. 1790). Another way to implement this approach is to measure attributes of care (such as primary care) that cross diagnostic categories. Access to, coordination of, and continuity of care have been seen as key potential areas of quality measurement. As McGlynn and colleagues note, "Measures of access to care or other areas of potential underuse will be important for children, particularly those without health insurance coverage" (1995, p. 366). In addition, a noncategorical approach to quality measurement implies a broad view of the health system. Because "child health care is delivered across these multiple service sectors, child health services research must not only focus on the point-of-service delivery, but also must include an integrative perspective across sectors" (Forrest et al., 1997, p. 1790; see also Homer, Kleinman, & Goldman, 1998).

Description of the Model

Given this rationale, how do vulnerable children access, use, and experience the health care system (in terms of care characteristics and technical and interpersonal competence; Stewart, Napoles-Springer, & Perez-Stable, 1999), what barriers prevent optimal quality, and what effect does this have on their HRQL? Figure 7.2 presents a model of health care quality and HRQL for vulnerable children that attempts to answer this question. This model refers to a health care system that could take any number of forms, such as the U.S. health care system, a pediatric integrated delivery system, a hospital, a community clinic, an office-based primary care practice, or a school-based health center. In this model, the health care system mediates, in part, the relationship between vulnerability and child health, especially for poor and minority children. Moreover, specific structures, processes, and outcomes occur within the health care system that relate to children's access to, use of, and experiences of care. Specific aspects of vulnerability give rise to potential barriers, which moderate children's access to, use of, and experiences with care. These in turn affect child HRQL.

We introduce this model, based on work by Seid, Varni, and Kurtin (2000), to help researchers organize a noncategorical approach to examining how health care structures and processes affect HRQL for vulnerable children. The more thoroughly applied child health services researchers understand the health care system, the more effective their interventions will be in improving that system. The conceptual model is framed in terms of Donabedian's structure, process, and outcome concepts (1966, 1988). Within this framework, the model borrows from Andersen and Aday's behav-

Figure 7.2. Conceptual Model of Quality of Care and Health-Related Quality of Life.

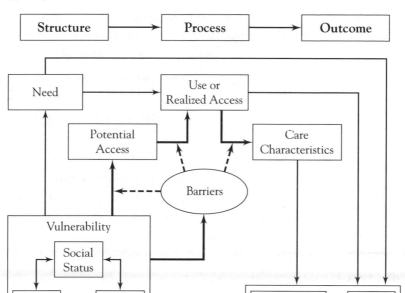

ioral model of health care access (Aday & Andersen, 1974; Andersen & Aday, 1978), Aday's model of vulnerability (1993, 1994), and the noncategorical approach to pediatric quality-of-care measurement. In addition, the model incorporates potential effects of barriers to care. The model illustrates the variables, grouped according to structure, process, and outcome, and their relationships. It makes explicit the chain of events that must occur to increase the likelihood of improved HRQL and the ways in which barriers to care might disrupt this chain.

Structure, Process, and Outcome Variables in the Model

Structural characteristics of the model include vulnerability, need, and potential access. "Vulnerability" is patterned after Aday's (1993) use of demographic (age, sex, ethnicity), human capital (socioeconomic status, language ability), and social capital (family, community) factors. "Need" refers to the child's need for health care services, measured by whether or not the child has a chronic health condition and by severity of illness. "Potential access" includes "structural indicators such as characteristics of the health care delivery system and enabling resources that influence potential care seekers' use of health services" (Andersen & Davidson, 1996, p. 17). Potential access encompasses insurance status, continuity of insurance coverage, the presence of a regular source of care, and provider availability.

Process measures include use of care and care characteristics. "Use of care" is similar to Andersen and Davidson's (1996) "realized access." The conceptual model draws from Andersen's work in distinguishing between potential access (for example, having an insurance card) and realized access (using that card to go to the pediatrician). In the model, use of care encompasses utilization, longitudinal continuity, and adherence to treatment. "Characteristics of care" include features of primary care such as coordination, comprehensiveness, communication, and contextual knowledge (Seid et al., 2001), as well as provider technical competence, which may be measured in terms of adherence to guidelines or the practice of evidence-based medicine. This technical competence variable is intentionally nonspecific in the model because it varies according to the condition being treated.

Outcomes in this model refer to physiological and clinical variables and HRQL.

Barriers to Care

The term **barriers to care** refers to a multidimensional construct, consisting of (1) expectations related to quality of care available from the health care system, (2) health-related knowledge and behavior, (3) pragmatic factors, and (4) the practical skills and knowledge needed to navigate the health care system. The four types of barriers to care, and the specific variables that each category comprises, are hypothesized to be related to SES and other vulnerability factors such as language ability, ethnicity, and nativity. For instance, all are mediated by individual language capabilities and institutional capacities for translation; if parents do not speak the native language (for example, English in the United States) and assistance for translation is not easily obtained, overcoming barriers to care will be very difficult. Barriers to care play a central role in the conceptual model, in that they have the capacity to disrupt the chain of events that must occur for the health system to affect a child's HRQL.

Of the four dimensions identified, the first three—expectations, health-related knowledge and behavior (often glossed as "health beliefs"; Good, 1994), and pragmatic factors—have received the most scholarly attention. A good deal is known regarding the expectations of care among African Americans whose historical experience of the health care system has included negative and exploitive encounters (Henry J. Kaiser Family Foundation, 2000; Sobo, 1995; Thomas & Quinn, 1991). Skepticism regarding medical care in general has also been examined (Fiscella, Franks, & Clancy, 1998), and low expectations (such as the perception that there will be many barriers to care) have been shown to correlate with delayed initiation of care and nonuse of care (Byrd, Mullen, Selwyn, & Lorimor, 1996).

The impact that certain sets of health beliefs (Good, 1994) have on certain kinds of medical care seeking has been fairly well documented. For instance, the understandings regarding *caida de mollera* (fallen fontanelle, a condition of infants) and the resulting **patterns of resort** in the southwestern United States have been documented (Trotter, Ortiz de Montellano, & Logan, 1989). Health beliefs regarding children's abdominal problems, such as *empacho* (Weller, Pachter, Trotter, & Baer, 1993), fright illness among Hmong children (Capps, 1999), and many other childhood ailments have been documented, as have the health beliefs that lead parents to resist procedures for their children, such as diagnostic and remedial heart care (Anderson, Toledo, & Hazam, 1982). Religion may figure prominently here, just as it may lead parents to seek alternative types of care for their children's ailments.

Health beliefs vary among the members of a given cultural or social group (Foster, 1994; Weller et al., 1993) and they are not monolithic or immutable. Research has shown that beliefs may shift according to context and may be fairly fluid, depending on available resources and short-term outcomes. They may be altered to accommodate the particular illness episode in question; they may serve to validate rather than proscribe action, surfacing in ex post facto rationalizations (Foster, 1994). Further, people are easily able to accommodate new information (such as health education messages) in terms of existing health beliefs (Sobo, 1995). This can sometimes mean that new information is applied in ways that might seem nonsensical to the people imparting it. Despite the research that has been done concerning expectations and health beliefs, we are far from fully understanding the impacts of these factors. We do know that expectations can be altered and health beliefs can be negotiated (Kleinman, Eisenberg, & Good, 1978).

Researchers are fairly well informed regarding the pragmatic factors, such as cost, financial resources, availability of time off from work, child care, proximity to a health service institution, transportation options, and an institution's open hours, that come into play when seeking care. Research has shown that such factors are associated with delay or failure in receiving necessary preventive care (Byrd et al., 1996) and also seem to militate against the receipt of proper treatment, hospitalizations, or prescriptions (Flores, Abreu, Olivar, & Kastner, 1998).

The practical skills and knowledge necessary for negotiating the health care system have received much less scrutiny than the other dimensions of barriers to care. Practical skills are the learned strategies or behaviors necessary for accessing and obtaining care and for making best use of the clinical encounter. Implementing these strategies involves variables such as functional literacy and organizational and planning skills, including the capacity to complete paperwork and follow through on health system communications, as well as biomedical literacy and knowledge of the health system itself. Possession of information on care availability, eligibility requirements, and so on (or knowledge about where and how to find it), and facility with the culture of the formal health care system are key.

The skills to move within the health care system and optimize the health care received can be thought of as **functional biomedical acculturation**, because these skills require that a person be *acculturated* to the world of the health care system in a way that allows him or her to function within it and achieve desired ends (Sobo & Seid, 2001). Notwithstanding the emphasis on functionality and minimal skills, "functional biomedical acculturation" is still a much broader construct than those that are commonly used to explain or understand barriers to care. Take, for example, "functional health literacy," a biomedical construct that focuses on reading-related comprehension, which research shows to be inadequate among English speakers and even more inadequate among Spanish speakers (Parker, Baker, Williams, & Nurss, 1995; Williams et al., 1995).

Functional biomedical acculturation, however, rests on the command of a whole set of skills, not just language. Further, while the functional health literacy construct locates the barrier to care squarely within the individual (Williams et al., 1995), our construct locates the barrier in the gap between cultures and in the health care system's own ethnocentrism.

Another construct that functional biomedical acculturation can replace is that of "acculturation," which in theory is a sophisticated, multidimensional concept but in practice simply means assimilation to Anglo-American culture. A good acculturation measure that is appropriate for use in naturalistic research settings has not yet been developed. Existing measures generally take too long to complete and analyze (Clark & Hofsess, 1998). Moreover, they come up short when scrutinized in terms of what they can tell us about a person's facility to navigate the various barriers to care. The functional biomedical acculturation construct corrects for that; furthermore, it avoids sending an implicit message about the virtues of a white middle-class U.S. lifestyle.

Barriers to care are conceptualized, in the present model, as intra- and interpersonal processes. The locus of measurement is at the level of the parent. Parents are in a unique position to report on the care their children receive (Crain, Kercsmar, Weiss, Mitchell, & Lynn, 1998; Dinkevich, Cunningham, & Crain, 1998; Garwick, Kohrman, Wolman, & Blum, 1998; Homer et al., 1999). They can provide both quantitative (how much, when) and qualitative (how come, why) information regarding their experiences in seeking care for their children. Some reported barriers to care (for example, expectations regarding care quality, knowledge, skills) will describe the parent's phenomenological experience. It is important to take the phenomenology of health seeking into account if we are to reduce the barriers to care that parents and children encounter.

This does not mean that barriers to care, as conceptualized here, are simply satisfaction ratings. A distinction has been made between patient or parent reports of experiences with the health care delivery system and ratings of satisfaction with health care delivery (Flocke, 1997; Starfield, Cassady, Nanda, Forrest, & Berk, 1998). Although reports of both experiences and ratings of satisfaction require the respondent to make evaluative responses, these two types of evaluations differ in the criterion against which the evaluation is made. Satisfaction ratings depend on an individual's expectations and preferences, which vary widely among individuals. High satisfaction may result when low expectations are met (Dougall, Russell, Rubin, & Ling, 2000). Therefore, satisfaction surveys ultimately do not suggest ways in which the health system can be improved (Starfield et al., 1998). In contrast, reports of experiences are evaluated against a specific prescriptive criterion—for example, that care be adequately communicated (Bindman, Grumbach, Osmond, Vranizan, & Stewart, 1996). Consequently, deviations from the criterion represent potential decrements in quality and hence areas for improvement.

The focus on parental reports does not imply that the locus for intervention must be at the individual level. Although barriers are encountered on the individual level, they are generated and maintained by, and organized according to, higher-order social structural arrangements (Loustaunau & Sobo, 1997; Singer, Valentin, Baer, & Jia, 1992). Although it is usually not possible for applied child health services researchers to alter macro-level social structures, it may be possible to identify modifiable barriers that have the potential to affect entire patient populations, not just individual families. For example, if parental reports indicate that people of color expect their care to be suboptimal (Snow, 1993), interventions may include systemwide attempts to ameliorate institutionalized racism.

Relationships Among the Variables

The model illustrates hypothesized relationships among the proposed variables. Vulnerability is shown as being directly linked to child health. In addition, vulnerability is also hypothesized to affect HRQL indirectly via the health care system. Poor children, children of color, and children whose parents do not speak English face substantial barriers to access to and use of the health system, and their care is less continuous and less well coordinated (Flores et al., 1998; Newacheck, Hughes, & Stoddard, 1996). Halfon and colleagues found in a study of Latino children in Los Angeles that many experienced discontinuity in insurance coverage and care, as well as barriers to access (Halfon, Wood, Valdez, Pereyra, & Duan, 1997).

Certain factors, including whether or not the child has a chronic health condition and the severity of that condition, will increase need for services. Children with special health care needs use the majority of health care services and are more likely to have worse health status (Ireys, Anderson, Shaffer, & Neff, 1997). Need is hypothesized to be related to vulnerability and enabling resources. Especially in managed care (Fox, Wicks, & Newacheck, 1993; Ireys, Grason, & Guyer, 1996; Newacheck, Stein, et al., 1996), variation in access to care and barriers to care exist, and these barriers are related to vulnerability factors such as poverty, ethnicity, and family structure (Aday et al., 1993).

Potential access is thought to have direct effects on use of care. For example, insurance status has been shown to be a major predictor of access to care for children (Aday et al., 1993; Burstin, Swartz, O'Neil, Orav, & Brennan, 1998; Henry J. Kaiser Family Foundation, 1995; Newacheck, Hughes, Stoddard, 1996; Newacheck, Stoddard, Hughes, & Pearl, 1998; Weissman, Witzburg, Linov, & Campbell, 1999). A child who does not have health insurance coverage is less likely to see a doctor when necessary. Insurance status and type of insurance have also been shown to affect continuity (Flocke, Stange, & Zyzanski, 1997; Newacheck, Hughes, & Stoddard, 1996; Weissman et al., 1999) and coordination of care (Reid, Hurtado, & Starfield, 1996). Children without health insurance face gaps in care and fragmented care.

Use and care characteristics are hypothesized to be interrelated (Forrest & Starfield, 1996; O'Malley & Forrest, 1996) and to have direct effects on HRQL. There is evidence linking access, continuity, and coordination with outcomes such as hospitalization (Billings et al., 1993; Bindman et al., 1995; Casanova & Starfield, 1995) and mortality rates (Larimore & Davis, 1995; Stolz & McCormick, 1998). Especially for children with special health care needs, coordination and continuity of care are predictors of health outcome (Ireys et al., 1996; Reid et al., 1996).

The conceptual model illustrates several ways in which barriers to care may moderate an individual's potential access, use of services, and care characteristics. Barriers to care might affect potential access to care. The types of barriers implicated can be found in all four categories of our barriers-to-care model: skills, pragmatic factors, health beliefs, and experience. For example, in our state children's health insurance program (S-CHIP) evaluation work (Landsverk et al., 2001), we found that despite the promise of translation services, a family may desire low-cost health insurance for its children but not have the linguistic ability to access insurance enrollment information or to complete enrollment forms (skills). Parents may not work in the formal economy and so may not have the required pay stubs as proof of income (pragmatics). Even if insurance is secured, the physicians who will accept it may be in a location not easily accessible by public transportation (pragmatics). Previous experience with the health system has taught some parents that actually using the health insurance card might provoke stigmatization, and this may keep them from accessing available care (expectations). Other research has shown that in certain circumstances, some parents may not want to participate in the formal U.S. health care system in any case, even when eligible, because their views on health lead them to dismiss the relevance of this system for their children (health beliefs), preferring instead to use home remedies (Boyd, Taylor, Shimp, & Semler, 2000; Snow, 1993).

Even when access to care is potential, it is not always realized. For example, a young mother interviewed by Loudell Snow during the course of her ethnographic research (1993) was advised to give expensive formula to her infant son. Lacking money (pragmatics), the young woman diluted the formula. This made the formula last longer and still allowed her to feed her son the correct prescribed number of fluid ounces each day. She knew that she was eligible for free formula, but she did not know how to navigate the bureaucracy in order to get it (lack of skills). In other cases described by Snow, people did not use the care that they had potential access to because of a history of negative experiences with the health system and a fear that clinicians will deliberately harm them or experiment on them (expectations). And many people did not adhere to physician advice because of a conflict with their own health knowledge (health beliefs). For example, one mother, concerned that the medical regime prescribed for her child was suppressing the red hives that needed to erupt for the child to heal, decided to take her own course of action to cure the child.

Using care does not guarantee that care characteristics, operationalized here as the patient's experience of care, is optimal. As just noted, barriers to optimal care can be found in all four categories of our model. For instance, a study of reported barriers to quality asthma care for inner-city children (Crain et al., 1998) showed that problems such as a long wait, lack of transportation, and the need to pay (pragmatics), rudeness of staff (expectations), and a lack language-concordant staff (skills) led to problems in accessing high-quality care. Lack of skill in negotiating the health system may also have been reflected in problems getting follow-up appointments, reported by some parents; alternately, this may have been due to system factors—factors related to the organization of the system set up to serve these inner-city children. The fact that some children with asthma are not identified as such by either parents or practitioners due to understandings about what constitutes asthma (health beliefs) can also have an effect on access, in that children without the diagnosis may not be able to access certain types of asthma care. Similarly, parent understandings about the links between certain types of medication, prevention activities, and the overall health of the asthmatic child can render doctors' orders inappropriate (Mansour, Lanphear, & De Witt, 2000). Satisfaction with care has been shown to be linked to both racial concordance between patient and physician (Saha, Komaromy, Koepsell, & Bindman, 1999) and diverse ethnic perspectives on interpersonal styles of clinicians (Stewart et al., 1999), as well as gender issues (Cooper-Patrick et al., 1999).

Implications for Applied Child Health Services Research

Although the goal of every child health system is to improve the health of the children it serves, it is a complicated task to understand how a health care system affects children's HRQL. Without a deep understanding of how a health system affects child health, it is very difficult for applied child health services researchers to guide that system in the right direction. Although no model is perfect, the model described in this chapter represents the first sketch of a road map to guide applied child health services researchers in understanding how their health systems (including integrated delivery systems, hospitals, community clinics, office-based primary care practice, and school-based health centers) might best improve the health of the children they serve.

Illustrative Example

Let us look at a hypothetical example to show how an applied child health services researcher might use this model. Joe Smith is a researcher working with a large integrated delivery system, Acme Pediatrics. The board of Acme Pediatrics is concerned by newspaper reports regarding the poor health of children in the urban center of their city. Because Acme Pediatrics is a nonprofit entity and the major provider of care to children in the city, the board directs Joe to find out why these children are doing so poorly and to formulate a plan for improving the health of these children in the most efficient way.

Joe first frames the problem in terms of structure, process, and outcome. He notes that certain characteristics of these children (chronic health condition status, poverty, minority status) are likely to be directly related to HRQL. Although Joe can't change these demographic and health status factors, there are ways that Acme Pediatrics can improve these children's health. Unfortunately, many of the children are uninsured, and there are few primary care offices in that part of the city, which limits the children's access to Acme Pediatrics. Joe's first suggestion to the board may be to try to enroll more of these children in government-sponsored health insurance programs and to enhance primary care outreach in these neighborhoods.

Joe realizes that a child's having an insurance card is no guarantee that the child will receive health care services when needed. Barriers to the use of care exist. Through his contacts in the community, Joe learns that there is distrust of formal health care in general, and Acme Pediatrics in particular, in certain segments of the community. Moreover, logistical factors such as time off from work, cost, and inconvenience of office locations and hours are preventing some parents from bringing their children in for care. Joe recommends that Acme Pediatrics develop a community outreach program to reduce the distrust and that existing or planned clinics have evening hours.

Another important aspect of care involves the actual health care encounter. Talking to physicians and patients in the existing neighborhood clinics, Joe realizes that language is sometimes a barrier and that even when the physician and parent speak a common language, the parent does not always have the necessary skills and knowledge to understand the physician's instructions or to know what questions to ask. Joe recommends hiring more translators and developing a series of community-based health education classes to increase parents' understanding of their children's health needs and of basic health maintenance skills.

Directions for the Future

The model illustrated here has been used in two related avenues of research. The first is an attempt to determine to what extent and under what conditions HRQL can be used as a noncategorical outcome measure of quality of care. The second is to understand what potentially modifiable factors mediate the links between vulnerability and HRQL. A noncategorical outcome measure of health care quality for children could be used to enhance accountability, support consumer choice, and develop, test, and implement quality improvement strategies in children's health care. Knowledge of which modifiable factors, for which children, affect HRQL will lay the foundation for designing effective interventions to improve the HRQL of vulnerable children.

Much work remains to be done. Two general areas of research are (1) developing measures and (2) testing the validity of the model in a variety of settings and for a variety of populations. Although measures exist for some of the constructs in this model—for example, the PedsQL to measure HRQL (Varni, Seid, & Kurtin, 2001; Varni, Seid, & Rode, 1999) and the P3C to measure care characteristics (Seid et al., 2001)—measures must still be developed for barriers to care and for some aspects of vulnerability, such as social capital. Further empirical work is also needed to test the usefulness of the model—whether it works as anticipated and for what types of children and problems—and the limits of the model's ability to describe the health care system. It is fully anticipated that this type of work will lead to revisions in the model as our knowledge of this area increases.

References:

Aday, L. A. (1993). *At risk in America: The health and health care needs of vulnerable populations in the United States*. San Francisco: Jossey-Bass.

Aday, L. A. (1994). Health status of vulnerable populations. *Annual Review of Public Health, 15*, 487–509.

Aday, L. A., & Andersen, R. (1974). A framework for the study of access to medical care. *Health Services Research, 9*, 208–220.

Aday, L. A., Lee, E. S., Spears, B., Chung, C. W., Youssef, A., & Bloom, B. (1993). Health insurance and utilization of medical care for children with special health care needs. *Medical Care, 31*, 1013–1026.

American Academy of Pediatrics, Committee on Pediatric Research. (2000). Race/ethnicity, gender, socioeconomic status—research exploring their effects on child health: A subject review. *Pediatrics, 105*, 1349–1351.

Andersen, R., & Aday, L. A. (1978). Access to medical care in the U.S.: Realized and potential. *Medical Care, 16*, 533–546.

Andersen, R., & Davidson, P. (1996). Access to health care: Measuring access and trends. In R. Andersen, T. Rice, & G. Kominski (Eds.), *Changing the U.S. health care system: Key issues in health services, policy, and management* (pp. 13–40). San Francisco: Jossey-Bass.

Anderson, B. G., Toledo, J. R., & Hazam, N. (1982). An approach to the resolution of Mexican-American resistance to diagnostic and remedial pediatric heart care. In N. J. Chrisman & T. W. Maretzki (Eds.), *Clinically applied anthropology* (pp. 325–350). Hingham, MA: Reidel.

Billings, J., Zeitel, L., Lukomnik, J., Carey, T. S., Blank, A. E., & Newman, L. (1993). Impact of socioeconomic status on hospital use in New York City. *Health Affairs* (Millwood), *12*, 162–173.

Bindman, A. B., Grumbach, K., Osmond, D., Komaromy, M., Vranizan, K., Lurie, N., et al. (1995). Preventable hospitalizations and access to health care. *Journal of the American Medical Association, 274,* 305–311.

Bindman, A. B., Grumbach, K., Osmond, D., Vranizan, K., & Stewart, A. L. (1996). Primary care and receipt of preventive services. *Journal of General Internal Medicine, 11,* 269–276.

Boyd, E. L., Taylor, S. D., Shimp, L. A., & Semler, C. R. (2000). An assessment of home remedy use by African Americans. *Journal of the National Medical Association, 92,* 341–353.

Burstin, H. R., Swartz, K., O'Neil, A. C., Orav, E. J., & Brennan, T. A. (1998). The effect of change of health insurance on access to care. *Inquiry, 35,* 389–397.

Byrd, T., Mullen, P., Selwyn, B., & Lorimor, R. (1996). Initiation of prenatal care by low-income Hispanic women in Houston. *Public Health Reports, 111,* 536–540.

Capps, L. L. (1999). Fright illness in Hmong children. *Pediatric Nursing, 25,* 378–383.

Casanova, C., & Starfield, B. (1995). Hospitalizations of children and access to primary care: A cross-national comparison. *International Journal of Health Services, 25,* 283–294.

Clark, L., & Hofsess, L. (1998). Acculturation. In S. Loue (Ed.), *Handbook of immigrant health* (pp. 37–59). New York: Plenum Press.

Cooper-Patrick, L., Gallo, J. J., Gonzales, J. J., Vu, H. T., Powe, N. R., Nelson, C., & Ford, D. E. (1999). Race, gender, and partnership in the patient-physician relationship. *Journal of the American Medical Association, 282,* 583–589.

Crain, E. F., Kercsmar, C., Weiss, K. B., Mitchell, H., & Lynn, H. (1998). Reported difficulties in access to quality care for children with asthma in the inner city. *Archives of Pediatric and Adolescent Medicine, 152,* 333–339.

Dinkevich, E. I., Cunningham, S. J., & Crain, E. F. (1998). Parental perceptions of access to care and quality of care for inner-city children with asthma. *Journal of Asthma, 35,* 63–71.

Donabedian, A. (1966). Evaluating the quality of medical care. *Milbank Memorial Fund Quarterly, 44*(3 Suppl.), 166–206.

Donabedian, A. (1988). The quality of health care: How can it be assessed? *Journal of the American Medical Association, 260,* 1743–1748.

Dougall, A., Russell, A., Rubin, G., & Ling, J. (2000). Rethinking patient satisfaction: Patient experiences of an open-access flexible sigmoidoscopy service. *Social Science and Medicine, 50,* 53–62.

Feinstein, J. S. (1993). The relationship between socioeconomic status and health: A review of the literature. *Milbank Quarterly, 71*, 279–322.

Fiscella, K., Franks, P., & Clancy, C. M. (1998). Skepticism toward medical care and health care utilization. *Medical Care, 36*, 180–189.

Flocke, S. A. (1997). Measuring attributes of primary care: Development of a new instrument. *Journal of Family Practice, 45*, 64–74.

Flocke, S. A., Stange, K. C., & Zyzanski, S. J. (1997). The impact of insurance type and forced discontinuity on the delivery of primary care. *Journal of Family Practice, 45*, 129–135.

Flores, G., Abreu, M., Olivar, M. A., & Kastner, B. (1998). Access barriers to health care for Latino children. *Archives of Pediatric and Adolescent Medicine, 152*, 1119–1125.

Flores, G., Bauchner, H., Feinstein, A. R., & Nguyen, U. S. (1999). The impact of ethnicity, family income, and parental education on children's health and use of health services. *American Journal of Public Health, 89*, 1066–1071.

Forrest, C. B., Simpson, L., & Clancy, C. (1997). Child health services research. Challenges and opportunities. *Journal of the American Medical Association, 277*, 1787–1793.

Forrest, C. B., & Starfield, B. (1996). The effect of first-contact care with primary care clinicians on ambulatory health care expenditures. *Journal of Family Practice, 43*, 40–48.

Foster, G. M. (1994). *Hippocrates' Latin American legacy: Humoral medicine in the New World*. Langhorne, PA: Gordon & Breach.

Fox, H. B., Wicks, L. B., & Newacheck, P. W. (1993). Health maintenance organizations and children with special health needs. A suitable match? *American Journal of Diseases of Children, 147*, 546–552.

Garwick, A. W., Kohrman, C., Wolman, C., & Blum, R. W. (1998). Families' recommendations for improving services for children with chronic conditions. *Archives of Pediatric and Adolescent Medicine, 152*, 440–448.

Gittelsohn, A. M., Halpern, J., & Sanchez, R. L. (1991). Income, race, and surgery in Maryland. *American Journal of Public Health, 81*, 1435–1441.

Good, B. J. (1994). *Medicine, rationality, and experience: An anthropological perspective*. Cambridge: Cambridge University Press.

Goodman, D. C., Stukel, T. A., & Chang, C. H. (1998). Trends in pediatric asthma hospitalization rates: Regional and socioeconomic differences. *Pediatrics, 101*, 208–213.

Gotay, C. C., Korn, E. L., McCabe, M. S., Moore, T. D., & Cheson, B. D. (1992). Quality of life assessment in cancer treatment protocols: Research issues in protocol development. *Journal of the National Cancer Institute*, 84, 575–579.

Gould, J. B., Davey, B., & LeRoy, S. (1989). Socioeconomic differentials and neonatal mortality: Racial comparison of California singletons. *Pediatrics*, 83, 181–186.

Gould, J. B., & LeRoy, S. (1988). Socioeconomic status and low birth weight: A racial comparison. *Pediatrics*, 82, 896–904.

Halfon, N., Inkelas, M., & Wood, D. L. (1995). Nonfinancial barriers to care for children and youth. *Annual Review of Public Health*, 16, 447–472.

Halfon, N., Wood, D. L., Valdez, R. B., Pereyra, M., & Duan, N. (1997). Medicaid enrollment and health services access by Latino children in inner-city Los Angeles. *Journal of the American Medical Association*, 277, 636–641.

Henry J. Kaiser Family Foundation. (1995). *Access to care: Is health insurance enough?* Washington, DC: Author.

Henry J. Kaiser Family Foundation. (2000). *Kaiser commission on key facts: Medicaid and the uninsured.* Washington, DC: Author.

Homer, C. J., Kleinman, L. C., & Goldman, D. A. (1998). Improving the quality of care for children in health systems. *Health Services Research*, 33, 1091–1109.

Homer, C. J., Marino, B., Cleary, P. D., Alpert, H. R., Smith, B., Crowley Ganser, C. M., et al. (1999). Quality of care at a children's hospital: The parent's perspective. *Archives of Pediatric and Adolescent Medicine*, 153, 1123–1129.

Howard, G., Anderson, R. T., Russell, G., Howard, V. J., & Burke, G. L. (2000). Race, socioeconomic status, and cause-specific mortality. *Annals of Epidemiology*, 10, 214–223.

Institute of Medicine. (1996). *Primary care: America's health in a new era.* Washington, DC: National Academy Press.

Institute of Medicine, Committee on Quality Health Care in America. (2001). *Crossing the quality chasm: A new health system for the 21st century.* Washington, DC: National Academy Press.

Institute on Race and Poverty. (1995). *Race and poverty: Our private obsession, our public sin.* Washington, DC: Author.

Ireys, H. T., Anderson, G. F., Shaffer, T. J., & Neff, J. M. (1997). Expenditures for care of children with chronic illnesses enrolled in the Washington State Medicaid program, fiscal year 1993. *Pediatrics*, 100, 197–204.

Ireys, H. T., Grason, H. A., & Guyer, B. (1996). Assuring quality of care for children with special needs in managed care organizations: Roles for pediatricians. *Pediatrics*, 98, 178–185.

Kleinman, A., Eisenberg, L., & Good, B. J. (1978). Culture, illness, and care: Clinical lessons from anthropologic and cross-cultural research. *Annals of Internal Medicine, 88*, 251–258.

Krieger, N., Williams, D. R., & Moss, N. E. (1997). Measuring social class in U.S. public health research: Concepts, methodologies, and guidelines. *Annual Review of Public Health, 18*, 341–378.

Kuhlthau, K., Walker, D. K., Perrin, J. M., Bauman, L., Gortmaker, S. L., New-acheck, P. W., & Stein, R.E.K. (1998). Assessing managed care for children with chronic conditions. *Health Affairs* (Millwood), *17*(4), 42–52.

Landgraf, J. M., Abetz, L., & Ware, J. E., Jr. (1996). *Child Health Questionnaire: A user's manual.* Boston: Health Institute, New England Medical Center.

Landsverk, J., Kurtin, P. S., Connelly, C., Simmes, D. R., Sobo, E. J., & Seid, M. (2001). *Evaluation of Outreach and Education Campaign for Healthy Families and MediCal for Children.* Sacramento: California Department of Health Services.

Larimore, W. L., & Davis, A. (1995). Relation of infant mortality to the availability of maternity care in rural Florida. *Journal of the American Board of Family Practitioners, 8*, 392–399.

Lohr, K. N. (1988). Outcome measurement: Concepts and questions. *Inquiry, 25*, 37–50.

Loustaunau, M., & Sobo, E. J. (1997). *The cultural context of health, illness, and medicine.* Westport, CT: Bergin & Garvey.

Mangione-Smith, R., & McGlynn, E. A. (1998). Assessing the quality of health-care provided to children. *Health Services Research, 33*, 1059–1090.

Mansour, M. E., Lanphear, B. P., & De Witt, T. G. (2000). Barriers to asthma care in urban children: Parent perspectives. *Pediatrics, 106*, 512–519.

Mayberry, R. M., Mili, F., & Ofili, E. (2000). Racial and ethnic differences in access to medical care. *Medical Care Research Review, 57*(Suppl. 1), 108–145.

McConnochie, K. M., Roghmann, K. J., & Liptak, G. S. (1997). Socioeconomic variation in discretionary and mandatory hospitalization of infants: An ecologic analysis. *Pediatrics, 99*, 774–784.

McGlynn, E. A. (1997). Six challenges in measuring the quality of health care. *Health Affairs* (Millwood), *16*(3), 7–21.

McGlynn, E. A., & Asch, S. M. (1998). Developing a clinical performance measure. *American Journal of Preventive Medicine, 14*(3 Suppl.), 14–21.

McGlynn, E. A., Halfon, N., & Leibowitz, A. (1995). Assessing the quality of care for children: Prospects under health reform. *Archives of Pediatric and Adolescent Medicine, 149*, 359–368.

Newacheck, P. W., Hughes, D. C., & Stoddard, J. J. (1996). Children's access to primary care: Differences by race, income, and insurance status. *Pediatrics, 97*, 26–32.

Newacheck, P. W., Stein, R.E.K., Walker, D. K., Gortmaker, S. L., Kuhlthau, K., & Perrin, J. M. (1996). Monitoring and evaluating managed care for children with chronic illnesses and disabilities. *Pediatrics, 98*, 952–958.

Newacheck, P. W., Stoddard, J. J., Hughes, D. C., & Pearl, M. (1998). Health insurance and access to primary care for children. *New England Journal of Medicine, 338*, 513–519.

O'Malley, A. S., & Forrest, C. B. (1996). Continuity of care and delivery of ambulatory services to children in community health clinics. *Journal of Community Health, 21*, 159–173.

Pappas, G., Hadden, W. C., Kozak, L. J., & Fisher, G. F. (1997). Potentially avoidable hospitalizations: Inequalities in rates between U.S. socioeconomic groups. *American Journal of Public Health, 87*, 811–816.

Pappas, G., Queen, S., Hadden, W. C., & Fisher, G. F. (1993). The increasing disparity in mortality between socioeconomic groups in the United States, 1960 and 1986. *New England Journal of Medicine, 329*, 103–109.

Parker, R. M., Baker, D. W., Williams, M. V., & Nurss, J. R. (1995). The test of functional health literacy in adults: A new instrument for measuring patients' literacy skills. *Journal of General Internal Medicine, 10*, 537–541.

Perrin, E. C., Newacheck, P., Pless, B. I., Drotar, D., Gortmaker, S. L., Leventhal, J., et al. (1993). Issues involved in the definition and classification of chronic health conditions. *Pediatrics, 91*, 787–793.

Reid, R. J., Hurtado, M. P., & Starfield, B. (1996). Managed care, primary care, and quality for children. *Current Opinion in Pediatrics, 8*, 164–170.

Saha, S., Komaromy, M., Koepsell, T. D., & Bindman, A. B. (1999). Patient-physician racial concordance and the perceived quality and use of health care. *Archives of Internal Medicine, 159*, 997–1004.

Schulman, K. A., Rubenstein, L. E., Chesley, F. D., & Eisenberg, J. M. (1995). The roles of race and socioeconomic factors in health services research. *Health Services Research, 30*, 179–195.

Sebastian, J. G., & Bushy, A. (Eds.). (1999). *Special populations in the community: Advances in reducing health disparities*. Gaithersburg, ND: Aspen.

Seid, M., Varni, J. W., & Kurtin, P. S. (2000). Measuring quality of care for vulnerable children: Challenges and conceptualization of a pediatric outcome measure of quality. *American Journal of Medical Quality, 15*, 182–188.

Seid, M., Varni, J. W., Olson-Bermudez, L., Zivkovic, M., Far, M. D., Nelson, M., & Kurtin, P. S. (2001). Parent's Perceptions of Primary Care measure

(P3C): Measuring parents' experiences of pediatric primary care quality. *Pediatrics, 108,* 264–270.

Singer, M., Valentin, F., Baer, H., & Jia, Z. (1992). Why does Juan Garcia have a drinking problem? The perspective of critical medical anthropology. *Medical Anthropology, 14,* 77–108.

Siu, A. L., McGlynn, E. A., Morgenstern, H., Beers, M. H., Carlisle, D. M., Keeler, E. B., et al. (1992). Choosing quality of care measures based on the expected impact of improved care on health. *Health Services Research, 27,* 619–650.

Snow, L. F. (1993). *Walkin' over medicine.* Boulder, CO: Westview Press.

Sobo, E. J. (1995). *Choosing unsafe sex: AIDS risk denial among disadvantaged women.* University Park: University of Pennsylvania Press.

Sobo, E. J., & Seid, M. (2001, November 30). *Cultural issues in pediatric medicine: What kind of "competence" is needed?* Paper presented at the 100th annual meeting of the American Anthropological Association, Washington, DC.

Starfield, B. (1992). Effects of poverty on health status. *Bulletin of the New York Academy of Medicine, 68,* 17–24.

Starfield, B., Cassady, C., Nanda, J., Forrest, C. B., & Berk, R. (1998). Consumer experiences and provider perceptions of the quality of primary care: Implications for managed care. *Journal of Family Practice, 46,* 216–226.

Starfield, B., Riley, A. W., Green, B. F., Ensminger, M. E., Ryan, S. A., Kelleher, K., et al. (1995). The adolescent CHIP: A population-based measure of health. *Medical Care, 33,* 553–566.

Stein, R.E.K., & Jessop, D. J. (1982). A noncategorical approach to chronic childhood illness. *Public Health Reports, 97,* 354–362.

Stein, R.E.K., & Jessop, D. J. (1990). Functional Status II-R: A measure of child health status. *Medical Care, 28,* 1041–1055.

Stewart, A. L., Napoles-Springer, A., & Perez-Stable, E. J. (1999). Interpersonal processes of care in diverse populations. *Milbank Quarterly, 77,* 305–339.

Stolz, J. W., & McCormick, M. C. (1998). Restricting access to neonatal intensive care: Effect on mortality and economic savings. *Pediatrics, 101,* 344–348.

Szilagyi, P. G., & Schor, E. L. (1998). The health of children. *Health Services Research, 33,* 1001–1039.

Thomas, S., & Quinn, S. (1991). The Tuskegee Syphilis Study, 1932–1972: Implications for HIV education and AIDS risk education programs in the black community. *American Journal of Public Health, 81,* 1498–1505.

Trotter, R. T., II, Ortiz de Montellano, B., & Logan, M. H. (1989). Fallen fontanelle in the American Southwest: Its origin, epidemiology, and possible organic causes. *Medical Anthropology, 10,* 211–221.

U.S. Department of Health and Human Services. (2000). *Healthy people 2010:*

Healthy people in healthy communities. Washington, DC: Government Printing Office.

Varni, J. W. (1983). *Clinical behavioral pediatrics: An interdisciplinary biobehavioral approach*. New York: Pergamon Press.

Varni, J. W., Seid, M., & Kurtin, P. S. (1999). Pediatric health-related quality of life measurement technology: A guide for health care decision makers. *Journal of Clinical Outcomes Management, 6,* 33–40.

Varni, J. W., Seid, M., & Kurtin, P. S. (2001). PedsQL 4.0: Reliability and validity of the Pediatric Quality of Life Inventory Version 4.0 Generic Core Scales in healthy and patient populations. *Medical Care, 39,* 800–812.

Varni, J. W., Seid, M., & Rode, C. A. (1999). The PedsQL: Measurement model for the pediatric quality of life inventory. *Medical Care, 37,* 126–139.

Vivier, P. M., Bernier, J. A., & Starfield, B. (1994). Current approaches to measuring health outcomes in pediatric research. *Current Opinion in Pediatrics, 6,* 530–537.

Wallander, J. L., Varni, J. W., Babani, L., Banis, H. T., & Wilcox, K. T. (1988). Children with chronic physical disorders: Maternal reports of their psychological adjustment. *Journal of Pediatric Psychology, 13,* 197–212.

Ware, J. E., Jr., & Sherbourne, C. D. (1992). The MOS 36-item short-form health survey (SF-36): I. Conceptual framework and item selection. *Medical Care, 30,* 473–483.

Weinick, R. M., Weigers, M. E., & Cohen, J. W. (1998). Children's health insurance, access to care, and health status: New findings. *Health Affairs* (Millwood), *17*(2), 127–136.

Weissman, J. S., Witzburg, R., Linov, P., & Campbell, E. G. (1999). Termination from Medicaid: How does it affect access, continuity of care, and willingness to purchase insurance? *Journal of Health Care for the Poor and Underserved, 10,* 122–137.

Weller, S. C., Pachter, L. M., Trotter, R. T., II, & Baer, R. D. (1993). *Empacho* in four Latino groups: A study of intra- and intercultural variation in beliefs. *Medical Anthropology, 15,* 109–136.

Williams, D. (1990). Socioeconomic differentials in health: A review and redirection. *Social Psychology Quarterly, 53,* 81–99.

Williams, M. V., Parker, R. M., Baker, D. W., Parikh, N. S., Pitkin, K., Coates, W. C., & Nurss, J. R. (1995). Inadequate functional health literacy among patients at two public hospitals. *Journal of the American Medical Association, 274,* 1677–1682.

World Health Organization. (1948). *Constitution of the World Health Organization*. Geneva: Author.

8

. . . .

Standardized Approaches
to Clinical Care
Pathways and Disease Management

Patricia J. Richardson, Elisa J. Sobo, Erin R. Stucky

A child with asthma arrives at the emergency department late one afternoon, clearly in distress. He is wheezing and having trouble catching his breath. Nurses quickly identify him as a child with asthma and immediately begin treatment. They know exactly how to treat the boy's problems not because they know all about pediatric asthma (which as experienced pediatric nurses they surely do) but because they have been trained in the use of a locally relevant asthma pathway. The pathway provides them with a specific set of sequential instructions complete with clear and concise decision-making criteria so that the care the child receives is standardized to the best possible evidence-based practices.

Pathways are standardized, evidence-based action sequence recommendations for providing specific diagnosis- or procedure-related health care services. They are developed locally, with high participation of end users. **Disease management (DM)** is the coordination of services that provide comprehensive approaches to chronic illness conditions (such as diabetes or asthma) and rely heavily on the pathway methodology.

In this chapter, we explain how applied child health services researchers develop and implement pathways and DM programs. We describe how the outcomes or impacts of pathways and DM may be measured. The pathway (and DM) process is not one that researchers alone can accomplish; the key to success is the active, informed engagement of end users. Clinicians and, in the case of DM, patients will ultimately put the pathways and DM plans to the test. Before discussing the details of the pathway and DM process and the secrets to successful pathway and DM implementation, we will review the context in which the national interest in guideline development developed.

Background: The Need for Standardization

Pathways are locally created; by contrast, guidelines are official practice recommendations generated by professional bodies such as the American Academy of Pediatrics. In 1989, the Agency for Healthcare Research and Quality (AHRQ) was asked by Congress to form a committee to begin developing health care guidelines in an effort to address the need for consistent, high-quality patient care. The committee's charge was to identify "best practices" for diagnoses and, using an expert panel, to develop nationally applicable guidelines for specific diagnoses and procedures. The guidelines would provide evidence-based recommendations on standardized action sequences. Since then, the committee has developed many sets of guidelines. AHRQ's efforts have facilitated local implementation of the guidelines and have motivated health service personnel to develop their own site-specific guidelines (that is, pathways) in many hospitals.

Cutting Costs

Unnecessary variation results in added costs, overuse of services, and lower quality of care (Kurtin, 1997). Guidelines can promote standardization of care, which counteracts these problems. They were of particular concern for health plan officials in the early days of guideline development. High cost and overuse were also issues from the end users' point of view. Health plan members expressed concern that physicians might be charging excessively for procedures or care, performing unnecessary surgeries for profit, and ordering unnecessary tests or follow-ups.

Simply promoting lower use rates for specialty services or tests and capping primary care services did little to help the health plans manage costs. The expense of newer, high-priced tests and medically necessary drugs remained a factor, and cost-reducing efforts frequently resulted in more testing at a later stage of illness, leading to higher costs than would have been necessary if the original patient care plan had not been reduced.

These high costs might have been avoided if health plans had promoted preventive approaches; with prevention, a little spending now can mean big savings later. Health plans, however, responsible for paying for the services rendered to their members, were usually not concerned about long-term outcomes or the care of a member over his or her lifetime because members move in and out of systems. Health plans therefore found the managed care approach appealing.

Managed care is a method originally designed by health insurers to compel caregivers, including clinics, hospitals, and physicians, to manage health in a cost-efficient manner. It is a system of health care delivery in which reimbursement influences the use and cost of services, and it also serves as a measure of performance (Coughlin & Long, 2000). Managed care systems aim to deliver cost-effective care through the adoption and dissemination of practice guidelines. Nonadherence by providers can negatively affect reimbursements.

Because health care costs were highest in the 1990s on the East and West Coasts (Kurtin, 1997), insurance companies and Medicaid targeted these areas for the implementation of managed care as a means of control. Physicians in these areas grew fearful of losing patients to managed care, and many decided to join such organizations themselves. Unfortunately, lacking an understanding of contract detail, they agreed to care for patients at rates that did not cover costs.

Managed care seemed to many physicians to mean more than severe financial constraints—it also meant an end to traditional doctoring. Managed care challenged physician control of which and how many patients could be seen, treatment options, and the way outcomes were measured, as well as how much should be charged.

It challenged the position of the physician as the expert on medicine. To succeed in the new business era of medicine would require, for physicians as well as for the organizations that employ them, a paradigm shift.

New Models for Care

Managed care has forced physicians and health systems to reevaluate how they think about health care delivery. They have been driven not only to incorporate (or at least try to incorporate) guidelines into practice but also to also develop methods for internal cost reporting so that real costs might be calculated and tracked. Guidelines and cost accounting may seem antithetical to traditional doctoring, but they do provide a way to reduce unnecessary variation and to improve (and track improvements in) cost effectiveness. Guideline adherence can also lead to quality improvements—a benefit that is now receiving equal attention. This more inclusive view of the benefits of guidelines has come about in part due to the growth of research clearly demonstrating quality improvement results (Diaz-Rossello, 1999; Kennedy, 1999), as well as sociopolitical shifts in the importance ascribed to the safety and effectiveness of health care (Institute of Medicine, 2001; see also Chapter One, by Kurtin).

But guidelines are not enough. Local adherence to externally generated guidelines (such as those AHRQ or other organizations have developed) is known to be problematic (Cabana et al., 1999; Ornstein & Jenkins, 1999). Physicians frequently resent guidelines, inferring a message that their skills in determining what is best for the patient are not valued (Christakis & Rivara, 1998). Excessive complexity and poor-quality evidence have been identified as barriers to adherence, as have organizational factors, such as contradicting policies (Katz, 1999). Guidelines that do not mesh well with local clinical workflow patterns may not be implemented (Sun et al., 1999), and those that are too general may actually result in increased mismanagement (Shekelle et al., 2000). Unclear or very restrictive inclusion and exclusion criteria can foster poor interobserver reliability in interpretation and implementation (Katz, 1999). This has been demonstrated, for example, in relation to pediatric asthma guidelines (Werk, Steinbach, Adams, & Bauchner, 2000). Pathway (and DM) programs, as we will show, help offset some of the barriers to adherence described, because the people who will use them actually build them.

Focused learning about new models for patient care delivery (such as the pathways model) must take place throughout health care. At Children's Hospital and Health Center in San Diego, senior leaders have strongly supported the goal of identifying best practices for patient care as a part of efforts to maintain or decrease costs. Children's experience with pathways provides a prime example of how quickly a culture of learning can help ensure a system's survival in an era of managed care. With the adoption of innovative programs such as pathways and DM and the willingness to share what has been learned and to promote innovation in other health care settings, Children's is paving the way for other health care systems to not only survive but also thrive.

Pathways

A clinical pathway is a locally developed care **algorithm**—a decision tree that leads the caregiver through a series of questions and so to the most appropriate care ("If X, do Y"). Pathways are designed to increase the likelihood of positive outcomes based on the effective (evidence-based) and efficient use of resources. Paul Kurtin (1997) has described the large gap between what is known to be best practice and actual practice. Clinical pathways provide care specifications or action sequence instructions for the management of specific patient conditions while also serving as a systematic approach to quality improvement through the limitation of unnecessary variation. Unlike guidelines, pathways are internally generated, with high participation from end users.

Pathway development and implementation require cultural change. A system capable of implementing pathways first requires an enabling social structure—including a team to carry the pathways out. The team must be stable enough to be dependable, with consistent member dedication and reliable resources. Team members must be given equal authority: physician members cannot and should not have complete, unquestioned control. Further, a physician member cannot act as a mere figurehead; physicians must be active and engaged as a pathway is built and implemented. The experience of Children's has shown that failure will occur if physicians are told about a pathway after data have been gathered and are being presented for review (the literature on guideline acceptance fully supports this observation).

The process of building each pathway using this core team structure is dynamic. Review of the literature, research, and integration of local best practices help members form the template for a pathway, but the actual use of a given pathway always leads to changes. This dynamic approach requires a culture shift away from reliance on retrospective patient chart reviews toward prospective and **continuous quality improvement (CQI)**. CQI methods differ from prospective clinical research methods; the latter have a definite endpoint and generally focus on single outcomes questions, such as if a particular medication is effective in treating a disease. CQI is a more fluid and, as the name implies, continuous process; further, it is meant to accommodate real-world situations, with their inherent messiness, whereas clinical research generally seeks to control for all variation (Shortell, Bennett, & Byck, 1998).

Plan, Do, Study, Act

The **plan, do, study, act (PDSA)** system of **rapid-cycle improvement**, promoted by the Institute for Healthcare Improvement (IHI), is the foundation for a clinical pathway process. PDSA is also known as the **Shewhart-Deming cycle**, after the individuals who pioneered it (Davidson, 1993). The IHI's version includes adaptations made by Thomas Nolan and colleagues (Berwick, 1996; Langley, Nolan, & Nolan, 1992).

The PDSA process is familiar to many clinicians because it provides the basis for most quality improvement efforts in hospitals and health systems today (Joshi & Bernard, 1999). At the same time, the idea of continuous quality improvement that PDSA is a part of has worked to raise the expectations of purchasers and consumers, increasing demand on health care systems to prove their value through better outcomes (Seid, Quinn, & Kurtin, 1996).

The steps of PDSA CQI are as follows:

1. Problem identification and planning (P)

2. Doing something to improve the process (D)

3. Studying the results (S)

4. Acting on the findings by making adjustments, as needed, to the original plan (A)

The PDSA cycle is repeated over and over as the process continues to improve.

The Planning Stage

A pathway is selected for development based on the use of both internal and external criteria, including those identified by Seid and colleagues (Seid, Stucky, Richardson, & Kurtin, 1999):

- High-volume and high-weighted cost

- Physician and other clinician interest and involvement

- Potential to reduce variation in costs

- Length of stay and resource use

- High-risk, problem-prone, or high-profile diagnoses or procedures

- External competitive drivers

"High-volume and high-weighted cost" refers to diagnoses that, although high in volume and low in individual cost, have high aggregate cost. An example of this type of diagnosis is bronchiolitis, in which the individual cost per case is fairly low but the number of cases is generally high, making it a high overall cost diagnosis.

The "physician or other clinician interest" criterion is used to identify a diagnosis or procedure that people are already convinced would lend itself to pathway development. The benefits of pathway development in this case are in diffusing the pathways and CQI processes. For example, the spinal fusion pathway was developed at Children's in San Diego because orthopedic surgeons were interested in using the pathway process to streamline patient care.

"Potential to reduce variation in costs" and "length of stay and resource use" refer to a diagnosis or procedure in which there is documented variation in practice related to costs, resources used, or length of stay. Children's neonatal intensive care unit (NICU) developed a blood gas protocol because analysis showed less than optimum use of monitoring equipment in conjunction with high numbers of blood gas determination tests being performed on neonatal patients. By building a protocol to improve the use of monitoring equipment at the bedside, the NICU team reduced variation and costs related to the number of blood gas determinations performed.

"High-risk, problem-prone, or high-profile" pathways are based on those types of diagnoses and procedures, such as complex open-heart surgery. Diabetes, which receives so much media attention and is increasing in prevalence, is a high-risk, high-profile diagnosis that is amenable to the pathway process.

An "external competitive driver" such as payer interest or managed care contract negotiations might also underwrite pathway development. For example, in 1993, Children's was in negotiations for a NICU contract, and the respiratory distress syndrome (RDS) pathway was developed to meet payer expectations. The use of comparative databases also fits here. The Office of Statewide Health Planning and Development (OSHPD) in California is one of the databases that can be used for comparing internal practices to other hospitals in the region or state. OSHPD compiles basic diagnoses, charges, and demographics that may indicate patterns that, when compared to other institutions, show a need or potential to improve clinical practice. These findings can lead to the development of a pathway. Two additional databases that are used for comparison purposes are the National Association of Children's Hospitals and Related Institutions (NACHRI) and the Pediatric Health Information System (PHIS).

Reviewing the Problem

Once a diagnosis or procedure has been chosen, baseline data are collected. For example, a run chart of direct costs by discharge date may be used to evaluate variation currently in the system and the level of opportunity for improvement. A *run chart* graphs changes in a process over time and helps identify unnecessary variations (see Figure 8.1). This type of chart is reviewed in terms of how much and what types of variation are occurring with the diagnosis or procedure. Patient chart review is also used to capture information on key branch points for the pathway. (Data collection and presentation are discussed further in our description of the study phase of PDSA.)

Variation indicates whether a diagnosis or procedure has inconsistencies in resource use or length of stay that are unrelated to individual patient need. **Common cause variation** is variation that is inherent to a process, such as an equipment limitation or lack of or inconsistent methods or procedures. **Special cause variation** is variation in a process that is unusual or unexpected, as may occur when using new equipment or implementing a new idea in patient care. Both types of variation can be improved (that is, reduced) through analysis and the use of pathways. Exploring the scope and causes of variations in given diagnoses or procedures helps in the identification of specific areas where there are opportunities for improvements (Brassard, 1989; Melum & Sinioris, 1992).

Figure 8.1. Run Chart of Direct Costs Before and After Pathway Implementation.

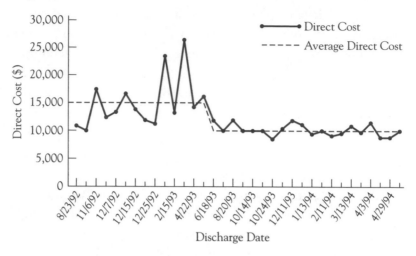

Reviewing the Literature

In addition to examining variation, a literature review must be done during the planning stage. This is because the practice of evidence-based medicine requires the conscientious, explicit, and judicious use of current best evidence in making decisions about individual patient care (Sackett, Rosenberg, Gray, Haynes, & Richardson, 1996).

The Cochrane Library houses many articles that use a meta-analytic approach in which the quantitative findings from a number of studies are themselves subjected to quantitative analysis. In addition to Cochrane Library searches, data gathering for a literature review should include a review of national and international medical databases, Association or Academy guidelines or statements (if available), and relevant literature from related disciplines (such as nursing or social work). Although older landmark articles should be included, searches should be focused on the most recent three to five years of published literature. Reference lists should be limited to ten to twenty items so that a reasonable review by pathway team members can be anticipated. Search strings can include such terms as *meta-analysis, review, guideline, consensus, overview,* or *evidence-based* and can exclude (using the search term BUTNOT) *editorial, comment,* and *letter* (Shojania, 2001).

The Pathway Development Team

The pathway team will review the literature, supported by the facilitator and the clinician who instigated (or was recruited to help instigate) the pathway in question. The facilitator must be an impartial party with the skills necessary to keep a group on track during and between meetings. The facilitator must be respected by the members of the group and must understand the data and the system under review.

The first meeting should be a one-on-one meeting between the pathway instigator and the facilitator to review group membership. They should then review the data and produce a first draft of the pathway, setting the stage for the larger group meeting. Multidisciplinary membership in this group (the "team") should include up to five of the top high-volume admitting physicians for the diagnosis or procedure in question, appropriate specialty physicians, nursing staff, social workers, local experts, and any other disciplines involved in the care plans for the diagnosis or procedure in question, such as pharmacists, laboratory technicians, business associates, and medical records clerks.

All members of the team provide important information and insight. In many cases, members will not have previously worked together and will not have shared patient treatment ideas, plans, or rationales for patient care. Team building is an essential part of successful pathway development. Individuals must be taught to think of themselves as part of a larger collective in which the whole is greater than the sum of its parts. Collaboration, insight, and cohesiveness develop as members of each discipline share information on their roles with other members of the group. A successful multidisciplinary development process can lead to enhanced systemwide teaming as individual change and organizational change reinforce each other.

Research suggests that when early adopters have higher status and larger social networks, they will be more influential in promoting the diffusion of an innovation; that is, "biased" cultural transmission is the dominant force in promoting individual (and, through this, organizationwide or culturewide) behavior change (Henrich, 2001). Therefore, carefully identified physician and nurse champions are crucial to a team's success. **Champions** should be individuals who both understand an innovation's importance and are well respected by their peers.

The physician champion leads the pathway development by providing both medical expertise and team leadership. The physician champion is chosen for the group on the basis of medical expertise, leadership skill, and level of interest (frequently, this is the same physician who instigated the project). Physician champion responsibilities include gaining other physician support, disseminating new ideas, educating peers, and maintaining momentum throughout the development and implementation process.

A *nurse champion* is a nurse who shows leadership ability, comprehensive knowledge of the diagnoses, and high commitment to the pathway process. Nursing leadership is responsible for providing valuable input to the development process on the teams as well as implementing and monitoring compliance with the pathway in day-to-day patient care. Nurses are critical to pathway support and compliance as educators, bedside experts, and patient advocates. Nurses also have training that emphasizes an understanding of the clinical and emotional needs of both patient and family (Manion, 1993). Other clinical specialists are also needed to champion the pathways when their services make up a large percentage of patient care, such as respiratory therapists in asthma cases.

Team membership of seven to ten individuals from diverse work areas ensures multidisciplinary input without inhibitory numbers of people; the facilitator and lead clinician should draw up the invitation list accordingly. Our experience at Children's suggests that there should be twice as many names on the list as required, to allow individuals to opt out if they wish. Requests for involvement should be sent to all potential participants, with follow-up phone calls as necessary. The first draft of the pathway (designed with the instigating clinician) and the list of references and copies of key articles should be sent to all committed team members before the first meeting so that they may review them prior to the meeting.

The Doing Stage

The initial pathway-building process can be accomplished with as few as three full-group meetings. Each meeting has a particular focus:

Meeting 1: Data presentation and decisions on questions to be answered from the first draft of the pathway

Meeting 2: Review of changes incorporated after members have completed the review reading and sent their comments to the facilitator

Meeting 3: Review of the final product, with last-minute detail changes; planning for implementation and education in all areas affected

Intervals of two to four weeks between full-group meetings are optimal to maintain enthusiasm and interest yet allow time for in-depth review of data and information (Melum & Sinioris, 1992; Scholtes, 1988).

At the first group meeting, the facilitator should review the team ground rules as well as the general rationale for the pathway. Any baseline data assembled by the facilitator (such as the run chart or cost and variation information) should be presented. After this, many questions will arise and ideas about other possible pathways will surface. Additional aims will be suggested, so limiting the team's attention to realistic, achievable goals is critical.

The first full-group meeting is followed by a period of informal communication during which a revised pathway is designed. The facilitator and the physician champion meet occasionally to review questions and details that arise. Subsequent full-group meetings are thereby limited to reviewing significant changes to the initial pathway's algorithm and implementation planning.

Although there may be only three meetings, each team member is expected to participate throughout the process. The physician champion and facilitator are responsible for ensuring that each part of the action plan is implemented. Key components are adherence to timelines and respect for what the literature reveals: each decision regarding the pathway algorithm should include references to the literature so that the resulting product is evidence-based.

When consensus has been reached regarding the pathway design, it is time for implementation. Most pathways require a three- to six-month pilot period. Pilot pathway implementation is most successful when overseen by a team with consensus. All team members are role models and should be considered champions for education, making themselves available for questions or comments (as so-called go-to people).

Acceptance of a new method beyond the team (that is, in the unit where the pathway is to be implemented) requires behavioral intervention and system simplification. Training programs are most effective when supported by invested core staff physicians who are present daily to educate the constant influx of new house staff (Seid et al., 1999). Concurrent monitoring of pathway acceptance and requesting feedback from all users allows for quick and simple modifications of aspects that might otherwise cause a pathway to fail (for example, creating computer drop-down menus when users find that typing in entries slows them down). Attention to process details, such as simplifying order sets and figuring out ways to have a pathway algorithm print automatically during registration, help immensely. The physical presence of team members in the affected department during the first few weeks of implementation for support and troubleshooting cannot be emphasized enough.

During the pilot phase, changes to a pathway may be made as necessary. Identifying areas that may be amenable to change by using the Pareto principle helps (Scholtes, 1988). According to the **Pareto principle**, also known as the *80–20 rule*, in any system, 80 percent of the trouble arises from 20 percent of the system. In other words, regardless of the process being examined, the majority of procedural failures will stem from a few specific breakdown points. For example, we found that extensive use of lab testing in neonatal patients was the primary variation from the respiratory distress syndrome pathway; when orders for certain lab tests were reduced, variation decreased.

The Studying Stage

Although many aspects of the pathway process can be studied real time, it is valuable to set aside time for formally scrutinizing the results. Adherence to the pathway, barriers to implementation, and ability to streamline care should be fully discussed. Financial data should be presented in parallel with clinical data, with before and after costs noted. Though efforts should remain focused on the initial pathway goal or issue and the original outcomes intended, opportunities for evaluating additional quality parameters may emerge, and incorporating them may add validity to the process.

For example, elimination of repeated urine cultures in a clinically improving child on appropriate antibiotics decreases cost and eliminates a delay in obtaining a voiding cystourethrogram (VCUG), which helps determine whether damage has occurred in the renal system. During the pilot phase of the VCUG pathway, parents noted that repeated urine cultures were a significant quality issue: they were emotionally stressful, and parents preferred to avoid them.

Data Display

Data obtained during (or in a review of) the pilot phase should be displayed in the same format as the baseline data to allow for easy comparison. Definitions of statistical terms used should be repeated when reviewing the baseline data, highlighting the areas in question and again acknowledging known limitations of the information system.

The format for reporting results varies, depending on the audience and the time from pathway implementation. The first analyses after implementation should include the current percentage of adherence to the pathway and average length-of-stay (LOS) reports. Quality measures such as readmission rates, transfers to higher level of care, or revisits to the emergency department after discharge are also reported. Charts that give quick, easy-to-read views of the initial pathway findings are recommended.

Data derived from a **decision support (DS) system** should be used to give team members the broad clinical picture. Decision support systems are information technology systems set up to track cost information that can be used as a basis for organizational decision making. They are essential for providing an evidence basis for the types of claims regarding resource use or adherence to standards of practice on which pathway development is based.

Before DS data are presented to team members, clinical outliers need to be removed. **Clinical outliers** are patients excluded from analysis because of **comorbid** conditions or a particularly difficult disease course that makes their data inappropriate for comparison with data for the more typical or more homogeneous group. Statistically, these outliers are defined as all patients two standard deviations above or below the mean for LOS if the difference is due to patient condition and not just variation in management.

One tool used successfully to document a pathway's performance is a *cumulative proportion chart* (see Figure 8.2). In this technique for data display, each mark is a patient, with cost per episode plotted on the x-axis and percentage of patients on the y-axis. The more vertical the line, the less variation there is in practice. In addition, a shift of the line to the left indicates a decrease in variation and cost. It is important to recognize that the lines will never be perfectly straight because there will always be some degree of patient variation due to individual variations of disease processes.

Figure 8.2. Cumulative Proportion Chart for Patients with Asthma.

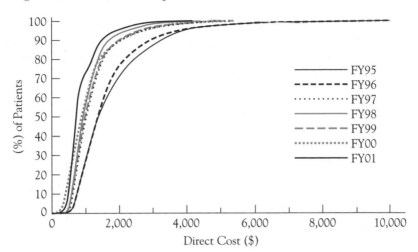

Other charts used to display data include bar charts (see Figure 8.3) and run charts (as in Figure 8.1). These charts give a quick, at-a-glance look at services and costs for the given pathway and show year-to-year comparisons as well as pre- and postpathway implementation costs.

Quality reporting is often more difficult to provide than cost, service, or compliance overviews because most medical information or DS systems are based on the accurate capture of charges. Future developments in information technology (IT), such as electronic medical records (EMRs), are promising as a means for collecting and analyzing patient interventions and quality. Enhancing the capability of IT systems is in fact crucial for improving the health care system. Nonetheless, even in the most limited DS systems, pre- and postpathway quality measures such as readmission rates, returns to emergency department (ED), and complication rates should be retrievable for use in making resource use comparisons. Resource use comparisons can be used to show that patients are getting better faster without revisits to the ED or readmission. This reporting

Figure 8.3. Bar Chart for Patients Treated for Bronchiolitis.

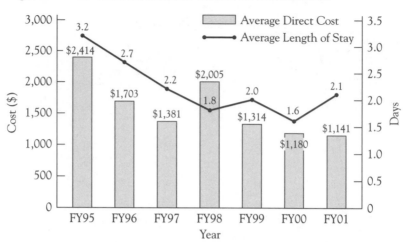

method may also be used to show that interventions that should be done as per the pathway occurred at higher rates while those that should not be done occurred at lower rates. This may result in faster resolution of clinical problems and hence a decrease in LOS.

When clinical data are available, they should be made use of, and this can often be done in tandem with cost data, such as for oxygen use. For example, during the development of our asthma pathway, a comparison of the number of hours asthma patients used oxygen on average to reach recommended safe oxygen saturation showed a dramatic decrease. Clinical data confirmed that patients reached recommended oxygen saturation at a much faster rate using the clinical pathway.

We are currently evaluating other tools for measuring quality and clinical outcomes using patient care data. These tools include recognizing zero charges for nonchargeable interventions (coding nonchargeable interventions as costing $0 so that data can be re-trieved from the DS database) as well as the ongoing development of a trackable clinical documentation system.

Fearless Use of Data

Clinicians generally want to improve their practice of care and will look for opportunities to do so. Data are often linked to physicians because of their authoritative role as care team members. *Blinded data* (in which the physician link is not revealed) allow for critical analysis of the outcomes obtained and any unforeseen barriers to change; fear of being the scapegoat abates when outcomes and global improvement, and not individual physicians, are the targets. At the same time, care must be exercised when data reveal problems among members of the health care team. Such information should be shared in a confidential manner with those individuals under the usual peer review and evaluation processes established at each step.

Confidentiality strictures also apply in regard to the patients whose data are being accessed for discussion. Data should be presented only in aggregate. Wherever the pathway process is implemented, care should be taken to apprise all team members of local, state, and federal regulations regarding patient data use so that patient privacy is respected. Regulations are controversial and evolving, so constant updates may be needed.

At the study stage, team members are frequently excited to present the data to their peers as well as administrators. Armed with data they understand and plans they have developed and can validate, team members can approach administrators, who reap the benefits of decreased cost and LOS, improved patient satisfaction, decreased medication error rates, and invested physicians and health care staff members. This last aspect cannot be emphasized enough, especially in an environment of change that has had business and clinical professions at odds with one another. The trust that must be maintained and nurtured between the two groups is critical to the survival of medicine as a respected profession. For example, physicians have a responsibility to use resources responsibly, but at the same time, administrators have a responsibility to support physician-directed care decisions. The pathway and algorithm process offers a unique method by which to achieve these goals with neither participant feeling disrespected.

The Acting Stage

Once the team has studied the pathway data collected over the course of the pilot phase, it is time for formal modifications. The algorithm is altered in keeping with findings, and a new version of the pathway (incorporating all of the modifications that tests proved efficacious) is approved. Once this version has been distributed, superseding any versions previously available to the care teams, the full cycle of PDSA has been run. The resulting pathway has generated quality patient care while eliminating redundant or unnecessary interventions and decreasing costs.

The newly approved pathway format becomes the working version for a new round of PDSA. The intense fine-tuning seen during the initial pilot (do) phase is rarely repeated, but the pathway remains open, as a living document, so that further modifications may be made as needed. Pathway data collection and monitoring are continuous, and as new issues arise due to the changing landscape of health care (perhaps a new test is introduced that should be incorporated, or patient volume decreases or increases, resulting in changed flow needs), pathway data must continue to be studied and acted on.

Long-Term Learning

In 1993, when Children's first initiated the pathways program, a single pathway took eight to ten meetings and about nine months to develop. As noted earlier, an initial pathway or template can now be designed in just three meetings and in no more than six months.

The original pathways primarily documented current practice; documenting best current practices was the desired outcome. At that time, we could identify cost components of patient stays associated with a given diagnosis or procedure; that is, we were limited to tracking data linked to a charge through our DS system. Due to the lack of clinical detail, randomly sampled chart reviews were required to obtain the necessary clinical detail.

When the pathway program was first started, most clinicians were not used to reviewing population-based data, such as analyzing the cases of more than four hundred children admitted with asthma in a single year. Data and information had to be given in small amounts, with plenty of explanation and guided interpretation. The evolution of the clinicians' capacity for data analysis has dramatically changed as team members moved from fearing data to demanding data. This change has been accompanied by a shift in the ownership of developing pathways from hospital administration to physicians and other clinicians, who generate ideas for pathway development rather than receiving them as requests from the administration. They now engage in peer-to-peer, physician-to-physician evaluation, improving pathway compliance.

In the early days, the information gleaned from the data review was mapped to a blank day-by-day form that described patient care activity, from diagnostic testing to milestones in management and patient recovery. These excessively detailed data were then collated into a pathway template outlining current practice. The team used this outline to assist with the development of the consensus-based, streamlined pathway.

Once the pathways were in template form, the team sought to improve the processes of care. Team members were encouraged to ask questions in regard to the processes mapped ("Why are we doing this? How could we do it differently while maintaining or adding or care quality?"). Answers facilitated streamlining the pathways and determining best local practices. The team was then encouraged to explore ideas beyond the usual experience, using available resources such as journals, benchmarking, and external expertise. Rather than focusing on the evidence, initial pathway work centered on building consensus.

These early pathways were extremely detailed, defining every intervention on a day-to-day or phase-to-phase grid (see Exhibit 8.1).

Exhibit 8.1. An Early Pathway.

Diagnosis _____ **Extreme Prematurity, 750–999 Grams** _____

Diagnosis Code _____

Procedure _____

Procedure Code _____

Unit/Acuity	Acute Unstable Phase
Consults	Social Services
Monitoring	Consider UAC, UVC, Continuous cardiorespiratory, TCM if skin cond. allows, Pulse oximetry, vital signs q1-2, wt. 2 x week or more, Head circumfer. q wk, Physical assessment q shift: breath sounds, pulse, capillary refill, skin integrity, heart & bowel sounds.
Non-Invasive Tests	CBC w/diff., H/H qd, clinically indicated: Lytes q 12-24 & Bilirubin days 2 & Ca qd, BUN, Cr q wk, New born screen as needed. Type & Coombs, Tox screen if meets high risk criteria Blood cult. x 1, ABG q 4-6, Glucose q 4-8 (chem strips) CXR/Abd. if clinically indicated and done at ref. hosp. Head US at day 1 & 7-10 days of life Check stools q shift for blood.
Respiratory	CPPV or HFV, Suction prn CPT if clinically indicated
Thermodynamic Regulation	Doublewalled isolette or radiant warmer or bubble isolette with servocontrol.
Hygiene	Inspect and debride skin. Bathe with water as tolerated.
Fluid Status	Occlusive skin covering require. > 200cc/kg/day to discontinue if < 150cc/kg/day. I & O
Diet	NPO with TPN started on day 3-7 if clinically indicated. Monitoring: calorie/kg/day, carbohydrate/kg/day, protein/kg/day.
Meds	Antibiotic levels/protocal before 4t dose. Amp/Gent x 72 Surfactant. Sedation (subgroup). Inotropic support. Immunizations.

Source: Children's Hospital San Diego. Reprinted by permission.

Stable Recovery Phase	Maintenance Phase
Consider Nutrition	Ophthalmology 4-6 wks
UAC or UVC discontinued Continuous cardiorespiratory, TCM, Pulse oximetry, vital signs q4, wt. 2 x week, Consider percutaneous/broviac line.	UAC discontinued, Continuous cardiorespiratory, TCM discontinued, Pulse oximetry, vital signs q3-4, wt. 2 x week, Peripheral blood pressure q shift.
H/H 2 x wk Lytes qd or QOD Ca qd or QOD ABG q shift, Freq. of chem screen 2 x wk. Head US at 7-10 days of life, Urine dipstick q shift.	H/H q wk. Lytes wkly. Ca wkly. ABG/CBG q 1-3 days, more frequent Clinically indicated. Glucose qd, Chem screen q week/ hyper alimentation.
CPPV	CPPV/CPAP
Doublewalled isolette or radiant warmer or bubble isolette with servocontrol.	Doublewalled isolette or radiant warmer or bubble isolette Thermo weaning.
Occlusive skin covering require. > 200cc/kg/day to discontinue if < 150cc/kg/day. I & O Bathing as toler. with HO or Cetaphil.	Occlusive skin covering require. > 200cc/kg/day to discontinue if < 150cc/kg/day. I & O
TPN/Start feeds.	Start feeds per protocal. Wean TPN
Amp/Gent discontinued. Sedation weaned. Inotropic support weaned. Consider steroids.	Consider steroids. Aminophylline/levels per protocal. Fer-n-sol at 4 wks when stable on feeds. Insulin Rx if clinically indicated.

Pathways have evolved from the detailed grid to a decision tree or algorithm. The decision tree is a much better analogue for the clinical thinking process than the grid, as it allows for the easier incorporation of naturally occurring changes or timing in the course of the diagnosis. For example, patients progress through the pathway based on their condition and results, outlined by the key indicators on the algorithm (see Exhibit 8.2).

Another major change is that a literature review (as described earlier) is now formally part of pathway development rather than an add-on and has assumed a predominant role. Each team member has homework to do between meetings and is expected to read literature, discuss findings and issues in his or her respective work area, and bring knowledge gained back to the pathway team meetings. After an evidence-based pathway is developed, any providers not wanting to use the pathway or even those disagreeing during development are asked to provide evidence to support their opposing practice opinions. This move to evidence-based development using medical and nursing literature made overall support from clinicians easier to achieve; in addition, it allowed the team to quickly reach agreement based on detailed and thoroughly reviewed literature.

Another factor behind the quicker pace of development has to do with increasingly sophisticated DS systems. The detailed clinical data they can provide include data on timing of interventions and cost-of-care processes. This added electronic information has greatly reduced the time-consuming chart review process. Now a smaller, more focused chart review is used to identify patterns of practice related to patient data not electronically captured. For instance, patient process markers such as a decrease in pain or a patient's ambulating are still captured only in chart review.

Experience has taught us that the pathway process should be as automated as possible. At Children's, the pathways, complementary order sets, and protocols print out with the patient's admission documentation forms, making implementation and adherence virtually seamless. This process supports departmental decisions making a pathway the default care standard. It is critical in providing a method for changing individual physician behavior in relation to a given procedure or diagnosis and as infrastructure support for the broader organizationwide culture change necessary for use and development of pathways.

Successful implementation of the pathways program required a major shift in individual clinician and support staff beliefs about what constitutes best patient care. The increase over time in familiarity with pathways was key here. As more pathways were developed and implemented, sharing the results worked to enhance the changing organizational culture in which CQI is valued. Now that the institution has many pathways in place, the initial training is not as lengthy, and many teams consist of people already using developed pathways. Further, organizational change supports individual change: as team work became part of the Children's culture, the organization began to provide training in the process of teaming. This in turn helped undergird our pathway-building efforts.

Results

Clinicians' initial compliance with pathway use was approximately 20 percent. The compliance figure has increased to over 90 percent in recent years. Not every patient should be placed on a pathway due to a complicated course of illness or comorbid condition; therefore, 100 percent compliance is never the goal. The dramatic change in compliance can be attributed to the cultural changes that occurred as more clinicians became involved and recognized the value of the pathways. Several critical steps occurred that helped make pathways the primary framework for patient care: the automation of the pathway and order sets and the approval of the pediatricians to make pathways the default for all patients with the given diagnoses. Physicians then had to order a patient off the pathways and give the rationale for doing so. This improved both pathway use and compliance and added to our impressive results (see Figure 8.4).

Exhibit 8.2. A New Algorithm Pathway.

Admit Criteria:

-Pt admitted with primary diagnosis of status
asthmaticus or recurrent wheezing or family hx of asthma
-No underlying disease (ie-CF, significant cardiac dx)
-Non-PICU pt

↓

Admit Orders: (RESPIRATORY)

SVN 0.03ml/kg of albuterol 0.5% diluted with 2cc
NaCL given Q2-4h
(can give up to 1cc albuterol)
Asthma Resp. Severity Score every tx
O2 to keep Sats 90-93%
Pre/Post PFMR if pt able
Begin Education Modules if strongly suspect asthma

↓

Admit Orders: (MEDICATIONS)

IV Hydration if clinically indicated by dehydration **OR** decreased
PO intake **OR** IV ABX needed
IV/IM Methylprednisolone (Solumedrol) for intital dose
1-2mg/kg **OR** PO Prednisone/Prednisolone 2mg/kg
THEN 1mg/kg Q6hrs (Max 120-180mg/day) until 50% personal
best PEFR or FEV1 then decrease to 1-2mg/kg/day divided BID
(Max 80mg/day)
ABX if clear evidence of bacterial infection
(ie sinusitis, pna-see pna algorithm)

↓

CONSIDER THE FOLLOWING:

Consider atrovent 250-500mcg mixed with albuterol Q4-6h prn X
24h (usually given Q20min X3 unless started in ER, then Q4-Q6prn)
         [OR until pt 50% personal best PEFR or FEV1]
Consider CBC if temp >101
Consider CXR if first wheezing episode or Temp >101 or Chest Pain
or Severe Resp. Distress
Consider ABG if indicated by: severe dyspnea or cyanosis or
prolonged hx of distress/patient tiring
Consider Electrolytes if frequent vomiting or dehydrated, or if
receiving frequent nebs over time, or co-existing cardiovascular
disease or on diuretics.
Consider Sinus XRAY if suspect sinusitis
Consider Anti-allergy medication if persistent nasal discharge.

Source: Children's Hospital San Diego. Reprinted by permission.

Monitoring

Continue to monitor and wean respiratory treatments
and oxygen as indicated by patient improvement
Wean and heplock IV when pt clinically improving and
able to take PO fluids and meds

If pt not clinically improving:

Consider: Continous Nebs per protocal
Consider: ICU, Asthma, Pulmonary or Allergy consult
Consider CXR

Discharge when pt meets discharge criteria:

Able to do peak flow meter if age appropriate
>70% predicted or personal best
Able to take PO fluids and meds
No oxygen requirement for at least 4 hours
Clinically responsive to bronchodilator-frequency no greater
than Q4hrs
No respiratory distress as indicated by: retraction, flaring, dyspnea
Discharge/Education Plan completed
Modules and Asthma Control Plan if suspect asthma
Homecare/PMD follow up scheduled
Consider referral to ADM program

Figure 8.4. Savings in the First Six Years of the Children's Hospital Pathways Program.

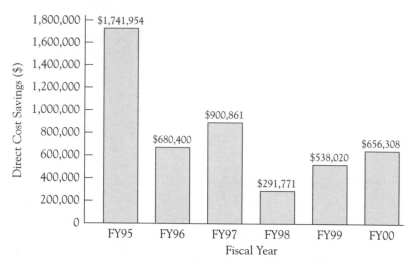

Children's pathways program has demonstrated its value through the continuous documentation of improved-quality patient care and decreased costs. In most instances, decreases in average length of stay also occur, although this is not necessarily a primary goal.

Disease Management

In addition to offering competitive pricing and documented high-quality care on a per-visit basis, hospitals, ambulatory care, and health care systems must now also document the quality of the services they provide over the course of the patient-system relationship. Disease management programs present an innovative approach to this dilemma. First, DM team members identify diseases that make extensive use of health care services. Comprehensive education and treatment (that is, DM) programs can then be developed targeting the patients most often seen for those specific diseases.

Due to its high and increasing prevalence in most pediatric care systems, asthma will be a high-utilization diagnosis, as it is at Children's. Our Asthma Disease Management (ADM) program was initiated in 1997 to address the needs of a large, severely asthmatic population. An asthma pathway was already in use, and through it we identified a subset of the asthmatic population ($N = 1,500$; $n = 144$) that had unacceptably high ED and in-patient encounter rates (more than two visits per year), and many of their inpatient stays were less than or equal to one day in length. Given these findings, all stakeholders involved in the care and follow up of severely asthmatic patients, including inpatient, outpatient, specialty care, and physician offices, were brought together to develop an action plan.

The DM Development Process

The ADM program's development illustrates the steps in the DM development process: steering committee formation, followed by program planning, testing, and modification, all according to the PDSA model. DM program development can be thought of as pathway development across time and place.

For ADM, a steering committee was formed, consisting of representatives from all areas of asthma care, including physicians, nursing, representatives from ancillary departments such as pharmacists, and community caregivers such as school nurses and home health visitors (a home visitor in our system is a layperson with at least a bachelor's degree in social work). The ADM program aimed to improve the health of the high utilizers.

Using *SWOT analysis*—in which participants are asked to identify their *strengths* and *weaknesses* and to examine the *opportunities* and *threats* that the process in question represents in order to facilitate the development of a strategic approach (Valentin, 2001)—the steering committee developed an integrated DM program. The program incorporated information systems linking parts of the continuum for patient care and tracking patient and family needs, resource allocation strategies, and DS-driven cost-benefit models. (SWOT can also be used for developing particularly complicated pathways.)

The ADM steering committee met weekly and aimed to initiate the first cohort within ninety days. Identification of the components, reimbursement, and outcomes tracking had to be designed, and it took four weeks to develop the program outline and begin to pilot the program on ten patients.

The DM program that emerged included assigning each of the severe asthmatics to a multidisciplinary care team consisting of a physician, a nurse case manager, a pharmacist, a home care nurse, and a home visitor. The nurse case manager coordinates all parts of the program, including the child's contact with the school nurses.

The program begins with an initial clinical screening during which the child and his or her primary caretakers are introduced to the care team. The child is trained in keeping an asthma diary (which helps monitor symptoms), educated regarding asthma, and assessed using two questionnaires, the PedsQL Health-Related Quality of Life Questionnaire (see Chapter Six, by Knight, Burwinkle, and Varni) and an asthma education assessment. The initial screening also includes allergy testing and the development of an actual plan for the child's care.

After this initial screening, home visiting begins and continues, weekly, for eight weeks. The first home visit includes a nurse as well as the home visitor, both assessing the patient's home environment and need for education or interventions. The home visitor alone completes the remaining seven visits. The home visitors are crucial because they are able to identify key nonmedical issues related to the specific patient's needs. In some instances, families face significant psychosocial or financial challenges, meaning that controlling the child's asthma is not their top priority. When this happens, the home visitors may link them up with resources beyond ADM.

In addition to the home visits, the child's assigned pharmacist calls the family weekly to check on medication refills and provide further medication education as needed. The ADM program, like all of our DM programs, is divided into three parts: the initiation or acute phase, the graduation phase, and the maintenance phase. For

ADM, the graduation criteria are categorized into three areas: physiologic, compliance, and quality of life. The time it takes to reach the graduation phase is generally eight weeks. Once a patient has met the criteria for graduation, he or she will enter the maintenance phase, which provides follow-up for the remainder of the year.

Key Success Factors for Pathways and DM

The success of Children's pathway and DM programs are due in large part to broad-based administrative and medical staff support. Administration, physicians, and clinical staff members now recognize the value of the clinical pathways and provide support in their respective areas.

Physician champions and nursing involvement have been essential for lending credibility to the pathways and DM projects and for providing support for collaboration around patient care. Reliable and consistent feedback from pathways and DM facilitators on both quality and cost has also been crucial to our continued success. Monthly, quarterly, and biannual reports regarding quality and cost-savings indicators are given to every pathway team, physician group, and department throughout the institution. Organizationally, Children's has explicitly chosen to be an outcome-driven institution, and resources have been explicitly dedicated to pathways and DM development, further ensuring success.

Culture Change

Children's has taken innovative steps to meet the challenges of the shifting health care environment. Culture change is the result of what leadership measures and pays attention to (Schein, 1992). The institutional incorporation of CQI principles has had a profound impact on CHSD culture. CQI, and the pathways and DM programs in which it is expressed, has become central to the institution's quality improvement program. Children's leaders began to pay attention to pathways and DM outcomes, and Children's staff followed suit.

As the high-quality, cost-efficient methods that we developed were shared with the public, Children's gained market share in areas not expected. Contracts were granted to Children's by hospitals and insurers in areas outside of California. This positive reinforcement lent further support to Children's goal of improving the culture of improvement.

Pathways have become part of Children's organizational culture. Diffusion is assured: as a teaching hospital, Children's has been able to use pathways and DM to give interns, residents, and medical students experience in and a full understanding of how to use evidence-based processes for patient care.

Next Steps

Success with clinical pathways and disease management has opened the door to ambulatory pathways (for use in the physician's office and other outpatient settings). For example, pathways have been developed for ambulatory diagnoses such as otitis media (ear infection) and asthma. However, ambulatory pathways are a challenge due to the fact that ambulatory settings such as individual physicians' offices may, for a complex set of reasons, lack the motivation to change that is seen in larger health care settings today. For instance, as Charles Homer notes, ambulatory settings provide less improvement infrastructure and fewer quality management resources than hospitals (Berman, 2002). Further, office physicians may be more isolated and have more years of practitioner experience than hospital physicians do and so may not be aware of (and in some cases may not be amenable to adopting) new or other ways of health care provision.

What is more, outpatient data are more difficult to collect for review than inpatient data. Inpatient settings generally have at least rudimentary DS systems (and the need for enhancement in this area has been noted), whereas ambulatory settings may have no electronic information systems at all. Teams may lack the ability to accurately track utilization and so to report on pathway progress without reverting to manual chart reviews. As technology improves, development and tracking of outcomes for ambulatory pathways will become easier, and the growth of ambulatory pathways should come to match that of hospital-based pathways.

Conclusions

Over the years, many changes in health care have occurred, including paradigm shifts relating to quality and cost reporting. At Children's, the shift toward pathways and DM has been a product of both external drivers and internal leadership. As managed care's impact on costs and the new focus on quality reporting took center stage, innovative pathways and DM solutions were devised. By involving all stakeholders and emphasizing true teamwork and the continuous nature of improvement, we helped make them well received and effective.

The benefits of pathways and DM go beyond individual programs. Leadership and physicians now play a less adversarial role with the entire hospital staff. This has led to a more focused, team-oriented approach, not only to patient care but also to all other aspects of Children's business. The overarching culture is one of cooperation, support, and teamwork. As Children's moves into the next era of health care, expectations are high that we will meet all new challenges in a way that supports our desire not just to survive but to thrive.

The process and development of pathways can work to help child health services research improve patient care in real time. Using the techniques described in this chapter can lead to the provision of high-quality, cost-efficient care, creating a platform for research as well as a start for contract negotiations with insurers. As information technology continues to evolve rapidly, integrating all areas of patient care becomes not only possible but even crucial to the future of patient care.

References

Berman, S. (2002). Improving children's health care: An interview with Charles Homer. *Joint Commission Journal on Quality Improvement, 28*, 139–147.

Berwick, D. M. (1996). A primer on leading the improvement of systems. *British Medical Journal, 312*, 619–622.

Brassard, M. (1989). *The memory jogger plus.* Methuen, MA: GOAL/QPC.

Cabana, M. D., Rand, C. S., Powe, N. R., Wu, A. W., Wilson, M. H., Abboud, P. A., & Rubin, H. R. (1999). Why don't physicians follow clinical practice guidelines? *Journal of the American Medical Association, 282*, 1458–1465.

Christakis, D. A., & Rivara, F. P. (1998). Pediatricians' awareness of and attitudes about four clinical practice guidelines. *Pediatrics, 101*, 825–830.

Coughlin, T. A., & Long, S. K. (2000). Effects of Medicaid managed care on adults. *Medical Care, 38*, 433–446.

Davidson, S. J. (1993). Closing the loop: Discard bad apples or continuously improve EMS? In R. A. Swor (Ed.), *Quality management in prehospital care* (pp. 55–69). St. Louis, MO: Mosby.

Diaz-Rossello, J. L. (1999). Evidence-based and value-based paediatrics. *Lancet, 28*, 354.

Henrich, J. (2001). Cultural transmission and the diffusion of innovations: Adoption dynamics indicate that biased cultural transmission is the predominate force in behavioral change. *American Anthropologist, 103*, 992–1013.

Institute of Medicine, Committee on Quality of Health Care in America. (2001). *Crossing the quality chasm: A new health system for the 21st century.* Washington, DC: National Academy Press.

Joshi, M., & Bernard, D. (1999). Classic CQI integrated with comprehensive disease management as a model for performance improvement. *Journal of Quality Improvement, 25*, 383–395.

Katz, D. A. (1999). Barriers between guidelines and improved patient care: An analysis of AHCPR's unstable angina clinical practice guideline. *Health Services Research, 34*, 377–389.

Kennedy, M. P. (1999). Implementation of quality improvement methodology and the medical profession. *Journal of Quality Clinical Practice, 18*, 143–150.

Kurtin, P. S. (1997). Assessing outcomes of care: Lessons learned at a CHHC hospital. *California Pediatrician, 15*(2), 14–21.

Langley, G. J., Nolan, K. M., & Nolan, T. W. (1992). *The foundations of improvement.* Silver Spring, MD: API.

Manion, J. (1993). Chaos or transformation? Managing innovation. *Journal of Nursing Administration, 23*(5), 41–48.

Melum, M. M., & Sinioris, M. K. (1992). Critical pathway. In *Total Quality Management: The health care pioneers* (pp. 305–314). Boston: American Hospital Association.

Ornstein, S. M., & Jenkins, R. G. (1999). Quality of care for chronic illness in primary care: Opportunity for improvement in process and outcome measures. *American Journal of Managed Care, 5,* 621–627.

Sackett, D. L., Rosenberg, M. C., Gray, J. A., Haynes, R. B., & Richardson, W. S. (1996). Evidence-based medicine: What it is and what it isn't. *British Medical Journal, 312,* 71–72.

Schein, E. H. (1992). *Organizational culture and leadership* (2nd ed.). San Francisco: Jossey-Bass.

Scholtes, P. R. (1988). *The team handbook*. Madison, WI: Joiner.

Seid, M., Quinn, K., & Kurtin, P. S. (1996). Hospital-based and community pediatricians: Comparing outcomes for asthma and bronchiolitis. *Journal of Clinical Outcomes Management, 4,* 21–24.

Seid, M., Stucky, E. R., Richardson, P. J., & Kurtin, P. S. (1999). Lessons learned from teaching clinical pathways at a pediatric hospital. *Seminars in Medical Practice, 2,* 16–20.

Shekelle, P. G., Kravitz, R. L., Beart, J., Marger, M., Wang, M., & Lee, M. (2000). Are nonspecific practice guidelines potentially harmful? A randomized comparison of the effect of nonspecific versus specific guidelines on physician decision making. *Health Services Research, 34,* 1429–1448.

Shojania, K. G. (2001). Evidence-based hospital medicine in real time: Using systematic reviews to keep up with the literature. *Hospitalist, 5*(1), 12–13.

Shortell, S. M., Bennett, C. L., & Byck, G. R. (1998). Assessing the impact of continuous quality improvement on clinical practice: What it will take to accelerate progress. *Milbank Quarterly, 76,* 593–624.

Sun, Y., van Wingerde, F. J., Kohane, I. S., Harary, O., Mandl, K. D., Salem-Schatz, S. R., & Homer, C. J. (1999). The challenges of automating a real-time clinical practice guideline. *Clinical Performance and Quality Health Care, 7,* 28–35.

Valentin, E. K. (2001). SWOT analysis from a resources-based view. *Journal of Marketing Theory and Practice, 9,* 54–70.

Werk, L. N., Steinbach, S., Adams, W. G., & Bauchner, H. (2000). Beliefs about diagnosing asthma in young children. *Pediatrics, 105,* 585–590.

Part IV

· ·

Child Health Outcomes

Broadening the Reach of Applied Research

9

Translating Research into Practice

Planning Research to Inform
Policy and Program Development

Kimberly Dennis

In Chapter Three, Elisa Sobo discussed the need for child health services researchers to understand a child's home and cultural environment, and in Chapter Five, Diana Simmes and I discussed the importance of knowing and working with the community to advance child health. There is another key stakeholder group in the **child health services research (CHSR)** field that applied researchers need to actively engage to improve child health and well-being: policymakers and practitioners. Just as applied CHSR investigators need to develop stronger relationships with the communities in which children and families reside, they also need to forge closer ties with the ultimate end users of their research findings. In this chapter, we broadly define *policymakers* to encompass the diverse group of individuals who have the ability to make or influence policy and program decisions at the national, state, and local levels. We use the term *practitioners* broadly as well, to include all who provide, administer, or manage child health programs and services.

Researchers, policymakers, and practitioners share the same underlying goal of improving children's lives. Yet there is a fundamental gap between these stakeholders that needs to be bridged, one that contributes to unnecessary variation in and poor quality of health care for children. This gap is best represented by the lengthy delay (at least one year) in getting research published and applying results to routine practice. For example, research has shown that for children with asthma, having a written asthma management plan lowers the risk of emergency department visits and hospitalizations (Lieu et al., 1997). However, we know that most children with asthma go home from the emergency department without such instruction. A community-based survey of children with asthma in inner-city New York found that only half of the children went home with written instruction (Warman, Silver, McCourt, & Stein, 1999). A group of researchers in Chicago studying children with asthma in three managed care organizations concluded: "Five years after the dissemination of national guidelines for care, the pattern of asthma therapy does not reflect guideline recommendations" (Donahue et al., 2000, p. 1108).

Early childhood development is an area that provides further example of this delay. Although scientists have known for more than two decades that the first few years are critical to a child's physical, emotional, and cognitive development, it is only in the past several years that this information has captured the attention of the public and policymakers (Sylvester, 2001).

As our understanding of how to strengthen child health and well-being deepens, researchers continue to struggle with how best to move insights "off the shelf" and into the "real world." Research rarely makes its way into the public debate on its own. Rather, researchers need to proactively determine who will learn about the research results, how they will learn about the results, how to ensure that useful information gets to people, and how to gain feedback from the community (Heymann, 2000). Researchers need to remember that "*how* evaluation information is used and disseminated is as important as *what* data are collected" (Woodbridge & Huang, 2000, p. 18; emphasis in original).

While researchers struggle to communicate their knowledge, policymakers, service providers, program administrators, and other practitioners actively search for appropriate, reliable, and effective science-based evidence to guide child health policy and program development. Malcolm Anderson and colleagues explain that not only are federal, state, and local policymakers searching for answers, but community-based agencies and organizations (CBOs) are also seeking out "much needed knowledge and analytical capacity from experienced researchers" to integrate research into their day-to-day operations (Anderson, Cosby, Swan, Moore, & Broekhoven, 1999, p. 1008). This is particularly true in the wake of *devolution*, as program control and accountability are shifted to the local level. Before researchers can effectively help CBOs, Anderson and colleagues assert, they need to develop a better understanding of the extent to which current research efforts meet the operational needs of CBOs, to what degree the transfer of research to local agencies actually occurs, and to what extent these agencies use research to inform policy and program development.

To address the needs of children and families effectively, a different kind of partnership must be forged among researchers, policymakers, and practitioners. In this chapter, we explore the nature of the gap between researchers, policymakers, and practitioners, why it is important to narrow the gulf, and how we can begin to do so. Our discussion focuses primarily on policymakers, though much of what is discussed applies to other users of research as well. We include an overview of the policy landscape so that applied CHSR personnel will better understand how to work within it.

Interdependence Among Researchers, Policymakers, and Practitioners

Researchers and policymakers each make their own important contribution to achieving the shared goal of improved child health outcomes. Researchers, for instance, can assess the need for new or different services, measure quality and outcomes of existing services, and identify the reasons why implemented programs succeed or fail (Zervigon-Hakes, 1995). Policymakers, for their part, can provide new funds or shift budget allocations as well as influence program effectiveness by establishing expectations and requirements concerning desired outcomes. The California Children and Families Act of 1998 (Proposition 10) is a good example of this. The act, which was intended to foster the physical, emotional, cognitive, and social development of children up to age five in California and enhance their school readiness, requires counties to identify desired outcomes and to document progress in achieving those outcomes.

Research on scientific, economic, social, and other issues is essential to framing public policy and contributing to public discourse. Policymakers are dependent on input from researchers and practitioners to understand the nature and extent of the needs of children and youth, as well as the benefits and drawbacks of the various options for meeting those needs. Indeed, in light of the rapidly changing nature of the health care system, policymakers and practitioners need access to well-grounded, evidence-based research (Sellors & Mitchell, 1998). For example, since the State Children's Health Insurance Program (S-CHIP) was created in 1997, states have been struggling with how to most effectively identify and enroll eligible children in no-cost and low-cost health insurance programs. Soon after S-CHIP went into effect, states learned that significant changes were needed. Indeed, in the past several years, states have streamlined application procedures, expanded coverage, and changed eligibility requirements. In an environment where policy is continually changing, policymakers and practitioners need to know, on a rapid-cycle basis, the effect of these changes on child health and well-being.

Philip Nyden and Wim Wiewel (1992) refer to research as a "political resource" that can be used to challenge and compel policymakers and institutions to bring about change that will benefit children and the larger community. They add, "Data that call into question a community organization's understanding of an issue, or its strategies in dealing with an issue, can be useful in providing a more accurate focus on the issue and developing more effective strategies" (p. 50).

While research should play an integral role in forming policy and program decisions, the reverse also is true: policies and programs should influence the questions researchers ask. Stryer and colleagues point out that researchers frequently need a deeper understanding of the type, quality, and quantity of evidence necessary to inform decision making (Stryer, Tunis, Hubbard, & Clancy, 2000). Further, as Michael Reich notes, "Health agencies tend to stress epidemiological and economic analyses, and they rarely use systematic political analysis in policy reform efforts" (1996, p. 2).

Efforts are under way to bridge this gap. Recognizing that the translation of research findings into sustainable improvements remains a significant barrier to improving the quality, efficiency, effectiveness, and cost effectiveness of health care, the Agency for Healthcare Research and Quality (AHRQ) committed funding for the development of researcher–health care system partnerships that can overcome this hurdle.

Key Reasons for the Gap

Partnerships among researchers, policymakers, and practitioners rarely emerge on their own because each group operates in a different culture with different demands, communication styles, and measures of success (Zervigon-Hakes, 1995). Although it is difficult to pinpoint all of the reasons associated with the divide, several common themes surface in the literature: relevance and usefulness of data, ineffective or limited communication and interaction, timeliness of research and policy implementation, and the general culture clash between researchers and policymakers regarding scientific rigor.

It is important to note that the following discussion of these elements is not exhaustive, nor are the various elements mutually exclusive. Rather, they come together to create a complex picture of the nature of the relationship between researchers and policymakers.

Anita Zervigon-Hakes (1995) captures this complexity: researchers can feel ineffective when their work does not result in immediate policy changes, and policymakers can be frustrated by researchers who overlook the important questions to study and present their findings with technical jargon and endless caveats.

Relevance and Usefulness of the Research

A resounding complaint of policymakers and practitioners is that studies done by outside researchers seldom reflect the needs of the agencies and organizations involved (see, for example, Anderson et al., 1999; Davis & Howden-Chapman, 1996). This problem can play out on several different levels. On one level, use of research findings has tended to focus on the larger policy environment or the clinical community and largely ignored the day-to-day operational needs of community-based health and social service agencies that serve children (Anderson et al., 1999). This seems to be changing as researchers are increasingly partnering with community organizations on studies (see Chapter Five) or are providing technical assistance to local organizations on how to use data for effective planning (see Chapter Four).

On another level, a good fit is often lacking between academic-driven research projects and an agency's service delivery mandate. For instance, research may be focused on high-profile issues that are not relevant to the development of an agency's core services. As a result, an agency's staff time and resources may be diverted from the primary focus of service delivery (Anderson et al., 1999). At still another level, programs or services may be planned, carried out, and evaluated without sufficient documentation of costs. Unless cost data are available and accurate, policymakers will have difficulty making decisions about which child health program or policy to adopt (Sechrest & Mabe, 1981).

Further complicating the issue of usefulness is uncertainty about and lack of guidelines indicating when data should lead to action. More than twenty years ago, Lee Sechrest and Paul Mabe pointed out that "we have no systematic way of deciding whether effects are large enough to warrant the development of policy" (1981, p. 67). Their case in point: even though research on a particular outreach program resulted in a statistically significant 12 percent increase in well-baby visits, it still did not answer the question of whether the program should or could be implemented regionally or nationally. Thus while statistical significance may be scientifically important, it may have little value in the clinical or direct service delivery world. This dilemma remains today, concur Kathleen McCartney and Eric Dearing: "Statistical significance tells you nothing about the size of the effect—that is, whether the program leads to meaningful differences in participants' lives. . . . There is no agreement on how to interpret effect size estimates" in the policy arena (2002, p. 4).

Still another dimension of the relevance question is the social and programmatic relevance of scientific rigor (Atwood, Colditz, & Kawachi, 1997). Managers and policymakers may be quick to ignore relevant research on the grounds that at key decision points, the conclusions that can be drawn from **randomized controlled trials (RCTs)** are too limited (Davis & Howden-Chapman, 1996). Further, policymakers' need to handle a broad range of issues that cut across disciplines is often in direct contrast to researchers' tendency to focus on a very limited, specialized area, in part to publish more frequently (Zervigon-Hakes, 1995). (See Chapter Five for further discussion of the need for CHSR to adopt innovative research methods.)

Ineffective or Limited Communication and Interaction

Traditionally, the researcher and the policymaker, program administrator, or other user of the research findings have been thought of as separate and independent, the communication among them linear and static, and the interactions between them few and far between. This is due in large part to the ostensibly objective way in which health research has been carried out in the past (Atwood et al., 1997). (See Chapter Five for a discussion of how this traditional researcher role is changing.)

An additional barrier to clear communication is the fact that researchers, policymakers, and practitioners do not always speak the same language. Researchers are trained to be analytical; their communications tend to take on a very academic or scientific voice; and they often focus on the details of the research process and its strengths and limitations, rather than on the implications for policy or program changes. Zervigon-Hakes explains: "Publishing in academic journals requires that researchers communicate their relatively esoteric knowledge using a technical language that is seldom understood by any but their peers" (1995, p. 180). This is in contrast to policymakers, who tend to favor far-reaching statements, gravitate toward the thirty-second sound bite or punchy headline, and weave points into stories that will resonate with the public.

Timeliness of Research and Policy Implementation

Timeliness is another obstacle to closing the gap between research and practice. Thomas Prohaska and colleagues note that even the most innovative behavioral research can become obsolete in the face of the rapidly changing health behavior issues in the community (Prohaska, Peters, & Warren, 2000). Researchers' practical understanding, they explain, changes far more rapidly than the speed with which they can communicate this knowledge, at least through the traditional research publication process, which can often take several years. In addition, changes in communities may not be communicated to researchers on a timely basis. Community practitioners are likely to observe and experience emerging health problems long before researchers and funders are aware of the problem.

S. Jody Heymann (2000) discusses a slightly different time-related challenge. He notes that long-term effectiveness is often the gold standard for researchers, and while it is the theoretical gold standard in policy programs as well, the practical reality is far different. Heymann explains that for policies to be passed, policymakers must believe the impact will be immediate—within the time frame of a political or budget cycle—so that benefits will be seen before the next election or budget negotiations. In the world of politics and budgeting, policies that take a long time to show results often do not last long enough to demonstrate their effectiveness.

Culture Clash

Although researchers, policymakers, and practitioners may share the same goals when it comes to improving the lives of children, their beliefs about the value and role that rigorous science plays in these efforts differ. Heymann (2000) describes several examples of this particular disconnection. In the research world, he explains, the technique of **multiple regression** tells us—holding everything else equal—what will likely happen if a given variable is changed. Yet in the policy or program world, rarely is a single, isolated change even possible. In many research fields, randomized controlled trials are highly regarded. Yet in the real world, where issues of cost and moral ethics may be more influential, it is difficult to convince a legislature to conduct a randomized controlled trial of social policy. And whereas randomized trials focus on program or service effectiveness in one defined setting, policy needs to be effective in a wide range of settings across the country. In some fields, particularly those that focus primarily on quantitative research methods, researchers look at measures of **central tendency** and may eliminate **outliers** or rare cases in calculating mean or average effects. Yet in the policy world, outliers can drive the debate, and individual stories are often used to capture media attention and symbolize the need for programs. (The influence of storytelling is discussed later in this chapter.)

Zervigon-Hakes (1995) and Sechrest and Mabe (1981) add that policymakers must often act on the basis of partial information or a few pilot studies to support a broad-based program. Research scientists, by contrast, tend to be more conservative and cautious, wanting instead to gather and analyze a preponderance of data and account for all mitigating factors before reaching a definitive conclusion. Interestingly, despite their differences, "policymakers still seek to wrap themselves in the legitimacy provided by researchers" (Zervigon-Hakes 1995, p. 181), using the perceived credibility of science to bolster their case.

Understanding the Policy Environment and the Role of Research

Not only is the real world "a moving target with treacherous currents," but children are "moving systems," too (Weiss, 1999, p. i). Thus the world of child health and public policy is dynamic, chaotic, serendipitous, and chock full of values—an environment in which "there are few dependable signposts or guideposts for translating research into policy" (Davis & Howden-Chapman, 1996, p. 869). Ron Haskins echoes this sentiment: "Like the planets, the current state of policy in a given domain exists in what might be called a dynamic equilibrium. Note that the operative word here is *dynamic*: this equilibrium can change" (1991, p. 617). Developing informed policy responses to problems and issues that reflect the insights and knowledge gained from applied CHSR is made even more difficult by the continuously shifting financial, political, and social context for both child health and the policy world (Grason, Minkovitz, Silver, Fountain, & Ashaye, 2001; Lewis, Saulnier, & Renaud, 2000).

Ann Kirwin (2001) argues that if CHSR professionals want policymakers to better understand the world in which children and their families live, they need to better understand the world of policy and politics. They need knowledge of the political landscape in which they are working (for instance, the community's or government's current priorities, policymakers' and the public's openness to change) and an awareness of the power structure with which they are dealing. This is increasingly important in the wake of devolution, as states, cities, counties, and other forms of regional government assume primary responsibility for financial administration and program control of children's services. Peter Pratt and colleagues add: "Depending on your location, the mayor's office may carry more weight in affecting policy change than the city council; or the majority party in the state legislature may be the first place to look for support or to introduce a bill" (Pratt, Floyd, Langley, Flynn, & McAuliffe, n.d., p. 81).

Further, the link between research and policy must be managed according to the given circumstances or situation. Peter Davis and Philippa Howden-Chapman (1996) point out that the translation strategy may differ, for instance, when dealing with policy change on a larger systems level (such as increasing access to care for children with special health care needs) compared to implementing new guidelines in a single clinical practice or unique community-based program setting (such as making sure that every child with asthma who comes into the local community clinic has a written asthma management plan). Davis and Howden-Chapman also suggest that researchers be more strategic in targeting desired policy areas by distinguishing between what they call the "policy core," which is rarely open to direct challenge and turnaround, and various "protective belts" of policy commitment, which are more open to change in light of research (p. 867).

Whatever the situation or audience, to effectively move findings into action and influence policy, applied CHSR investigators need to identify an achievable and viable solution to the given problem and determine what resources and assets are available to tackle a given issue. They need to know what motivates and drives the target audience of decision makers and present their case convincingly.

The next section is intended to help applied CHSR investigators better understand the policymaking environment so that they may design and undertake more policy-relevant research and effectively translate findings into action. It provides a brief overview of what policy is, who the key players are, and the dynamics that characterize the environment.

The Many Nuances of Policy

Policy can mean different things to different people. As Chapter Four points out, CHSR must negotiate a common frame of reference around outcomes and indicators. The same holds true for policy. Table 9.1, based on an article by Toby Citrin (2000), outlines how academics, practitioners, and community residents and organizations think about policy. Applied CHSR investigators need to understand the different vantage point of these diverse audiences if they are to design, carry out, and communicate research that will ultimately effect policy and program change.

Though the specific nuances of policy may differ according to group, the end goal of effective policy is essentially the same: to maximize the positive benefits of particular programs or interventions. Public policies affect the health and well-being of children and their families by determining what services we can provide, to whom, for how long, and at what cost (Kirwin, 2001). Consequently, policy-relevant CHSR should serve to answer such fundamental questions as: "Who shall receive the resources?" "Who shall deliver the resources?" "What is the nature of services to be delivered?" "What are the conditions under which the services will be delivered?" and "How did children's health and well-being improve as a result of these services?"

In conducting CHSR that seeks to bridge the gulf between research and policy, researchers should also be aware of the key principles of child health policymaking, as outlined by Stephen Berman (2000): integrity, credibility, fairness, and responsibility. *Integrity* involves gaining as complete an understanding of the issue as possible, communicating an unbiased assessment, and acknowledging both what is known and what is not. *Credibility* involves issues of conflict of interest and the belief that policymakers are serving the best interests of the children rather than the special interests of pediatricians, governmental agencies, or special industry. *Fairness* addresses the need to develop policy recommendations that result in

Table 9.1. Perspectives on Policy.

Policy Issue	Academics	Practitioners	Community Residents and CBOs
How to define "policy"	Recognized academic discipline involving the study of the processes by which institutions and organizations develop and adopt laws, rules, guidelines, and standard practices that govern their future activities.	Articulation of the rules, financing patterns, and guidelines within which they formulate and implement programs and deliver services.	Abstract concept not clearly related to the quality of life of the community. While the *effects* of policy decisions raise concerns or trigger actions in the community, the terms *policy* and *policy development* are rarely used to describe these actions.
How to view policy	From the perspective of those who study and teach.	From the perspective of their role as implementers.	From the perspective of personal experience (theirs or their friends and neighbors).
Starting point	The university or place where the research and teaching take place.	Public health department or health care organization.	Daily lives of people in the community.
Primary concerns	Tend to be research-oriented; search for factors that lead to success or failure of policy adoption and implementation.	Rules, guidelines, and budgets of those to whom they report and those who fund their activities.	Problems encountered in earning a decent living, maintaining a clean and safe environment, and improving the quality of life for themselves, their children, and their neighbors.
Scope and timing	Focus on the macro level—federal, state, and, less frequently, local and institutional policymaking; over large time spans.	Focus on the level of their own jurisdiction; over budget periods or terms of office.	Focus on the immediate, personal level; centers on local government and immediate tasks that need to be addressed in daily challenges they face.

Source: Based on "Policy Issues in a Community-Based Approach," by T. Citrin, 2000, in T. A. Bruce & S. U. McKane (Eds.), *Community-Based Public Health: A Partnership Model* (pp. 83–90), Washington, DC: American Public Health Association. Copyright © 2000 by the American Public Health Association. Adapted with permission.

one uniform standard of care for all children, rather than multiple standards that may be influenced by family income, insurance status, or other sociodemographic factors. Finally, *responsibility* entails recognizing how the consequences of the policy might have unintended effects detrimental to the public good. The design and conduct of applied CHSR needs to reflect an understanding of these principles, and researchers, as individuals, need to be able to address these issues when conveying their findings to policymakers.

Different Policymakers, Different Research Needs

Like researchers, policymakers are not a homogeneous bunch. Whether they are appointed, elected, or hired civil servants, and whether they act on the local, state, or national level, has implications for the amount and kind of research they need and how they will use it. Zervigon-Hakes (1995) provides an extensive overview of the different types of policymakers, how their roles and responsibilities influence their use of data, and guidelines for how researchers might best engage and reach them with important findings. What follows is a brief summary of the three types of policymakers she identified—elected officials, appointed legislative and executive branch staff members, and career policymakers—in addition to a discussion of key differences among state policymakers, the benefit of connecting with local officials, and the importance of staffers and nontraditional policymakers.

Elected Officials

Elected officials propose and approve the development, continuation, and expansion of publicly funded programs; they establish program goals and funding levels. Elected officials are driven by their constituents' interests, which means they often have a very specific agenda or concern for one particular issue.

When it comes to research, elected officials respond to publicly presented information. It is unlikely that they will read research directly in an academic journal; they will more likely learn about a new study from the media, a constituent, or an advocacy group. Elected officials want studies that provide information about constituent opinion and that show that new policies will lead to beneficial change for a number of groups. They also tend to focus on the broad brushstrokes of a program rather than the underlying detailed, complex components.

Elected officials' interest in changing policy is more often prompted by anecdotal data offered by a concerned constituent than by hard evidence presented by a researcher. For them, reality is the public's perception of the issue or problem.

Appointed Legislative and Executive Branch Staff Members

This group of policymakers resembles elected officials in many ways (and in fact they generally remain steadfastly committed to the elected officials who appointed them). Appointed legislative and executive branch staff members are driven to accomplish tasks within the same short budget and electoral time frames as elected officials. They are equally motivated to avoid controversy, to seek positive press coverage, and to undertake activities that will result in quick, positive outcomes. However, because they are responsible for managing the implementation of an administration's programs (and thus its goals and priorities), they have a greater need for detail and seek out more information about areas of concern than elected officials.

Career Policymakers

Career policymakers are a somewhat different group who view the world through a more defined and narrow lens. They are responsible for the more detailed program operations and the drafting of rules and regulations that govern the programs. Consequently, they gravitate toward research that evaluates program effectiveness or is designed to help improve program quality, and they may be especially interested in longitudinal studies and research that can be replicated in other settings. They are the policymakers who will read and understand fairly detailed research reports, using research findings to obtain increased budgets to improve the quality and scope of current programs. Career policymakers tend to be wary of large-scale change or rapid, massive shifts in programs.

The Challenge of Informing All State Policymakers

Not only are policymakers, as a whole, a heterogeneous group, but also within more discrete groups of policymakers, important differences exist in how they use information. In a study of state policymakers, Cynthia Jackson-Elmoore and colleagues found that while national policymakers tend to look to universities, think tanks, research reports, and journals to inform their efforts, state policymakers generally turn more to grassroots organizations, their own staff, statewide lobby groups, and national ethnic associations as their key sources of information (Jackson-Elmoore, Knott, & Verkuilen, 1998). This means that applied CHSR professionals must develop effective dissemination strategies to these sources, in addition to communicating their research findings directly to the policymakers. Even among state policymakers, differences exist. Jackson-Elmoore and colleagues further found that a policymaker's ethnic background and the type of district he or she represents affect what information sources are used. For example, state policymakers representing communities of color rate ethnic associations as one of their most important sources of information, while policymakers from rural districts rate the local offices of national associations as more important and those from upper- and upper-middle-class districts tend to prefer the media.

The Benefit of Connecting with Local Officials

Investigators seeking to translate their research into practice should also consider the value of linking to local officials. Joan Twiss (2001) outlines several reasons why local officials may be poised to take effective action on research: (1) city officials are positioned to be more responsive to local needs, values, and interests; (2) they have the ability to rally broad constituencies; (3) their personal values are more likely to be representative of the communities they serve; (4) increasing local control over programs and services makes the local level an obvious center of community engagement and primary prevention; and (5) less bureaucracy means implementation can happen more quickly.

The Importance of Staffers and Nontraditional Policymakers

Applied CHSR investigators must also look beyond the typical stakeholders to individuals behind the scenes who may also influence policy. These include, according to Pratt and colleagues (n.d.), staffers and nontraditional policymakers, such as leaders of the faith community; political consultants; members of business, labor, and community groups; professional association leaders; and the media. Pratt and colleagues urge researchers not to underestimate the role and importance of staff at any level—not only congressional staff and staff of other elected officials, but also those in various city, county, and state agencies and commissions; they write, "Staffers provide continuity and relative stability in a tumultuous political world where elections, hirings, firings, and other events can upset your best-laid plans overnight" (p. 152).

How Research Is Used in the Policy Environment

The relationship between research and policy is not always direct. Davis and Howden-Chapman (1996) indicate that models of the research-policy relationship range from one where empirical research rationally informs decision making to research that incrementally affects policy to an "enlightenment" or "infiltration" model. This last model, in which concepts and ideas infiltrate policymaking in a diffuse and indirect manner, is believed to be a more authentic and accurate reflection of the policy-research relationship than other models.

In essence, policymakers and practitioners use data in a variety of ways, some of which are not immediately apparent to researchers, such as to evaluate pending legislation, share information with colleagues, or identify contacts for further information (Bogen-schneider, Friese, & Balling, 2002). In fact, we can think of research being used along a policy development continuum. Along this continuum, researchers may play a number of different roles or strike a certain type of relationship with policymakers, such as consensual, contentious, or paradigm-challenging (Davis & Howden-Chapman, 1996).

Uses of data vary. At one end of the continuum, for example, data may be used for general education and awareness. Research is used to describe a problem, explain why an issue is important, and force the attention of policymakers. In this way, data can be a powerful asset in promoting a cause and making the case for policy change, as in the example of the Carnegie Corporation of New York's 1994 report, *Starting Points: Meeting the Needs of Our Youngest Children*. This report provided evidence-based research on the importance of addressing the fundamental needs of children in the first three years of life and received substantial news coverage. In addition, its findings contributed to the legislation that established the Early Head Start program for pregnant woman and infants and toddlers (Levine & Smith, 2001). Data used for educational purposes can help people gain a deeper understanding of the relevance of certain issues in their lives and contribute to a change in attitudes and thinking. Results may also show that solutions will take time and significant investment or that continued research is needed before implementing policy change (Sechrest & Mabe, 1981). Although clear research findings are not always "a passport to policy," researchers can reframe the way child health policy issues are seen, and collaboration with policymakers initially can enhance implementation later (Davis & Howden-Chapman, 1996, p. 865).

Further along the continuum, research can play a role in getting an issue on a policymaker's agenda and weighing alternatives in formulating policy. Sechrest and Mabe (1981) maintain that one of the most useful consequences of good data is that such data help set the stage for debate rather than affecting policy directly. They note that even studies showing no effects of interventions can affect policy by gradually forcing the attention of policymakers to more appropriate or more effective alternatives.

Still further along the continuum, at the opposite end of general education and awareness, research is instrumental in evaluating the effectiveness and efficiency of existing policies and justifying current policy and programs. For example, Head Start is a federally funded child development program that serves low-income children and their families. Begun in 1965, the Head Start program still receives policymakers' support and funding, in part due to research demonstrating that the program makes a difference in the lives of children, families, and communities. From 1987 to 2001, Head Start funding increased fivefold, from $1.13 billion to $6.2 billion (U.S. Department of Health and Human Services, 2002).

Key Characteristics of Policy-Relevant Research

Wherever research may fall on the continuum, there is a set of basic criteria that policymakers and practitioners use to weigh research. They must ask if research is authentic, actionable, relevant, and generalizable (Anderson et al., 1999; Davis & Howden-Chapman, 1996; Grason et al., 2001; Shriver, de Burger, Brown, Simpson, & Meyerson, 1998; Stoddard, 1997).

Authenticity

Policymakers and practitioners look for authenticity. Does the research ring true, and is it compatible with their knowledge, experience, and values? If so, researchers are more apt to receive community, agency, and political support regarding their findings and recommendations. Practitioners are more likely to adopt innovations in research when they are consistent with the value system of the practitioner and organization (Prohaska et al., 2000).

Actionability

Policymakers and practitioners also judge whether research is useful and actionable; that is, can the results be used to produce effective changes in public policy and current practice? As Stoddard has noted, "Research can perhaps have its greatest impact when it moves beyond incremental additions to knowledge into the realm of fundamentally altering our understanding of major issues" (1997, p. 326). To increase the likelihood that research will have an impact on policy, "research needs to have a 'real world field test' component that demonstrates that the particular program . . . is politically and operationally feasible," as well as economically feasible (Grason et al., 2001, p. 15). Applied research is more likely to be translated into policy if the research addresses questions of resource allocation.

Being *actionable* means that the research offers a viable solution and addresses who is really responsible for the problem, what can be done to fix it, who has the power to do that, and how much it will cost. Researchers need to redefine problems in a way that points to the underlying causes and the institutions and organizations (not individual victims) responsible (James, 2001). In the political sense, operationalizing the theory means providing policymakers with concrete ideas for what they can fund to help young children (Sylvester, 2001).

Relevance

Policymakers and practitioners want to know if research findings are relevant and meaningful to their programs, target populations, or constituents. Mike Shriver and colleagues (1998) note that practitioners are not looking for perfect research but rather for data that have meaning to them and that can be replicated to the benefit of their communities. Indeed, a common complaint of decision makers about research findings is a mismatch between the selected conditions or outcome measures (chosen by researchers) and the local conditions or outcome measures of immediate and local interest (Sechrest & Mabe, 1981). In short, research must "view child health broadly in terms of health needs and consequent system challenges, but simultaneously provide results that are local and that can be applied by local constituents to community contexts" (Grason et al., 2001, p. 17).

Although policymakers may at times seem to favor massive number crunches using existing large-scale national data sets, such analyses are rarely applicable to community populations or settings. Further, as Stephen Bell points outs, "the standard practice in large-scale evaluations of asking policymakers to wait years for usable findings will become increasingly untenable" (1999, p. 23). In contrast, applied CHSR provides the multidisciplinary perspective needed to help policymakers, practitioners, and the larger community understand the local implications and learn about local strategies for change (Sylvester, 2001). In this way, applied research provides a much clearer linkage among research, policy, and practice.

Yet the ability to translate research findings for the local setting is a major difficulty researchers face. Findings are often based on an agency that offers similar services but differs on several levels, such as population served or size of budget (Anderson et al., 1999).

Generalizability

Finally, policymakers and practitioners are looking for research that can be taken out of the lab, out of the initial community studied, or off the research paper and applied to other settings. This ability to generalize can be a challenge, as applied CHSR tends to be tailored to the specific needs and issues of a particular setting or community. Although applied research findings may not be completely generalizable to all settings, such research is valuable in that it can identify guiding principles and key lessons that can inform similar efforts. For instance, there is no unequivocal best health care delivery model for school-based health centers. Even as researchers and practitioners gain more knowledge and experience, "it is unlikely that there will ever be one or two models that could or should be reproduced 'cookie cutter' style" (Levy & Shepardson, 1992, p. 46). Deciding which model will work best in a given situation must be a local decision based on an analysis of that community by that community. Various local dynamics, including the community's history, student needs, available resources and funding, local preferences, the strengths of particular leaders, the politics of agency relationships and government entities, and key stakeholders' views, all influence what type of school-based health program will ultimately succeed in a given community.

Other Factors Influencing the Use of Research

Policy development and implementation is usually a complex, multidimensional process in which program effectiveness is only one of a host of factors that will be taken into account (Sechrest & Mabe, 1981). Project D.A.R.E. (Drug Abuse Resistance Education), for example, remains a popular drug education program for children despite studies showing it has no long-term effect on drug use. Its popularity may be due to the "feel-good" nature of a program that everyone can support (Lynam et al., 1999). The demise of President Clinton's health care reform plan in 1994 has been primarily attributed to political factors. The $17 million "Harry and Louise" television ad campaign was recognized as instrumental in changing the level of the health care debate, much more than careful research on the costs and benefits of various systems of health care finance and delivery. In short, this experience "shows that politics affects the definition of a policy problem as well as the origins, formulation, acceptance, and implementation of public policy" (Reich, 1996, p. 1).

The lesson for CHSR is that we need to ask and answer a number of questions: What is the context in which messages will be delivered? At what policies or behaviors will the messages be directed? What is the policy environment for those issues at the time? What events might be happening in the target area at the time the messages will be delivered? What other messages have recently been delivered to those audiences? (Lake & Oliphant, 2001). Researchers need to be aware of and sensitive to other influencing factors, several of which will be highlighted shortly, understanding that all have a bearing on whether policymaking will be influenced by findings of systematic research (Davis & Howden-Chapman, 1996).

Values, Beliefs, and Public Opinion

The public's concern for children and policymakers' motivation to take action are often shaped by complicated, multifaceted, and sometimes conflicting values and beliefs. Much of policy process involves debates about values masquerading as debates about facts and data (McDonough, 2001). These value systems, which Steven Lewis and colleagues say are "not easily shaken by data" (2000, p. 515), may influence health policy far more profoundly than evidence-based research. Haskins agrees: "Most members of Congress have a set of values that determines their position on most issues. These values are relatively impervious to facts" (1991, p. 630).

Welfare reform is a good example showing the importance of values. Sylvester (2000) explains that a new era of thinking about family, work, and fairness began in the 1980s and emerged fully during the national debate over welfare reform in the 1990s. Indeed, every social policy question of the 1990s was debated against a backdrop of public concern about the larger issue of so-called family values. The successful passage of S-CHIP, or the State Children's Health Insurance Program in 1997, Sylvester notes, was due in part to its emphasis on working families; it also succeeded because of a focus on the most vulnerable segment of the low-income population. Further, Sylvester maintains that because children are "blameless" (p. 12), policy changes that target them will probably enjoy more political success than those that also help their parents. Indeed, while many states have succeeded in expanding eligibility levels for children under S-CHIP, to date only a few select states have been able to extend coverage to the uninsured parents of these children.

Because the public's values and opinions critically influence policy formation, child health services researchers need to understand what shapes values and opinions on issues critical to child health and well-being if they hope to see changes in policies affecting child health. Applied CHSR investigators need to spend more time thinking about how their work reaches the public domain. Heymann argues that "stopping with writing an article in an academic journal . . . is like throwing seeds into the wind. They may land, they may bear fruit, but taking the time to till the land and to plant them is far more likely to reap results" (2000, p. 376).

Political Climate

The political climate, which includes such things as political will, policymakers' authority to facilitate change, and their political motivations, is a major factor influencing how and to what extent research is translated into policy. Katharine Atwood and colleagues (1997) explain that political will represents a society's desire and commitment to develop and fund new programs or to support or modify existing programs. Unfortunately, we have little understanding of how to successfully build political will. Although knowledge creates political will and vice versa, Atwood and colleagues recognize that the magnitude of risk posed by a public health problem often bears little relation to amount of political will and resources generated by the issue. For example, research shows that childhood obesity is reaching epidemic proportions and juvenile diabetes is on the rise. Though no one disputes the importance of good nutrition, many schools still sell soda and junk food on campus to generate much-needed revenue to support other school services. A Public Health Institute study on districtwide beverage contracts in California's largest school districts found that health recommendations are rarely integrated into negotiations with soda companies and that "many beverages sold at school conflict with the mission of schools to promote the health and welfare of students" (Purcell, 2002, p. 3).

The policymakers' limited scope of authority is another dimension of the political climate that affects political will. Sechrest and Mabe point out that policymakers "can do only what the community will accept and pay for, only what the unions will allow, only what local conditions of geography, demography, and economics will really permit, and only what their political rivals and the exigencies of time will tolerate" (1981, p. 70). The timing of California's Proposition 10, the California Children and Families Act of 1998, is an example of this. Greater public awareness and understanding of the importance of child development in the early years won out over concerns about taxing a specific group of individuals (those who use tobacco products) to benefit an entirely different group (children to age five). A decade earlier, this might have played out quite differently.

A third aspect of the political climate that researchers need to consider in translating their findings is the political motivations driving a policymaker's actions. "Logic and data will not overcome an agreement between powerful politicians," notes Haskins (1991, p. 628). Researchers need to not only identify the key political players but also assess their power and position and consider how the different program or strategies will affect these key players. Political motivations may also be shaped by changes or transitions going on in the broader political environment or within the organization, agency, department, or other entity that is responsible for implementing the policy (Reich, 1996). "Successful policy formation will need to rely not only on understanding the problems targeted by social epidemiologic research but [also] on developing meaningful policy responses and building political support for these responses" (Heymann, 2000, p. 373).

Broader Social Forces

Broader social forces—including social, economic, and market factors—cannot be overlooked or ignored when it comes to public policy development (Sechrest & Mabe, 1981). These social forces help determine child health priorities and dictate what issues receive available resources. Heymann (2000) offers two examples of how such social forces may affect policy formation. Programs designed to move mothers from welfare to work, for example, may enjoy great success in a strong economy with record low employment but fail miserably in a recession or otherwise weak economy.

Similarly, programs for children with learning disabilities may be highly politically successful and effective when schools have ample resources and are flush with money yet turn into political pariahs when legislation cutting property taxes results in tighter constraints on how local school dollars are spent.

Presumed costs and benefits, Heymann adds, can play as big a role in political decisions as known consequences do. Policymakers must consider whether an intervention costs more than it is worth or than is currently available or if it will generate other new and different problems because of redistribution of resources (Sechrest & Mabe, 1981). Budget cuts, too, will always be a deciding factor, as every level of government seeks to do more with less money. Cost-benefit or cost-effectiveness analysis may not be directly tied to measuring child health outcomes. Yet, as Judy Baker (2000) explains, it enables policymakers to measure program efficacy by comparing alternative interventions on the basis of the cost of producing a given output. Such analysis can greatly enhance the policy implications of outcomes research, and researchers are urged to include it when possible. Baker acknowledges, however, that for many programs, it is not possible or appropriate to measure all benefits in financial terms. A school readiness program, for example, is likely focused on increased learning rather than financial outcomes.

We have sought here to provide some basic guidance to CHSR investigators seeking to jump into the policy world by describing the nature of the policy environment and the role research plays in policymaking. In the next section, we shift our focus to exploring how researchers can more effectively communicate their findings to policymakers.

Communicating the Research: A Necessary but Often Overlooked Link in the Research-Policy Chain

The mere act of doing research will not shape public policy. Further, policy does not always parallel available scientific evidence. Indeed, Shriver and colleagues contend that policy discussions typically take place in what others have deemed "data-free zones," meaning that evidence-based research rarely comes into play and that there is a need "to translate research data so that policy discussions can be based on science and not science fiction, on fact and not persuasion" (1998, p. 193). Haskins, then a Republican staff member, examined the role that research played in the development of the Family Support Act of 1988 in the U.S. House of Representatives and found that "given the rich base of research evidence reviewed during subcommittee meetings, and the direct bearing of this research on the precise issues members were debating, it is disappointing that members did not base more of their arguments on research as they debated how the bill should be written" (1991, p. 624).

Data, on their own and especially in their raw form, are seldom sufficient to sway decision makers to take action. The usefulness of data is ultimately determined by how researchers interpret and report them, meaning that researchers have a responsibility to communicate effectively. As Grason and colleagues note, "It is important to ensure that social science research studies are used appropriately and not misinterpreted as part of the political process" (2001, p. 6). Effective presentation of findings is a key element of any overall applied CHSR initiative and essential for researchers.

Dissemination, one dimension of a strategic communications strategy, is an important aspect of translating research into policy or practice. During the formulation of the Family Support Act of 1988, the Manpower Demonstration Research Corporation, a nonprofit, nonpartisan social policy research organization, testified on five different occasions and conducted ten briefings to a diverse set of groups (Haskins, 1991). When appropriately produced and disseminated, data can provide "powerful tools for improving service delivery, marshalling public support, validating managerial decisions, and sustaining emotional and financial involvement in the service systems" (Woodbridge & Huang, 2000, p. 11).

The key phrase here is "appropriately disseminated," in terms of both target audience and style of presentation. The Urban Institute's Stephen Bell notes that "*how* information is circulated—and its accessibility to the vast and growing state and local audience—will determine the influence of individual research projects as much as a study's content or institutional affiliation. As a result, researchers can no longer assume that doing the right work, then releasing it through standard channels, will place their findings in front of the key decisionmakers" (1999, p. 22; emphasis in original). Dissemination, Peter Levesque and Jill Chopyak explain, is "more than publishing in journals or writing reports. It includes presentations that [laypeople] can understand, ask questions about, and relate back to their particular circumstance" (2001, p. 29). In addition, effective communication of CHSR to policymakers will require researchers to understand and navigate the differing cultures of practice, research, and the political process (Kirwin, 2001).

In short, one size does not fit all; applied CHSR professionals will have to learn to communicate in various ways to different people using numerous dissemination strategies. A key challenge is to contextualize and simplify results and actively disseminate those findings without directly advocating for them (Grason et al., 2001).

Helping Policymakers Find a Needle in a Haystack

Jacqueline Dugery of the Pew Partnership for Civic Change states, "We live in an information age that is set to transform the prospects of communities. In-boxes, both real and virtual, overflow with research" (2001, p. 5). However, she adds that simply increasing the quantity of information and the means by which we receive it is no guarantee that individuals seeking knowledge can locate it and find it useful. If research results are to benefit policy and program development, the results must be accessible and easy to find. CHSR investigators need to provide policymakers and practitioners with timely updates of the latest scientific evidence in user-friendly, easy-to-digest formats to ensure timely application of research findings (Grason et al., 2001).

Typically, research does not get widely communicated to the broader community or community-based organizations and providers serving children (Shriver et al., 2000). Instead, changes within agencies often occur because someone stumbles onto research findings. Anderson and colleagues maintain, "If agencies had a structured approach to reviewing research, an increase in positive, evidence-based change could be anticipated" (1999, p. 1014).

Packaging CHSR for Application

There are several overarching techniques that CHSR professionals should employ to help ensure that their findings are presented and received so as to maximize their impact on policymakers. Understanding one's audience and properly framing one's message are key.

Understand the Audience

Cultural competence and relevancy is a prevailing topic of discussion in child and adult health care services delivery. Elisa Sobo explains in Chapter Three that pediatric health care providers need to understand a family's cultural context and adjust the way they deliver care accordingly. Similarly, applied CHSR investigators need to convey their findings in a manner that is sensitive to and reflective of a deep understanding of the backgrounds and experiences of the intended audience. Researchers need to steer clear of jargon. They need to tailor and present their research in a context and language that will be understood and used not only by those they want to influence but also a wider variety of audiences (including people who are not "experts"). For example, in initially defining the problem, researchers need to be multilingual, using the language of the economist, the legislator, the chief financial officer, the constituent, and the families directly affected by a particular problem (Fox, 1999).

Developing a message that fits also requires researchers to consider who is interested in the issue and why and what the political motivations likely to drive a policymaker's actions might be. Researchers should be aware that they may be entering an environment where people already have ways of understanding an issue.

Indeed, how policymakers and practitioners perceive an issue may be an obstacle that researchers must overcome (Bohan-Baker, 2001).

Frame the Message Properly

A key principle in effective communication is proper framing of the issue. Framing, as explained by Susan Bales (Bohan-Baker, 2001), involves the way the issue is presented and who delivers the message, in addition to the visuals and metaphors used to convey the idea. Effective framing allows us to bridge the differences across various disciplines. To enhance the development of effective public policy and program delivery, it is essential that applied CHSR investigators provide context and a broad frame of reference so that the message is not about a single problem involving one child and one family. For instance, rather than an episodic story with a narrow frame of reference and focused on a single child committing a violent act, one might provide a broader, thematic story about neighborhood conditions and what alternatives to violence are available to children. Instead of a story about a particular child suffering from abuse and neglect, one could recount a more expansive tale about the supports and resources families need to help raise healthy, happy, and safe children.

Using Anecdotes and Stories: Benefit or Barrier?

Policymaking is not simply a scientific exercise in data analysis. McDonough (2001) explains that most policymakers (especially legislators) have not had training in research methods and share the general public's suspicion of statistical analysis. Even if policymakers are well versed in research, he says, most of their decisions cannot wait for a randomized controlled trial to take place. As a result, and because of the value stories have for stimulating emotions that can motivate action, policymakers often gravitate toward anecdotal information to help make their case. In tracking the role of research in the development of the Family Support Act of 1988,

Haskins also found that during the most intense and pivotal phases of policymaking, the most important arguments were not always empirical. He concluded, "Here, as often happens in congressional debate, anecdote was the enemy of scientific evidence" (1991, p. 622).

McDonough (2001) notes that stories are central to policymaking because they are central to the way we make meaning in our lives. Stories enable us to select certain nuances and details to drive home our message and engage our audience. We craft stories to make sense of the various events, data, and stimuli in our lives. Narrative knowledge in medicine, as Trisha Greenhalgh and Brian Hurwitz explain, "provides meaning, context, and perspective for the patient's predicament. It defines how, why, and in what way he or she is ill" (1999, p. 48).

Contextually appropriate stories used in the policy environment can identify important problems with existing programs or policies that have been unrecognized or insufficiently understood. They can also provide evidence that a program or law is working as intended or even producing additional, unanticipated benefits. Stories assist policymakers in thinking about the consequences of rival policy choices and the potential impact of policy decisions.

However, as McDonough cautions, storytelling also can have adverse effects when false or out-of-context stories provide the basis for public policies or are presented in a context that distorts their relevance to the policy matter at hand: "One compelling anecdote (true or false) at a crucial moment in a floor debate can vaporize a mountain of data and careful policy analysis" (2001, p. 209). McDonough recounts the example of how President Ronald Reagan's reference to a fictional Chicago "welfare queen"—collecting her monthly check while sitting at home—fundamentally changed the way Americans think about recipients of government assistance and set the tone for a backlash in the 1980s against helping families in need.

Storytelling is "oxygen to the process and cannot be eliminated," McDonough further explains (2001, p. 212); the challenge is to raise everyone's skill level so that we can be more intelligent consumers of stories. The question is how applied CHSR can craft a more appropriate role for stories in the policy process. Stories should be to policymaking what suitable case studies are to empirical research; using stories to inform policy requires the same standards of validity as those applied to case study. However, developing more sophisticated criteria for evaluating stories is a difficult task because, although stories may not resonate with all audiences, they have authenticity and validity for the teller and fellow sufferers. As Greenhalgh and Hurwitz note, "In contrast with a list of measurements or a description of an experiment, there is no self evident definition of what is relevant or what is irrelevant in a particular narrative" (1999, p. 48).

In essence, as Shriver and colleagues surmise, policymakers and practitioners look for "the powerful mixture" (1998, p. 192) of anecdotal information and research data when developing policy and program priorities. The challenge in using personal stories to affect health policy is to effectively combine the personal and emotional aspects of stories with objective evidence. Several key questions emerge: What are the criteria for making judgments about stories as a basis for generalizing public policy? How do we distinguish among competing stories when all are compelling? Is it possible to move to a different level of storytelling, one that transcends competing stories? (Sharf, 2001).

Selecting Partners Who Can Help Bridge the Gap

Researchers do not have to fight the communication battle alone; joining forces with others can complement researchers' strengths and minimize weaknesses. The greater the collective membership, the more likely researchers are to get policymakers' attention. But in teaming up with other stakeholders, who may have their own agendas, researchers are cautioned to be mindful of their reputation and credibility (Pratt et al., n.d.).

Zervigon-Hakes (1995) identifies several players with whom researchers can collaborate to help get the word out and more effectively translate findings into policy and program development. These include the media, local program administrators, advocacy organizations, and foundations.

Media

The media, like policymakers, are interested in the meaning of research, not the process. They are adept at using everyday language to communicate and are able to influence public perception of policy issues through both presentation style and content, primarily presenting problems as snapshots of individual lives (Heymann, 2000). How the media frame and present an issue influences public opinion; public opinion seems to follow, not lead, the agenda set by the press.

Lewis and colleagues point out that although "many broad policy or programmatic interventions have been successful, the public is not always aware of them. The competition for public allegiance is staged in the media" (2000, p. 519). Researchers who effectively present their findings to the media will likely find it easier to convince policymakers of needed reform (Zervigon-Hakes, 1995).

Local Program Administrators

Local program administrators are likely to be consumers of applied CHSR, using studies to determine best practices, train staff, learn about new effective services, and advocate for change. They are also a stakeholder group to whom policymakers are likely to turn for reactions to research and can thus legitimize and validate research findings by confirming that the results ring true and match their experiences. Local program administrators can also share stories to help translate technical jargon into everyday language that resonates in real-world settings.

Advocacy and Professional Organizations

Policymakers listen to advocacy and professional organizations, which play an important role in the formulation of child health policy. The most sophisticated of these organizations, such as the

Children's Defense Fund or the American Academy of Pediatrics, frequently conduct and summarize research to validate their calls for more funding or different regulations. The Advocacy Initiative, a project of the Research Forum on Children, Families, and the New Federalism, highlights for researchers the key research needs of advocates and stresses the importance of collecting state- and county-level data for advocacy (Lawrence, 2001). Congress often relies on representatives of advocacy and professional organizations to testify as experts on child health issues. When testifying, these representatives typically use research to make their case. Advocacy and professional organizations may also collaborate with policymakers in other ways to push child health policy and program change. In May 2001, for example, Marion Wright Edelman, founder and president of the Children's Defense Fund, teamed up with congressional representatives to unveil the Act to Leave No Child Behind, a bill that would help ensure all children in the United States grow up safe, healthy, and educated.

Foundations

Foundations are another valuable asset in creating links among researchers, policymakers, and practitioners. To facilitate communication, foundations can convene meetings of research and policy teams to discuss specific issues of concern. The Harvard Family Research Project (HFRP), for example, held its first After School Evaluation Symposium in Washington, D.C., in 2001 to bring together researchers, evaluators, practitioners, policymakers, and funders to advance the knowledge base about after-school programming and evaluation by sharing insights and experiences. HFRP is also posting recordings of the plenary sessions on its Web site (http://www. gse.harvard.edu/hfrp/index.html), accompanied by question-and-answer sessions during which the public can submit questions to the presenters. The Promising Practices Network is a partnership of four state-level foundations that serve as intermediaries between researchers, policymakers, and practitioners. Its Web site, operated by

RAND, "highlights programs and practices that credible research indicates are effective in improving outcomes for children, youth, and families" (http://www.promisingpractices.net).

Research emerging from foundation-supported projects is often presented in brief, well-written reports and distributed widely to technical journals, media outlets, and policymakers (Zervigon-Hakes, 1995). For instance, the David and Lucile Packard Foundation's publication *The Future of Children* produces guides for policy-makers and press to complement journal articles that summarize issues and ideas, describe innovative programs, and list relevant Web sites, experts, and reports. In addition, many foundations, as well as advocacy and professional organizations (such as the California HealthCare Foundation, the Henry J. Kaiser Family Foundation, the American Academy of Pediatrics, and Families USA), maintain listserv discussions and electronic newsletters that provide timely synopses of research findings and often discuss their implications for policy and program reform.

Moving Forward

The field of CHSR has only begun to characterize and test the design principles of translational research—research that takes place in the real world, where part of the researcher's role is to provide information to facilitate change and improve practice (Weiss, 1999). Translating research into policy and program development is indeed a challenge, but it can be done. "Effective analysis, interpretation, and presentation of . . . data elements require a blend of science, art, technology, and communication skills," write Woodbridge and Huang (2000, p. 11). To understand and effectively navigate the policy environment, applied CHSR investigators need to broaden the way they think about CHSR—considering what impact the answers to their research questions may have on child health policy and practice and not just patient outcomes, for example—and fundamentally expand their core skills to include relationship building and communication.

Involve Policymakers and Practitioners in the Research Process

Like community-based researchers (see Chapter Five), CHSR investigators are much more likely to have an impact when they involve policymakers, program developers, and practitioners in the research process and deliberately respond to their needs. Researchers can enhance their credibility by engaging in direct regular contact with policymakers, increasing their visibility in the policy arena, and providing a clear and consistent image to the parties responsible for policy and program development. Researchers, policymakers, and practitioners can work together at various stages—for example, in developing the framework for and focus of the research, during ongoing review of interim findings, and before the final presentation of the results. Such collaboration reduces the chance that policymakers and practitioners will misuse or misinterpret important research. Haskins notes, "Most politicians, especially when engaged in political fights, have little regard for quality control: They want support for their position and they take whatever they can get" (1991, p. 629).

A systematic approach that provides opportunities for these exchanges is lacking. More opportunities are needed for policymakers and practitioners to meet and talk with research scientists to understand how research insights can be adapted and adopted in a target community (Shriver et al., 1998).

Act as a Knowledge Broker

For most policymakers and practitioners, direct one-on-one contact with someone they trust is the preferred method for accessing needed information. Each applied CHSR professional should network with advocates, program administrators, and policymakers and their staff to establish an identity as a person with expertise in the general field of child health or in a specific child health issue area. In doing so, researchers can play the role of knowledge broker with both providers and policymakers. In this role, researchers can serve as a trustworthy local source who has access to the best and most current information on child health and well-being, as well as the ability to sort through, synthesize, and translate information tailored to an organization's or policymaker's interests and needs. As knowledge brokers, researchers can also develop a process that supports continual, rather than piecemeal and erratic, learning. They can gain a deeper understanding of an organization's or policymaker's operating environment, including time constraints, budget issues, and priority community concerns (Dugery, 2001). Knowledge brokering is not about researchers acting as advocates; rather, it is about establishing credibility and relationships so that researchers become known and trusted sources of child health information.

In sum, applied CHSR professionals have a critical role to play in ensuring that public policies and investments contribute to improved child health and well-being. They have a responsibility to move beyond the narrow walls of the research community and actively immerse themselves in the policy environment to make certain that important research findings are translated into action.

References

Anderson, M., Cosby, J., Swan, B., Moore, H., & Broekhoven, M. (1999). The use of research in local health service agencies. *Social Science and Medicine, 49,* 1007 1019.

Atwood, K., Colditz, G. A., & Kawachi, I. (1997). From public health science to prevention policy: Placing science in its social and political contexts. *American Journal of Public Health, 87,* 1603–1606.

Baker, J. L. (2000). *Evaluating the impact of development projects on poverty: A handbook for practitioners.* Washington, DC: World Bank.

Bell, S. H. (1999). *New Federalism and research: Rearranging old methods to study new social policies in the states.* Washington, DC: Urban Institute.

Berman, S. (2000). Child health policymaking. *Pediatrics, 105,* 638–640.

Bogenschneider, K., Friese, B., & Balling, K. (2002). Connecting good research and ideas with policymaking. *Evaluation Exchange, 8*(1), 12–13.

Bohan-Baker, M. (2001). A conversation with Susan Nall Bales. *Evaluation Exchange, 7*(1), 10–11.

Carnegie Corporation of New York. (1994). *Starting points: Meeting the needs of our youngest children*. New York: Author. Retrieved from http://www.carnegie.org/starting_points

Citrin, T. (2000). Policy issues in a community-based approach. In T. A. Bruce & S. U. McKane (Eds.), *Community-based public health: A partnership model* (pp. 83–90). Washington, DC: American Public Health Association.

Davis, P., & Howden-Chapman, P. (1996). Translating research findings into health policy. *Social Science Medicine, 43*, 865–872.

Donahue, J. G., Fuhlbrigge, A. L., Finkelstein, J. A., Fagan, J., Livingston, J. M., Lozano, P., et al. (2000). Asthma pharmacotherapy and utilization by children in 3 managed care organizations. The Pediatric Asthma Care Patient Outcomes Research Team. *Journal of Allergy and Clinical Immunology, 106*, 1108–1114.

Dugery, J. (2001). Coming of age in the information age. *Evaluation Exchange, 7*(1), 5–6.

Fox, D. M. (Moderator). (1999, May 12). Summary, Plenary Session I: Health Services Research in Policy-Making, at the first national conference of the Center for Health Policy and Health Services Research, Columbia University School of Nursing, New York. Retrieved from http://cpmcnet.cpmc.columbia.edu/dept/nursing/institute-centers/chphsr/index.html

Grason, H. A., Minkovitz, C. S., Silver, G. B., Fountain, M., & Ashaye, O. (2001). *Building bridges for child health research, policy, and practice: New concepts and paradigms*. Baltimore: Johns Hopkins Bloomberg School of Public Health, Women's and Children's Health Policy Center.

Greenhalgh, T., & Hurwitz, B. (1999). Narrative-based medicine: Why study narrative? *British Medical Journal, 318*, 48–50.

Haskins, R. (1991). Congress writes a law: Research and welfare reform. *Journal of Policy Analysis and Management, 10*, 616–632.

Heymann, S. J. (2000). Health and social policy. In L. F. Berkman & I. Kawachi (Eds.), *Social epidemiology* (pp. 368–381). New York: Oxford University Press.

Jackson-Elmoore, C., Knott, J. H., & Verkuilen, J. V. (1998). *An overview of the State Legislators Survey: Sources of information and term limits impacts*. Battle Creek, MI: W. K. Kellogg Foundation. Retrieved from http://www.wkkf.org/pubs/Health/Pub636.pdf

James, T. (2001). The media: A tool for change? *Evaluation Exchange, 7*(1), 13.

Kirwin, A. (2001, June-July). The art of the possible: Getting involved in policy change. *Zero to Three*, pp. 9–15.

Lake, K., & Oliphant, G. (2001). "Ask the experts." *Evaluation Exchange, 7*(1), 17, 20.

Lawrence, S. (2001). Advocacy and research: A reciprocal relationship. *Forum*, 4(3), 1–5.

Levesque, P. N., & Chopyak, J. M. (2001, April). *Managing multi-sector research projects: Developing models for effective movement from problem identification to problem solving*. Paper presented at the Fifth International Research Symposium on Public Management, Barcelona, Spain.

Levine, M. H., & Smith, S. V. (2001). Starting points: State and community partnerships for young children. *Future of Children, 11*, 143–149.

Levy, J. E., & Shepardson, W. (1992). A look at current school-linked service efforts. *Future of Children, 2*, 44–55.

Lewis, S., Saulnier, M., & Renaud, M. (2000). Reconfiguring health policy: Simple truths, complex solutions. In G. L. Albrecht, R. Fitzpatrick, & S. C. Scrimshaw (Eds.), *Handbook of social studies in health and medicine* (pp. 509–523). Thousand Oaks, CA: Sage.

Lieu, T. A., Quesenberry, C. P., Jr., Capra, A. M., Sorel, M. E., Martin, K. E., & Mendoza, G. R. (1997). Outpatient management practices associated with reduced risk of pediatric asthma hospitalization and emergency department visits. *Pediatrics, 100*, 334–341.

Lynam, D. R., Milich, R., Zimmerman, R., Novak, S. P., Logan, T. K., Martin, C., et al. (1999). Project D.A.R.E.: No effects at 10-year follow-up. *Journal of Consulting and Clinical Psychology, 67*, 590–593.

McCartney, K., & Dearing, E. (2002). Evaluating effect sizes in the policy arena. *Evaluation Exchange, 8*(1), 4, 7.

McDonough, J. E. (2001). Using and misusing anecdote in policy making. *Health Affairs* (Millwood), *20*, 207–212.

Nyden, P., & Wiewel, W. (1992). Collaborative research: Harnessing the tensions between researcher and practitioner. *American Sociologist, 24*, 43–55.

Pratt, P., Floyd, V. D., Langley, W. M., Flynn, K. H. & McAuliffe, J. (n.d.). *Sustaining community-based initiatives: Module 2. Communicating with Policy Makers*. Battle Creek, MI: W. K. Kellogg Foundation. Available online at http://www.wkkf.org/Pubs/CustomPubs/SusComBasedInits/sustainingcommunitybasedinitiatives2.pdf

Prohaska, T. R., Peters, K. E., & Warren, J. S. (2000). Health behavior: From research to community practice. In G. L. Albrecht, R. Fitzpatrick, & S. C. Scrimshaw (Eds.), *Handbook of social studies in health and medicine* (pp. 359–373). Thousand Oaks, CA: Sage.

Purcell, A. (2002). *Prevalence and specifics of district-wide beverage contracts in California's largest school districts: Findings and recommendations*. Sacramento, CA: Public Health Institute.

Reich, M. R. (1996). Applied political analysis for health policy reform. *Current*

Issues in Public Health. Retrieved from http://www.polimap.com/applied. html

Sechrest, L., & Mabe, P. A., III. (1981). Translating evaluation research findings into health policy. *Health Policy Quarterly, 1*, 57–72.

Sellors, J. W., & Mitchell, C. (1998). Restructuring health services delivery research: Community-based model. *Clinical and Investigative Medicine, 21*, 203–208.

Sharf, B. F. (2001). Out of the closet and into the legislature: Breast cancer stories. *Health Affairs* (Millwood), *20*, 213–218.

Shriver, M., de Burger, R., Brown, C., Simpson, H. L., & Meyerson, B. (1998). Bridging the gap between science and practice: Insight to researchers from practitioners. *Public Health Reports, 113*(Suppl. 1), 189–193.

Stoddard, J. J. (1997). Translating research into practice and policy. *Ambulatory Child Health, 3*, 322–328.

Stryer, D., Tunis, S., Hubbard, H., & Clancy, C. (2000). The outcomes of outcomes and effectiveness research: Impacts and lessons from the first decade. *Health Services Research, 35*, 977–993.

Sylvester, K. (2001). *Listening to families: The role of values in shaping effective social policy*. Washington, DC: Social Policy Action Network.

Twiss, J. M. (2001). Cities as partners in community-based public health. *Community-Based Public Health Policy and Practice, 2*, 1–4.

U.S. Department of Health and Human Services. (2002). *2002 Head Start fact sheet*. Retrieved from http://www.acf.dhhs.gov/programs/hsb/research/ factsheets/02_hsfs.htm

Warman, K. L., Silver, E. J., McCourt, M. P., & Stein, R. E. (1999). How does home management of asthma exacerbations by parents of inner-city children differ from NHLBI guideline recommendations? *Pediatrics, 103*, 422–427.

Weiss, K. (1999, June 26). *Translating research into practice: Quality, measurement, and improvement*. Presentation at the Improving Children's Health Through Health Services Research meeting, Chicago. Retrieved from http://www.ahrq.gov/research/chsrtrip.htm

Woodbridge, M. W., & Huang, L. N. (2000). Using evaluation data to manage, improve, market, and sustain children's services. *Systems of care: Promising practices in children's mental health* (2000 Series, Vol. 2). Washington, DC: Center for Effective Collaboration and Practice, American Institutes for Research.

Zervigon-Hakes, A. M. (1995). Translating research findings into large-scale public programs and policy. *Future of Children, 5*, 175–191.

10

Looking to the Future

The Need for Applied Child Health Services Research

Paul S. Kurtin, Blair L. Sadler

Existing at the intersection of clinical services, health policy, and the marketplace, **applied child health services research (CHSR)** is uniquely situated to shape the future of health services for children and families. Looking to the future, we believe there are five important points to make about the potential of applied CHSR to affect the overall health care agenda for children. Applied CHSR can and should do all of the following:

1. Increase the ability of consumers, medical groups, and health plans to make informed choices about care based on quality

2. Support organizational improvement work and develop effective, widely usable measures of quality for a variety of purposes (including the transformation of health care organizations when embedded in the core fabric of decision making)

3. Assist hospitals and medical groups in reducing and controlling costs

4. Improve communitywide health status when used in tandem with traditional public health interventions

5. Educate and train the caregivers of today and tomorrow in the science and practice of quality improvement

Improving Consumer Choice Based on Quality

Informed choice about quality requires reliable, valid, and understandable information. Such is currently unavailable to most health care consumers. Applied CHSR outcomes assessments of health services for children and families can go a long way toward meeting this need. However, to be effective, information derived from outcomes assessments must be communicated in clear, understandable language that consumers can understand. The measures must also address and assess illnesses, conditions, and procedures that are important to consumers.

Supporting Organizational Improvement and Developing Measures for Use by Accrediting and Regulatory Organizations

Applied CHSR can form the basis of organizational improvement work. If embedded in the core fabric of decision making in an organization, applied CHSR can also help transform that organization's culture over time to fully embrace continuous quality improvement. Used in this way, outcomes become a part of the **plan, do, study, act (PDSA)** cycle of improvement (see Chapter Eight, by Richardson, Sobo, and Stucky). In PDSA, a specific outcome becomes the starting point for the next cycle of improvement, for which outcomes will again be assessed and inserted into the subsequent improvement cycle. For example, if an immunization rate for a population of children managed by a single practice is lower than it should be, that outcome can be used to drive change in office processes in order to better identify children in need of vaccinations. By again assessing the immunization rate, another cycle of improvement can be undertaken, if needed. By providing useful outcomes information to consumers while also providing hospitals, medical groups, and doctors with information needed to continuously improve their services, applied CHSR can help support a health care system based on consumers' choosing between providers who are competing on the quality of their outcomes.

Under the leadership of the National Quality Forum (http://www.qualityforum.org), a welcome and unprecedented momentum for developing widely accepted measures of health care quality has arisen. These measures will be adopted and used by Medicare and Medicaid agencies, the Joint Commission on Accreditation of Healthcare Organizations (JCAHO), the Leapfrog Group, and others. Applied CHSR can significantly contribute to the development of measures for children, whether they receive care in doctor's offices, clinics, or hospitals.

Applied CHSR investigators must be actively involved in national efforts to define and measure quality of care for children. As noted, these definitions and measures must be meaningful to children and families. They must be reliable and valid so that they meet the scrutiny of providers. They must be relevant to payers so that a business case for quality can be made. Finally, the measures must be able to inform and support performance improvement.

Assisting in Cost Control and Quality Improvement While Developing a Business Case for Quality

Applied CHSR can be very effective in helping hospitals, medical groups, and doctors make informed decisions about reducing unnecessary or improper care and increasing necessary, appropriate care. This will make hospitals, medical groups, and doctors provide more effective and efficient care. By using clinical pathways and standardizing to excellence, unnecessary variation is reduced or eliminated, and that will result in improved outcomes and lower costs. In addition, reducing wasted health care resources will help control rising costs without significantly reducing choice or services. In some cases, this approach will help providers differentiate their care from others in their market by demonstrating superior levels of quality.

However, few provider organizations will make the needed financial commitment to major sustained quality improvement without receiving appropriate financial rewards for doing so. That is, applied CHSR's full financial benefit to providers will not be realized without an effective business case for quality that shares investment costs and benefits between payers and providers. As long as provider organizations bear most of the costs of health care improvement while the financial benefits of improvement remain with the payers, there will be little or no incentive to improve services by using the knowledge gained and lessons learned via applied CHSR. So far, a compelling business case for quality has yet to be built.

Applied CHSR can help make the business case for quality by demonstrating to consumers and payers that there are differences in quality between providers, that these differences are important to the health and well-being of children, and that in some cases, high-quality services actually save payers money. Applied CHSR investigators within an organization must share this information with their business and contracting colleagues for the development of contracting models that reward high-quality providers and can be adopted by payers.

Improving Communitywide Health Status

Applied CHSR can positively affect care provided to individual patients. It can have equally profound positive effects at the community health or public health level. Most of the tools and techniques described in this book are readily applicable to improving communitywide conditions and closing the gap between best practice and everyday practice in delivering public health services. Imagine the power of health care leaders throughout a community joining together and committing to implement and measure best practices of care for children and families regardless of their insurance status, health plan, or provider system. We believe that applied CHSR is a significantly underutilized resource for helping communities systematically and substantially improve their overall health status. This can and must change.

Educating and Training Caregivers of Today and Tomorrow

The full long-term potential of applied CHSR will not be realized without a significant and sustained investment in training and education. And such must not be limited to researcher training alone. The science and methods of quality improvement can differ greatly from traditional scientific approaches and are still unfamiliar to most current practitioners. However, this is changing as individual practitioners take on the challenge and responsibility of applied CHSR. Organizations are also beginning to efficiently and effectively develop the skills needed throughout their workforce to make widespread and lasting change possible.

Whereas many recent applied CHSR training efforts affect professionals already well into their careers, preprofessional training too must change. Medical schools and residencies are just starting to address the challenge of effectively embedding new quality improvement and outcomes-related skills into an already crowded learning experience.

Nursing and the other caring professions face the same challenges as medical practitioners. These challenges can be met in part through teaching and training the knowledge and skills of applied CHSR.

In conclusion, applied CHSR is on the threshold of a new age of opportunity and impact on the lives of our children. If this book has a bias, it is a bias to action. By fully engaging in the issues of quality, choice, and cost, will we, as applied CHSR investigators, look back twenty years from now not only on the papers we have published but also on the dramatic improvements in child health that our work will have helped bring about? That is our hope. The children and families we serve deserve no less.

Glossary

· ·

Accountability: Active acceptance of responsibility for one's outcomes; includes documenting the quality of a system's outcomes with quantifiable, comparable measures.

Acculturation: The process of learning a second or new culture on top of one's native culture.

Adaptive system: A system that can learn from its environment and change its behavior based on that new knowledge.

Adaptive warning signal: A useful signal, such as acute pain, that directs the individual to an injured part or disease condition or alerts the individual of the need to seek help.

Adherence: The extent to which a patient takes medications at the dosage and frequency prescribed or the completeness and frequency with which a patient engages in behavioral or psychosocial components of treatment.

Algorithm: A decision tree that leads the caregiver through a series of questions to determine the most appropriate care.

Alpha coefficient: A statistical model of an instrument's internal consistency reliability, based on the average inter-item correlation; conceptually, the alpha coefficient is a reflection of how well items on the same scale measure the same construct.

Applied child health services research: Research conducted with the proactive purpose of improving the health and well-being of children; research in which findings have immediate impact on service design, delivery, and outcomes.

Assimilation: To reject and replace one's culture with another, generally the dominant culture of the society in which one is living.

Barriers to care: A multidimensional construct, consisting of expectations related to the quality of care available from the health care system, health-related knowledge and behavior, pragmatic factors, and the practical skills and knowledge needed to navigate the health care system. Barriers to care may exist in accessing the health care system, in using necessary health care, or in experiencing an optimal health care encounter.

Benchmark: The best performance of a specific process or outcome.

Biomedicine: Conventional allopathic medicine, as taught in U.S. medical schools.

Central tendency: The middle or center of distribution. Mean, median, and mode are typical measures of central tendency.

Champions: Key individuals, usually physicians or nurses, who are committed to an innovation and held in high regard by their peers. Champions assume primary responsibility for a process or innovation and advocate for its acceptance.

Child health services research (CHSR): See *health services research*, and *applied child health services research*.

Children with special health care needs (CSHCN): Children who have chronic physical, developmental, behavioral, or emotional conditions and require health and related services of a type or amount beyond that generally required by children.

Clinical outliers: Patients at least two standard deviations above or below the mean who, upon review, are found to have complicating diagnoses or procedures that make them unlike the rest of the measured population; they are generally dropped from the population for review purposes.

Clinical pathways: An algorithmic process of care designed to increase the likelihood of positive outcomes based on the effective and efficient use of resources. The goals of the clinical pathways are to maintain or enhance quality of care, maximize cost effectiveness, and establish a collaborative approach for patient care delivery.

Collaboration: Action-oriented partnering in which various stakeholders create an interdependent system as a means to achieve the larger goal; collaborators have clearly defined roles and responsibilities, complement and support one another's efforts, and share a sense of community.

Common cause variation: Variation that is inherent to a process, such as an equipment limitation, lack of methods or procedures, or inconsistent methods or procedures.

Community: A group that shares a common interest such as living in the same geographical area, sharing a similar ethnic or cultural background, speaking the same language, experiencing the same history, or sharing the same profession.

Community-based research: Research that emphasizes active involvement of the community in all aspects of the research process to help enhance the relevance and usefulness of the research findings.

Community health report card: A document that provides a snapshot of the community's health by presenting objective information about past trends and current realities through the use of indicators.

Community indicators: Measures of well-being tied to local community areas.

Community-level social indicator: A social indicator that can be collected, reported, and meaningfully interpreted for geopolitical units such as neighborhoods, towns, cities, metropolitan areas, or regions.

Comorbid: Two or more diagnoses occurring simultaneously; dual diagnosis.

Complementary or alternative medicine (CAM): Medical interventions that are neither taught widely in U.S. medical schools nor generally available in U.S. hospitals or physicians' offices.

Conceptual model: A set of informed assumptions that scientists make about their focus of study, including definitions of variables, a description of the relationships among the variables, and delineation of the limits of the phenomena of interest.

Construct validity: The extent to which scores on an instrument assess a theoretical construct; the extent to which an instrument assesses what it purports to assess.

Continuous quality improvement (CQI): A management strategy focusing on the continuous improvement of processes through continuous critical appraisal, monitoring, and benchmark comparison making; see also *rapid-cycle improvement* and *plan, do, study, act (PDSA)*.

Control group: A group that serves as a point of comparison, having not experienced the condition (treatment, intervention) in question; see also *randomized controlled trial (RCT)*.

Cross-informant variance: The variance (difference in scores) found between multiple informants (parents, teacher, child).

Cross-sectional research design: Data are collected at one point in time from a cross-section of individuals.

Cultural competence: Techniques or practices promoting equity in health care, including interpreter services, recruitment and retention policies aimed at enhancing diversity in the workforce, training programs for staff, culturally relevant health promotion, and the inclusion of household and community members in health care planning.

Culture: The learned, shared practices and knowledge of a group of people.

Decision support (DS) systems: Information technology systems that collect data and allow for data extrapolation of procedures, interventions, medications, and so on; DS systems track cost information as a basis for organizational decision making.

Demographics: The statistical profile of a given population, such as children receiving health care.

Dependence: Relying on parents and other adults and on systems (school, social services) for such things as accessing and receiving care.

Descriptive community indicators: Community indicators that allow for the naming and quantification of problems to create an understanding of the current situation.

Developmental change: Growth and change over time; for children, this occurs at a rapid rate, and their development in numerous areas (cognitive, emotional, social, physical) affects their ultimate health status.

Devolution: A shift in the responsibility and accountability of programs from the federal or national level to state and local levels.

Differential epidemiology: Differences in disease frequency between segments of the population; in child health services research, this refers to the fact that children are affected by more low-prevalence conditions than adults are.

Disease: A biomedically measurable lesion or irregularity in a person's physiology or anatomy.

Disease management (DM): An innovative approach to patient management for a specific disease using a comprehensive education and treatment program that targets a single disease and is intended to reduce symptoms, increase quality of life, and decrease admissions and emergency visits.

Disease-specific measures: Measures intended to assess symptoms of disease, treatment effects, and other relevant factors not sufficiently covered by generic measures.

Enculturation: Being socialized into or learning one's native culture.

Epidemiology: The study of the distribution and determinants of disease frequency in human populations.

Ethnicity: A facet of the self that is tied to notions of shared origins that contrast with those of people with whom one shares borders (such as household, neighborhood, or national borders); a subset of culture.

Ethnocentrism: The belief that one's own culture's values and customs are the best.

Ethnography: The descriptive study of an individual culture, often undertaken through long-term participant observation that includes living with the people under consideration and immersing oneself in their way of life as much as possible.

Family: A kinship term that references biological (for example, genetic or blood) or legal ties as they relate to lines of descent and ancestry.

Functional biomedical acculturation: Learned, practical skills and knowledge necessary for negotiating the health care system and getting the most out of the health care received.

Functional status: An individual's ability to perform physical activities, as influenced by the presence or absence of disease.

Generic measures: General or nonspecific measures that reflect constructs such as physical, psychological, and social functioning, regardless of disease or treatment.

Geographic information system (GIS): A computer software system capable of assembling, storing, manipulating, and displaying geographically referenced information (data identified according to their location).

Health disparities: Differences in the incidence, prevalence, mortality, and burden of diseases and other adverse health conditions that exist among distinct population groups.

Health-related quality of life (HRQL): An individual's health-related physical, psychological, and social functioning and illness symptoms, all of which can be measured or classified.

Health-seeking process: The dynamic, cumulative, and often pluralistic process by which people seek better health; it often begins with symptom recognition and involves constant reevaluation of the sick person's condition in the quest for healing or a cure.

Health services research (HSR): A multidisciplinary field of inquiry that examines the use, costs, quality, accessibility, delivery, organization, financing, and outcomes of health care services to increase the knowledge and understanding of the structure, process, and effects of health services for individual and populations.

Health status: The overall health of an individual, as characterized by the extent of physical disability and overall well-being.

Hierarchy of resort: The ordered pattern by which people try and sometimes exhaust various health care options; generally, people try the most familiar or simplest and cheapest treatment first and then seek more expensive, complex, or unfamiliar treatments as necessary.

Household: A group of people who share living space at a given point in time; an economic unit that jointly produces goods or pools money and purchases commodities like power and water or food. Household members sleep in the same complex and generally share food

Human capital: Resources that reside within the individual, such as education, skills, and knowledge.

Hypothetical construct: An abstract phenomenon or concept, such as trust, satisfaction, or health-related quality of life, that cannot be measured directly but must instead be measured by intermediate variables; a concept that is assumed to exist because it gives rise to measurable phenomena.

Illness: The lived experience of being unwell or suffering.

Indicator: A measure for which data are available that helps quantify the achievement of a desired outcome.

Internal consistency reliability: The extent to which items on a measure produce consistent scores; measured by the alpha coefficient.

Longitudinal research design: Research employing data collected over time to track actual change in real time.

Managed care: A health care system that focuses on the coordination of all services to avoid overuse, overlap, and duplication as well as to reduce the overall cost of health care.

Microsystem: A particular group of personnel, with their associated technology, work processes, and information resources, who are working to meet all the needs of a specific group of patients; a preferred unit of analysis and improvement for the delivery of health services.

Modular assessment: An assessment approach involving administration of a generic instrument to healthy patients and patients with acute or chronic illnesses, as well as disease-specific modules designed for use in identified illness populations.

Multiple regression: A statistical technique that aims to find a linear relationship between a response variable and several predictor variables.

Needs assessment: The process of identifying the problems and needs of a target population.

Noncategorical approach: An approach to child health services research that does not depend on a particular diagnosis or diagnostic category but on illness burden; seeks to identify underlying features of health, illness, chronic health conditions, or health care that cross diagnostic boundaries and thus can describe phenomena for large segments of children.

Operational definition: A specific statement about how a researcher intends to measure a hypothetical construct; an explicit and detailed definition for a variable making that variable measurable in specific terms.

Outcomes: The health results of the interaction between providers and patients within the health care system; a change, either positive or negative, in the health status of the individual, group, or population as a result of previous or concurrent care. There are three types of health outcomes: clinical, patient-based, and financial.

Outlier: An observation in a data set that is unusually large or unusually small compared to the other values in the data set.

Parallel forms: Data collection instruments with congruent items and domains.

Pareto principle: This contention that in all systems, 80 percent of the trouble encountered arises from 20 percent of the problems; also called the *80–20 rule*.

Pathway: An algorithmic process of care designed to increase the likelihood of positive outcomes based on the effective and efficient use of resources.

Patient-centered care: Care that is responsive to the needs and preferences of patients and families.

Patterns of resort: The patterns people follow when resorting to curing or healing practices or professionals.

Pediatric care triad: The central trio of people involved in a child's health care, consisting of the dependent patient (child), empowered intermediary (parent or guardian), and practitioner (in biomedicine, the practitioner is the authoritative figure).

Performance measure: A measure of how well agency or program service delivery is working.

Plan, do, study, act (PDSA): A process for planning and changing a given practice; directs individuals to identify a problem, design a solution, test and study the solution, and then act to make the solution widespread. See also *rapid-cycle improvement*.

Prescriptive community indicator: A community indicator that helps identify root causes and the impact of existing assumptions on which potential policy decisions are based.

Primary data: Data collected in the field, directly for the project at hand, by and for those who will analyze it.

Process: The nature and dynamics of service delivery; what is done and how it is done. Processes of care include technical competence of the provider and the interpersonal or humanistic aspects of the patient-provider relationship.

Proxy: A respondent who provides information about the health or well-being of another subject (for example, physicians, parents, and teachers can provide proxy reports about a child's health).

Psychometric properties: Properties such as reliability and validity that ensure that instruments consistently measure the constructs that they are intended to measure.

Quality of care: The degree to which health services increase the likelihood of desired health outcomes and are consistent with current professional knowledge. High-quality care occurs when needed care is obtained, skillfully provided, delivered in a manner consistent with patient (or parent) preferences, and leads to the best possible outcomes.

Quality of life (QOL): A broad construct that typically encompasses many aspects of an individual's life, including housing, environment, work, and school.

Race: In theory, a biological subspecies of the human species distinguished by differentiated anatomical or physiological traits (such subspecies do not actually exist); in practice, a social construct involving categories of human beings differentiated by visually identifiable traits.

Randomized controlled trial (RCT): A research design in which groups of participants are matched according to a variable that the experimenter wishes to control. In the simplest type of experiment, two equivalent groups are created; one group undergoes an intervention, and the other group (the control group) does not.

Rapid-cycle improvement: Rapid, sequential cycles of quality improvement efforts involving highly focused, small-scale projects that aim for real-time improvement; allows for the incorporation of needed changes, thereby increasing project effectiveness.

Recall interval: The time interval to be used as a frame of reference by the respondent when completing the questionnaire items (e.g., in the past 7 days).

Reliability: Consistency of a measurement; the extent to which an instrument will generate the same answers from the same respondents every time it is administered (assuming there are no changes in the respondent's status).

Risk adjustment: Mathematical techniques that make comparisons possible across cases despite differences, such as illness severity.

Secondary data: Large data sets, generally assembled from surveillance systems, that are made available for use by others.

Shewart-Deming cycle: See *plan, do, study, act (PDSA)*.

Social capital: A community's norms, relationships, networks, and social trust, which shape the quality and quantity of the community's social interactions.

Social indicators: Quantitative data that serve as indexes to important conditions in society.

Society: An interdependent group of people who interact together, usually within a specific geographical area.

Sociodemographic variables: Individual factors, such as gender, age, social class, and marital status.

Special cause variation: Variation in a process that is unusual or unexpected, such as may occur when using new equipment or implementing a new idea in patient care.

Stakeholder: Any individual or organization with a vested interest in child health (for example, families, community organizations, nongovernmental groups, health care providers, or government agencies).

Structure: Components of a health service delivery system (facilities, staff, licensure) necessary for processes to occur; who delivers services, where services are delivered, and who receives services.

Systems thinking: Thinking holistically in terms of processes and the interconnected systems of staff, technology, workflow, and information that underwrite them (as opposed to thinking that places the individual at the center of events).

Unnecessary variation: Variation in the care of patients with similar conditions that is not due to patient need or preference but rather to provider preference and habit; such variation can be seen in costs, diagnostics, and treatment choices.

Validity: Accuracy of a measure; how well it measures what it purports to measure.

Value: Quality per unit of cost.

Vulnerability: Susceptibility of an individual or a group to negative events; risk for poor physical, psychological, and social health or adverse health outcomes.

Name Index

A

Aaronson, N. K., 211, 218
Abetz, L., 222, 226, 248
Abrams, B., 146
Abreu, M., 258
Achenbach, T. M., 219
Acorn, S., 99
Adair, J., 86
Adams, J., 175
Adams, W. G., 279
Aday, L. A., 45, 47, 249, 255, 262
Alaimo, K., 84
Aligne, C. A., 221
Allen, R. I., 101
Altamore, R., 89
Altman, D. G., 172, 173, 175, 176,
  177, 190, 196
Ambler, A. B., 80
Andersen, R., 255, 256
Anderson, B. G., 258
Anderson, G. F., 261
Anderson, M., 188, 315, 318, 331,
  333, 341
Anderson, R. T., 250
Andrulis, D., 222
Ansley, F., 174, 192, 193
Antoniou, G., 216
Asch, S. M., 252
Ashaye, O., 322
Atkinson, P., 108

Atkinson, S. S., 217
Atkisson, A., 125, 128, 136, 139, 141
Atwood, K., 319, 336
Auinger, P., 221
Axel-Lute, M., 188
Ayanian, J. Z., 30

B

Babani, L., 216, 253
Bader, B. S., 187
Baer, H. A., 68, 76, 261
Baer, R. D., 257
Bailey, L., 141, 160
Baker, D. W., 259
Baker, J. L., 338
Balling, K., 330
Banis, H. T., 216, 253
Barnett, C., 86
Barrera, M., 222
Bartholomew, L. K., 219
Barton, L., 92
Batalden, P. B., 9
Bates, D. W., 30
Bates, J., 13
Bauchner, H., 10, 50, 251, 279
Bauer, R., 124
Bayer, I. S., 174
Beaudoin, D. E., 80
Becher, E. C., 94
Becker, A. B., 178

Becker, M., 89
Behrman R. E., 102
Bell, R., 39, 93
Bell, S. H., 159, 180, 333, 339
Ben-Arieh, A., 121, 126, 129, 147
Bender, B., 223
Bennett, C. L., 280
Benson, B. A., 224
Berk, R., 260
Berkowitz, B., 164, 171
Berman, S., 306, 324
Bernard, D., 281
Bernier, J. A., 252
Bernstein, I. R., 230
Berwick, D. M., 9, 19, 30, 31, 213, 214, 281
Besleme, K., 126, 128
Betancourt, J. R., 54, 96, 97
Beuf, A. H., 35
Bhrany, V., 39
Bibace, R., 86
Biderman, A., 122
Billings, J., 128, 262
Bindman, A. B., 260, 262, 264
Birch, L. L., 84
Bjordal, K., 218
Blaszcak, M. R., 139
Blum, R. W., 260
Bocian, A. B., 13, 18
Bogenschneider, K., 330
Boggs, S. R., 217
Bohan-Baker, M., 342
Boissin, M., 217
Bordo, S., 84
Bottigheimer, H., 53
Bouman, N. H., 215
Bowen, N. L., 139
Boyd, E. L., 263
Boyd-Pringle, L. A., 222
Boyle, C. A., 40
Boyle, M., 216
Brach, C., 54, 95
Brassard, M., 283
Braveman, P., 146
Brennan, T. A., 31, 262
Breslau, N., 220

Brewis, A., 90
Brindis, C., 132
Bringewatt, R. J., 20
Broekhoven, M., 188, 315
Broide, E., 92
Brook, R. H., 52
Brown, B., 122, 125, 126, 127, 130, 133, 146
Brown, C., 331
Brown, P., 184, 190
Brown, R. T., 216
Bruner, C., 181, 187, 188
Brunner, W., 196
Bubolz, T. A., 9, 31
Buhi, L., 199
Bullers, S., 221
Burdine, J. N., 141
Buring, J., 122, 146
Burke, G. L., 250
Burke, J., 95
Burstin, H. R., 30, 262
Burwinkle, T. M., 209, 212
Bush, P. J., 86
Bushy, A., 249
Butler, J., 130
Butler, J.V.B., 212
Byck, G. R., 280
Byrd, R. S., 221, 258
Byrd, T., 257

C

Cabana, M. D., 278
Cadman, D., 216
Calkins, D. R., 213
Calman, K. C., 222
Cameron, M. E., 216
Campbell, E. G., 262
Campbell, K., 85
Canam, C., 99
Capps, L. L., 257
Carrillo, J. E., 54, 96, 97
Carson, C. A., 133
Carter, W. B., 211, 214
Carver, L. J., 191, 193
Casanova, C., 262
Cassady, C., 260

Cepeda, M., 216
Chang, C. H., 250
Charlton, A., 216–217
Charney, E., 45, 54
Chassin, M. R., 52
Cheadle, A., 189, 195
Chesley, F. D., 250
Chesney, R. W., 18
Cheson, B. D., 210, 248
Chilcoat, H. D., 220
Chopyak, J. M., 178, 192, 193, 340
Chrisman, N. J., 88, 89, 91
Christakis, D. A., 278
Christakis, N. A., 94
Christie, M. J., 217
Citrin, T., 324
Clancy, C., 9, 35, 93, 248, 257, 317
Clark, L., 54, 70, 96, 259
Cleary, P. D., 211
Clinch, J. J., 219
Cluss, P. A., 221
Cobb, C., 123, 124
Codman, E. A., 27, 28
Coffman, J., 176
Cohen, J. W., 45, 49, 251
Cohen, W. I., 93
Coid, J., 83
Colditz, G. A., 319
Colegrove, R., 219
Connell, J. P., 171, 185, 186
Contreras, J. M., 83
Cooper-Patrick, L., 264
Cope, D. W., 39
Corbett, T., 121, 125
Cordes, C., 189, 192
Cornell, F. A., 79, 175
Corrigan, J. M., 9
Cosby, J., 188, 315
Coughlin, T. A., 277
Coulton, C., 121, 135
Cowley, S., 128
Coye, M. J., 20
Crain, E. F., 260, 264
Crits-Cristoph, P., 209
Cull, A., 218
Culross, P. L., 102

Cummings, P., 40
Cummins, S. K., 83
Cunningham, P. J., 50
Cunningham, S. J., 260
Czyzewski, D. I., 219

D

Dahlquist, G., 74
Daniel, M., 166
Davey, B., 250
Davidson, P., 256
Davidson, S. J., 280
Davis, A., 262
Davis, P., 318, 319, 322, 323, 329, 330, 331, 334
Davison, K. K., 84
Davodi Far, M., 243
de Baca, R. C., 54, 96
de Burger, R., 331
de Groot, M., 218
De Guire, M. J., 222
De Witt, T. G., 222, 264
Dearing, E., 319
Decoufle, P., 40
Demers, R., 89
Deming, W. E., 10, 17, 29
Dennis, K., 121, 155, 313
Deuschle, K., 86
Devers, K., 180
Deyo, R. A., 211, 214
Diamond, J., 71
Diaz-Rossello, J. L., 278
Dickinson, P., 212
DiClemente, R. J., 83
Dinkevich, E. I., 260
Dishuck, N. M., 209
Dobkin, P. L., 223
Dolgin, M., 219
Donabedian, A., 33, 251, 252, 254
Donahue, J. G., 314
Donaldson, M. S., 9
Dore, C. J., 217
Dougall, A., 260
Drotar, D., 106
Duan, N., 261
Dugery, J., 340, 349

Duggan, A. K., 93
Durch, J., 141, 160
Dworkin, P. H., 43

E
Edelman, M. W., 346
Edwards, J., 94
Einstein, A., 22
Eisenberg, D. M., 91, 92, 93
Eisenberg, J. M., 250
Eisenberg, L., 258
Eiser, C., 210, 217, 219
Elixhauser, A., 47
Elliott, M., 96
Emmons, K. M., 83
Epstein, A. M., 221
Epstein, L. H., 221
Ergil, M. C., 107
Ernst, E., 91

F
Faden, R., 213, 223
Fadillioglu, B., 48
Faier-Routman, J., 216
Farmer, P., 68
Farr, W., 122
Farrow, F., 159
Fawcett, S. B., 163, 171, 179, 180
Feeny, D. H., 210, 219
Feinstein, A. R., 50, 219, 251
Feinstein, J. S., 250
Felix, M. R., 141
Ferrie, P. J., 219
Field, M. J., 25
Fielding, J. E., 130, 138, 141
Fielding, S. L., 221
Finucane, M., 136
Fireman, P., 221
Fiscella, K., 257
Fisher, G. F., 250
Flegal, K. M., 84
Flexner, A., 28
Flocke, S. A., 260, 262
Flores, G., 10, 50, 54, 251, 258, 261
Floyd, V. D., 323
Flynn, K. H., 323

Forrest, C. B., 9, 35, 36, 37, 39, 93,
    103, 248, 253, 254, 260, 262
Foster, G. M., 96, 109, 258
Fountain, M., 322
Fowler, M. G., 217
Fox, D. M., 341
Fox, H. B., 217, 261
Franklin, B., 26–27
Franklin, M., 141
Franks, P., 257
Fraser, I., 54, 95
Freeman, J. L., 9, 31
French, D., 217
Friday, G., 221
Friedman, M., 126, 129, 130, 131
Friedson, E., 90
Friese, B., 330
Frongillo, E. A., 84

G
Galanti, G.-A., 98
Galvin, R. S., 20
Galvin, R. W., 52
Galvis, S. A., 221
Gambone, M. A., 185
Gardner, S., 159, 164, 168, 171
Gardner, W., 13, 18
Garralda M. E., 217
Garro, L., 107
Garwick, A. W., 260
Gaventa, J., 174, 192, 193
Gergen, P. J., 48
Gibbs, D., 122, 126, 127, 130, 133
Gidwani, P., 25
Gielen, A. C., 223
Gill, T. M., 219
Gillman, M., 84
Gittelsohn, A. M., 250
Gladis, M. M., 209
Godfrey, C., 92
Goerge, R., 121, 126, 129, 147
Golden, W. E., 213
Goldman, D. A., 13, 254
Gomby, D. S., 102
Good, B., 72, 97, 257, 258
Good, M.-J. D., 72, 97

Goodman, A., 136
Goodman, A., 55
Goodman, D. C., 250
Goodman, M. H., 81
Goodwin, D., 217
Gosch, E. A., 209
Gotay, C. C., 210, 248
Gould, J. B., 250, 251
Gould, S. J., 71
Graham-Pole, J., 217
Grant, K., 92
Grason, H. A., 261, 322, 331, 332, 339, 340
Graunt, J., 122
Gray, J. A., 284
Greaney, M. L., 147
Green, A. R., 54, 96, 97
Green, L., 155, 166, 192, 193, 194, 195
Greene, J. W., 210
Greenfield, S., 52, 214
Greenhalgh, T., 343, 344
Grey, M., 216
Griffin, C., 174
Griffith, L. E., 219
Groenvold, M., 218
Gross, D. R., 73
Grossman, D. C., 40, 79
Grumbach, K., 260
Gustafson, K. E., 220
Guyatt, G. H., 210, 219
Guyer, B., 261
Guyver, A., 92

H

Haapasalo, J., 83
Hadden, W. C., 250
Hahn, R. A., 39, 86, 93, 97
Halfon, N., 36, 37, 48, 49, 132, 136, 138, 217, 248, 250, 261
Halpern, J., 250
Hamlett, K. W., 220
Hanson, C. L., 222
Harper, G. W., 191, 193
Haskins, R., 322, 335, 337, 339, 343, 348
Hassin, J., 81

Hay, T. C., 82
Haynes, R. B., 284
Hays, R. D., 96, 214
Hayward, S., 161, 179, 181
Hazam, N., 258
Heberden, W., 26
Helman, C. G., 103, 109
Hemstreet, M. P., 217
Hendricks, A., 53
Hennekens, C., 122, 146
Henrich, J., 286
Hernandez, D. J., 45
Hernandez, J. T., 83
Hernandez, M., 164
Herzlinger, R. E., 53, 54
Heymann, S. J., 178, 314, 320, 321, 335, 337, 345
Hibbard, J., 136
Hill, J., 181
Hislop, T. G., 223
Hodges, S., 164, 165, 168, 169, 171
Hoff, T. J., 183
Hofsess, L., 70, 259
Hojer, B., 74
Holland, B., 156
Hollister, R. G., 181
Homer, C. J., 13, 254, 260, 306
Horbar, J. D., 13
Horsch, K., 182, 184
House, J. S., 223
Howard, G., 250
Howard, V. J., 250
Howden-Chapman, P., 318, 319, 322, 323, 329, 330, 331, 334
Howell, C. T., 219
Huang, L. N., 186, 314, 339, 347
Hubbard, H., 317
Hubner, W., 92
Hufford, D. J., 70
Hughes, D., 132, 261, 262
Hunt, L., 39, 93
Hunt, S., 209, 210
Hurtado, M. P., 262
Hurwitz, B., 343, 344
Hutchins, V. L., 123
Hymel, K. P., 82

I

Iezzoni, L. I., 30
Illig, D., 142
Imrie, J., 178
Ingersoll, G. M., 217
Inglis, A. D., 221
Inkelas, M., 250
Innes, J., 124, 126, 128, 137
Ireys, H. T., 261, 262
Israel, B. A., 174, 178, 183, 194, 195, 198
Ivarsson, J. I., 74

J

Jackson, R. J., 83
Jackson-Elmoore, C., 328
Jacobs, J., 210, 221
Jacobson, A. M., 218
Jain, A., 85
James, T., 332
Jameson, E., 94
Jameson, J., 37
Janz, N., 89
Jenkins, R. G., 278
Jenney, M.E.M., 210
Jenny, C., 82
Jessop, D. J., 210, 227, 248, 253
Jia, Z., 68, 261
Johnson, J. H., 68
Johnson, M., 87
Johnson, M. P., 217
Johnston, B. D., 79, 80
Johnston, M., 109
Jones, R., 155
Jordan, C., 174, 189, 195
Joshi, M., 281
Jossy, R., 199
Julian, J., 82
Juniper, E. F., 219
Juran, J. M., 17

K

Kalk, C. E., 29
Kan, L., 223
Kane, R. L., 210
Kantor, D., 222

Kaplan, S., 52, 56, 213
Kaska, S. C., 27
Kass, B., 47
Kastner, B., 10, 258
Katz, D. A., 278, 279
Katz, E. R., 212, 219, 224
Kaufman, J., 83
Kawachi, I., 319
Kelly, J., 175
Kennedy, M. P., 278
Kercsmar, C., 260
Kerr, L., 84
Kessel, D., 13
Kessner, D. M., 29
Khaw, K. T., 222
King, C. R., 26, 27
Kingsley, T., 123, 125, 126, 128, 146
Kirk, J., 92
Kirste, T., 92
Kirwin, A., 322, 324, 340
Klein, J. D., 92, 93
Kleinman, A., 75, 76, 89, 97, 258
Kleinman, L. C., 13, 254
Kline, E., 128
Knight, T. S., 209
Knott, J. H., 328
Koepsell, T. D., 79, 264
Kohn, L. T., 9, 11
Kohrman, C., 260
Kolterman, O. G., 222
Komaromy, M., 264
Koné, A., 177
Koot, H. M., 215
Korbin, J., 81, 82, 83, 109
Korn, E. L., 210, 248
Kornblum, W., 82
Korsch, B. M., 39
Kot, V., 188
Kozak, L. J., 250
Krafft, L. J., 98
Krafft, S. K., 98
Krauss, H. H., 92
Kravitz, R. L., 39, 93
Kretzmann, J. P., 147
Kreuter, M. W., 170, 171, 185
Krieger, N., 249

Kubisch, A. C., 171, 175, 179, 185, 186
Kuhlthau, K., 9, 252, 253
Kurtin, P. S., 3, 7, 10, 13, 25, 93, 98, 130, 139, 210, 218, 220, 222, 228, 248, 254, 267, 276, 277, 279, 281, 353

L

Laessle, R., 84
Laguerre, M., 107
Laine-Ammara, G., 92
Lake, K., 334
Lakoff, G., 87
Land, K., 123
Landgraf, J., 214, 222, 226, 248
Landrigan, P. J., 83
Landsverk, J., 53, 262
Langley, G. J., 281
Langley, W. M., 323
Langveld, J. H., 219
Lanphear, B. P., 222, 264
Lansky, D., 9, 212, 213, 214
Larimore, W. L., 262
Lasker, R. D., 169
LaValley, J. W., 93
Lavigne, J. V., 216
Lawrence, S., 346
Lazar, J. S., 92
Le Compte, S. H., 219
Leake, B., 39
Lee, M., 10
Lee, P., 174
Lee, P. R., 147
Leibowitz, A., 37, 248
Lenaway, D. D., 80
Leonard, W., 85
Leonardi, D., 89
Leplege, A., 209, 213
LeRoy, S., 250, 251
Leventhal, J. M., 82, 99
Levesque, P. N., 178, 192, 193, 340
Levine, M. H., 330
Levy, J. E., 333
Lewin, K., 191
Lewis, B. L., 222
Lewis, S., 322, 335, 345

Lezin, N. A., 170
Lieu, T. A., 314
Lim, L. F., 121
Lindberg, C., 5
Lindel, B., 84
Lindsley, C. B., 217
Ling, J., 260
Linov, P., 262
Lipman, T. H., 216
Liptak, G. S., 251
Lock, M., 94
Loda, F. A., 217
Lodico, M., 83
Logan, M., 109, 257
Lohr, K. N., 218, 252
Long, S. K., 277
Long, T., 216
Lorimor, R., 257
Loustaunau, M., 54, 261
Lowes, L., 99
Lundeberg, T., 92
Lunsky, Y., 224
Lurie, N., 210
Lynam, D. R., 334
Lyne, P., 99
Lynn, H., 260
Lyon, M., 92

M

Mabe, P. A. III, 318–319, 321, 330, 332, 334, 337, 338
Maciel, T. L., 40, 94
Mahoney, P., 53
Maiman, L., 89
Mainland, D., 33
Mangione-Smith, R., 253
Manion, J., 286
Mankud, V., 216
Mansour, M. E., 222, 264
Mariotto, M. J., 219
Mark, J., 92
Marrero, D. G., 217
Martin, E., 87, 107
Maser, E., 126
Mather, C., 26–27
Matsui, D. M., 221

Mayall, B., 35, 86
Mayberry, R. M., 251
Mays, N., 182, 184
McAuliffe, J., 323
McCabe, M. S., 210, 248
McCarthy, T., 33, 34
McCartney, K., 319
McConaughy, S. H., 219
McConnochie, K. M., 251
McCormick, M. C., 47, 49, 262
McCourt, M. P., 314
McCubbin, H. I., 222
McDonnell, K. A., 223
McDonough, J. E., 335, 342, 343
McGlynn, E. A., 36, 37, 52, 132, 248, 251, 252, 253
McKnight, J., 147, 148, 177, 182
McManus M. A., 217
Mears, B., 223
Mechanic, D., 86
Meeske, K., 212
Meeuwesen, L., 39, 40, 94
Meigs, A., 107
Melum, M. M., 283, 287
Metzner, H. L., 223
Meyer, J., 136, 178, 191
Meyer, M., 90
Meyerson, B., 331
Mili, F., 251
Miller, R., 13, 169
Milstein, A., 21, 31
Minkler, M., 191
Minkovitz, C. S., 322
Mitchell, C., 316
Mitchell, H., 260
Mohr, J. J., 9
Moore, H., 188, 315
Moore, K., 122
Moore, T. D., 210, 248
Moorehouse, M., 133
Morales, L. S., 96
Moss, N. E., 249
Muhib, F. B., 181
Mullen, P., 257
Muller, A., 84
Mullin, M., 128
Mustin, H., 89

N

Nair, P., 81
Najman, J. M., 220
Nanda, J., 260
Napoles-Springer, A., 254
Narang, D. S., 83
Neal, J. H., 222
Neff, J. M., 261
Nelson, E. C., 11, 213, 214
Nelson, M., 243
Nesman, T., 164
Neuhouser, M. L., 40, 94
Neumann, M. S., 175
Neumark-Sztainer, D., 40, 94
Newacheck, P., 43, 48, 132, 136, 217, 261, 262
Nguyen, U. S., 50, 251
Nichter, M., 18
Nickel, R. E., 92
Nkinsi, L., 199
Nolan, K. M., 281
Nolan, T. W., 19, 281
Noll, R. B., 216
Nordahl, U., 92
Norris, T., 125, 128, 136, 139, 141, 160
Northam, E. A., 216
Novick, L., 166
Nunnaly, J. C., 230
Nurss, J. R., 259
Nyden, P., 174, 177, 180, 316

O

O'Campo, P., 223
O'Connor, B. B., 76, 92
Offord, D. R., 216
Ofili, E., 251
Olds, D. L., 102
Oliphant, G., 334
Olivar, M. A., 258
Olson, C. M., 84
O'Malley, A. S., 262
O'Meara, S., 85
O'Neil, A. C., 262
Orav, E. J., 262
Ornstein, S. M., 278
Ortiz de Montellano, B., 257
Osmond, D., 260

Ottolini, M. C., 93
Owleny, L. M., 219

P

Pachter, L. M., 54, 57, 257
Padur, J. S., 216
Pappas, G., 250
Park, M. H., 50
Parker, E. A., 178
Parker, R. M., 259
Pate, R., 84
Patrick, D. L., 210
Patterson, J. M., 222
Patton, M. Q., 176
Payer, L., 103, 109
Payne, D., 13
Pearl, M., 146, 262
Peddecord, K. M., 7, 130
Pedro, L., 223
Pelto, G. H., 18
Pelto, P. J., 18
Pereyra, M., 261
Perez-Stable, E. J., 254
Perkins, D., 174, 190
Perrin, E. C., 253
Perrin, J. M., 37
Petaja, S., 83
Peters, E., 136
Peters, K. E., 320
Petr, C. G., 101
Pincus, T., 214
Pittman, M., 160
Pless, B., 92
Plsek, P., 5
Pope, C., 182, 184
Pratt, P., 323, 329, 344
Price, C., 216
Proenca, E. J., 156, 160
Prohaska, T. R., 320, 331
Prussing, E., 98, 99
Purcell, A., 336
Purviance, M. R., 217

Q

Queen, S., 250
Quinn, K., 281
Quinn, S., 257

R

Radley-Smith, R., 216
Rapoff, M. A., 217, 221
Ray, N. F., 48
Reagan, R., 343
Rebchook, G., 175
Reich, M. R., 317, 334, 337
Reid, R. J., 262
Reidy, K., 54, 96
Reidy, M., 133
Reinert, S. E., 82
Renaud, M., 322
Rice, M., 216
Richards, J. M., 217
Richardson, P. J., 10, 275, 281
Richardson, W. S., 284
Riley, P. L., 199
Ritzen, A., 82
Rivara, F. P., 40, 278
Rixford, C., 123, 124–125
Robbins, C., 223
Robinson, J. C., 21
Rock, C. L., 40, 94
Rodat, C. C., 187
Rode, C., 210, 248, 267
Rogers, E. M., 12
Roghmann, K. J., 251
Romanucci-Ross, L., 91
Rosenberg, M. C., 284
Rosko, M. D., 160
Ross, R. K., 139
Roter, D. L., 39, 52, 56
Rotheram-Borus, M. J., 175, 179
Roussos, S. T., 163, 171, 179, 180
Royce, S. W., 147
Rubenstein, L. E., 250
Rubenstein, L. V., 214
Rubin, G., 260
Rundall, T., 180
Russell, A., 260
Russell, G., 250

S

Sabbeth, B. F., 99
Sackett, D. L., 284
Sadler, B. L., 7, 10, 13, 130, 353
Saha, S., 264

Samson, J. A., 218
Sanchez, R. L., 250
Sargent, C., 35, 101
Saulnier, M., 322
Saunders, F., 222
Sawyer, M. G., 216
Scammell, M. L., 156
Scheff, D., 29
Schein, E. H., 305
Scheper-Hughes, N., 35, 101
Schinkel, A. M., 222
Schipper, H., 219
Schmidt, K. L., 90
Scholtes, P. R., 287, 289
Schön, D. A., 155
Schor, E. L., 40, 222, 226, 247
Schorr, L., 121, 143, 148, 156, 161,
    162, 163, 171, 180
Schulman, K. A., 250
Schulz, A. J., 174, 178, 181, 192, 194,
    195
Schuster, M., 36, 52, 132
Sclove, R. E., 156, 188, 191, 195
Sebastian, J. G., 249
Sechrest, L., 318–319, 321, 330, 332,
    334, 337, 338
Seid, M., 7, 10, 14, 25, 38, 54, 70,
    130, 210, 211, 218, 219, 220, 221,
    225, 228, 243, 248, 254, 256, 259,
    267, 281, 288
Selig, S. M., 174
Seligman, M., 100
Sellors, J. W., 316
Selwyn, B., 257
Semler, C. R., 263
Setoguchi, Y., 219
Shaffer, T. J., 261
Shah, A., 216
Shapiro, E., 174
Sharf, B. F., 344
Sharpe, P. A., 147
Shekelle, P. G., 278
Shelton, R. M., 9, 31
Shepardson, W., 333
Sherbourne, C. D., 210, 248
Shimp, L. A., 263

Shojania, K. G., 285
Shortell, S. M., 280
Shriver, M., 331, 332, 338, 341, 344,
    348
Shryock, R. H., 28
Sibinga E. M., 93
Silberstein, J., 126
Silver, E. J., 314
Silver, G. B., 322
Simmes, D. R., 121, 139, 155
Simpson, H. L., 331
Simpson, L., 9, 35, 48, 93, 248
Singer, J., 29
Singer, M., 68, 261
Sinioris, M. K., 283, 287
Siu, A. L., 252
Skocpol, T., 123
Slater, C. H., 128, 149
Slora, E. J., 13
Slovic, P., 136
Smith, S. V., 330
Snow, J., 146, 195
Snow, L. F., 107, 261, 263
Sobo, E. J., 14, 25, 38, 40, 54, 67, 70,
    81, 90, 93, 94, 98, 107, 243, 257,
    258, 259, 261, 275
Sockrider, M. M., 219
Sofaer, S., 180, 183
Sowden, A., 217
Spigelblatt, L., 92
Spilerman, S., 123
Spilker, B., 209
Spock, A., 220
Sprangers, M.A.G., 218
Spritzer, K., 96
Stacey, R. D., 5
Stafford, A., 107
Stange, K. C., 262
Starfield, B., 29, 44, 227, 248, 252,
    260, 262
Stein, R.E.K., 210, 227, 248, 253,
    261, 314
Steinbach, S., 279
Stephenson, J., 178
Sterky, G., 74
Stern, R., 221

Stewart, A. L., 254, 260, 264
Stewart, M. A., 52, 56
Stoddard, J. J., 261, 262, 331
Stolz, J. W., 262
Stone, E. M., 53
Stoto, M. A., 141, 160
Stryer, D., 317
Stucky, E. R., 275, 281
Stukel, T. A., 250
Sturge, C., 217
Sumbler, K., 222
Summerbell, C., 85
Sun, J., 92
Sun, Y., 278
Sutherland, C. E., 130, 138
Svedberg, L., 92
Swan, B., 188, 315
Swartz, K., 262
Sylvester, K., 314, 332, 333, 335
Szatmari, P., 216
Szilagyi, P. G., 247

T

Tates, K., 39, 40, 94
Taylor, S. D., 263
Tengvald, K., 74
Thamer, M., 48
Their, S. O., 211, 214
Thomas, S., 257
Thompson, J., 48
Thompson, R. J., Jr., 220
Thurber, F. W., 216
Toledo, J. R., 258
Toogood, I., 216
Torres, M. I., 178, 191
Townsend, M., 217
Troiano, R. P., 84
Trost, S., 84
Trotter, R. T. II, 257
Trupin, E., 155
Tumlinson, A., 53
Tunis, S., 317
Turner, M., 54, 96
Tusler, M., 136
Twiss, J. M., 328

U

Uhl, H., 84

V

Valdez, R. B., 261
Valentin, E. K., 303
Valentin, F., 68, 261
Valentine, W., 36, 132
Van Gils, A., 215
van Ryn, M., 95
Vander Stoep, A., 155, 176, 189, 195, 199
Vandivere, S., 146
Varni, J. W., 209, 210, 212, 213, 216, 217, 218, 219, 220, 221, 224, 225, 228, 248, 253, 254, 267
Veatch, T., 187
Verhoef, M. J., 93
Verhulst, F. C., 215
Verkuilen, J. V., 328
Vivier, P. M., 252
Vranizan, K., 260

W

Wagner, E., 52
Waitzkin, H., 103
Walco, G. A., 224
Wald, D. L., 30
Waldman, M. L., 29
Walker, E., 93, 98
Walker, L. S., 210
Wall, S., 74
Wallander, J. L., 216, 253
Waller, F. T., 212
Walsh, M. E., 86
Wandersman, A., 174, 190
Ward, D., 84, 100, 103
Ware, J. E., Jr., 52, 210, 217, 226, 248
Warman, K. L., 314
Warren, J. S., 320
Warwick, W. J., 222
Wasserman, R. C., 13
Wasson, J., 214
Waters, E., 85
Waters, M., 71
Waxler-Morrison, N., 223

Wazana, A., 80
Weech-Maldonado, R., 95
Wehr, E., 37, 94
Weigers, M. E., 49, 251
Weinick, R. M., 45, 49, 54, 251
Weinstein, J. N., 27
Weiss, C. H., 171
Weiss, E. S., 169
Weiss, K. B., 260, 322, 347
Weissman, J. S., 221, 262
Weitzman, M., 221
Weller, S. C., 54, 257, 258
Welshimer, K. J., 217
Wennberg, J. E., 9, 10, 31, 34
Werk, L. N., 279
West, A., 217
White, K. L., 33, 34
Wicks, E., 136
Wicks, L. B., 261
Widlund, G., 74
Wiewel, W., 174, 177, 180, 316
Wilcox, K. T., 216, 253
Wilkes, M. S., 39, 93
Williams, B., 97
Williams, D., 249
Williams, M., 155, 259
Williamson, J. W., 29
Wilson, I. B., 211, 213
Wilson, K. M., 92, 93
Wilson, M. H., 93
Wilson, R., 29
Witt, L. C., 183
Witzburg, R., 262

Wolfe, F., 214
Wolman, C., 260
Wong, V., 92
Wong, W., 92
Woo, P., 217
Wood, B. L., 216
Wood, D. L., 250, 261
Woodbridge, M. W., 186, 314, 339, 347
Woodgate, R. L., 223
Wray, J., 216
Wu, A., 223

Y

Yacoub, M., 216
Yang, Y. M., 216
Yeargin-Allsopp, M., 40
Young, J., 107
Young, L. A., 170

Z

Zervigon-Hakes, A. M., 315, 317, 318, 319, 320, 321, 322, 326, 344, 345, 347
Zigler, E., 83
Zill, N., 221
Zimmerman, B., 5
Zinn, J. S., 160
Zivkovic, M., 243
Zucconi, S. L., 133
Zuvekas, S. H., 45
Zyzanski, S. J., 262

Subject Index

• •

*Boldface numbers indicate pages on which glossary terms appear in **boldface** in discussions in the text.*

A

A.B. 1741 Collaboratives (California), 167
Academy for Health Services Research and Health Policy (AHSRHP), 34
AcademyHealth, 34
Access to care: conceptual model of, and HRQL, 244–245, 246; as concern of CHSR, 49–51; and health insurance, 49–51, 262; as influence on HRQL, 222. *See also* Barriers to care
Accountability: defined, **130**; demand for, **14**; outcomes-based, 125, 161–163; as purpose for using indicators, 125, 126
Acculturation, **69–70**; functional biomedical, 70, **259–260**
Act to Leave No Child Behind, 346
Action research, 191
Actionability of research, 331–332
Acute care visits, for children vs. adults, 40
Adaptive systems, **5**
Adaptive warning signals, **225**

Adherence, as influence on HRQL, **221**
Adults, differences between children and, 37–47, 248
Advocacy Initiative, 346
African Americans: health care expectations of, 257; health disparities among, 47–48. *See also* Minority children
Agency for Healthcare Policy and Research (AHCPR). *See* Agency for Healthcare Research and Quality (AHRQ)
Agency for Healthcare Research and Quality (AHRQ), 36, 50; asked to identify best practices for diagnoses, 276; Consumer Assessment of Health Plans Study (CAPHS) sponsored by, 32; establishment of, 34; funds researcher–health care system partnerships, 317
Algorithms, **279**
Alpha coefficients, **226**
Alternative medicine. *See* Complementary or alternative medicine (CAM)
American Academy of Pediatrics (AAP), 37, 346; Committee on Children with Disabilities, 93; Committee on Injury and Poison

Prevention, 78; Committee on Pediatric Research, 250; Committee
on School Health, 72, 80; Pediatric
Research in the Office Setting
group, 13

American College of Surgeons, Hospital Standards program, 28

American Hospital Association,
Community Care Networks
(CCNs) promoted by, 160

American Medical Association
(AMA), Council of Medical Education, 28

American Public Health Association,
134

Annie E. Casey Foundation: child indicator newsletter, 146; Kids Count
initiative, 131–132

Applied child health services research
(CHSR), 3; benefits of using
HRQL instruments in, 212–215;
and complex adaptive systems, 4–6;
examples of, 3; future potential of,
353–357; methodological orientation of, 18–20; mission of, 6–9; and
model of quality of care and HRQL
for vulnerable children, 264–267;
settings for, 3–4; sustainability facilitated by, 172; training in, 357;
units within organizations devoted
to, 14–18. See also Child health services research (CHSR)

Assessment: benefits of, of health-related quality of life (HRQL),
212–215; modular, 218; needs,
130. See also Evaluation

Assimilation, 69

Association for Health Services Research (AHSR), 34, 37

Asthma: African American children's
experience with, 48; disease management program for, 302–305; gap
between research and practice related to, 314

"At Last, Good News on the Family,"
73

Attention deficit hyperactivity disorder (ADHD), cultural tolerance of,
90

Authenticity of research, 331

B

Balance, health beliefs about,
108–109

Bar charts, 291, 292

Barriers to care, 256–261, 262–264;
and functional biomedical acculturation, 259–260; health beliefs as,
257–258, 263, 264; pragmatic factors as, 258–259, 262–263. See also
Access to care

Beliefs. See Health beliefs

Benchmarks, 129; state of Oregon,
142

Best practices: identification of, 276;
spread by collaboratives, 12–14

Biomedicine, 39

Blinded data, 293

Blood, health beliefs about, 109–110

Body fluids, health beliefs about,
109–110

Boost4Kids program, 167

Breastfeeding, and obesity, 83–84

C

C. S. Mott Foundation, 193

California Children and Families Act
(Proposition 10), 142, 316, 337

California Department of Education,
165

California Office of Statewide Health
Planning and Development
(OSHPD), 282–283

California Public Employee Retirement System (CalPERS), 31

California Youth Pilot Project, 167

Carnegie Corporation, 193, 330

Carnegie Foundation, Flexner Report
commissioned by, 28

Causation, web of, 178–180

Center for AIDS Prevention Studies,
188, 199

Center for Child Health Outcomes (CCHO): establishment of, 14; objectives of, 15, 22; Pathways Program, 16, 17; research of, demonstrated to organizations, 15–17. See also Children's Hospital and Health Center (San Diego)

Center for Mental Health Services, 167

Center for Studying Health System Change, Community Tracking Study, 158

Center for the Study of Social Policy, 158–159, 166

Centers for Disease Control and Prevention (CDC), 133, 156, 189, 192

Centers for Medicare and Medicaid Services, 33

Central tendency, **321**

Champions, **286**, 305

Change: as characteristic of children's health policy environment, 322–323; complexity of, in communities, 184–187

Charts: bar, 291, 292; cumulative proportion, 290–291; run, 283, 284, 291

Child abuse, 81–83, 102

Child Health Accountability Initiative (CHAI), 12–13

Child Health and Illness Profile (CHIP), 227

Child Health Initiative, 132

Child Health Questionnaire (CHQ), 226–227

Child health services research (CHSR), **3**, **25**, **67**, **313**; agenda for, 48–57; community as focus of, **155–156**; and community indicators movement, **127–128**; emergence of, 35–37; implications of collaboration for designing, 172–187; suggestions for future communication of, 347–349; trends affecting, 157–163. See also Applied child health services research (CHSR); Health services research

The Child Indicator: The Child, Youth, and Family Indicators Newsletter, 146

Child Trends, 146

Childhood Cancer Research Institute (CCRI), 156

Children: causes of death in, 41; differences between adults and, 37–47, 248; with disability or chronic illness, 98–100, 215–217; health services utilization by, 40, 42, 43, 45. See also Children with special health care needs (CSHCN); Minority children

Children Now: guide to producing community report cards, 137; indicator data used by, 141–142

Children with special health care needs (CSHCN): CAM medicine for, 92–93; health services utilization by, 45; number of, **43**, **44**

Children's Bureau, 123

Children's Defense Fund, 142, 346

Children's Health Act of 2000, 198

Children's Health Insurance Program (CHIP). See State Children's Health Insurance Program (S-CHIP)

Children's Hospital and Health Center (San Diego): Center for Child Health Outcomes (CCHO) at, 14, 15–17, 22; disease management at, 302–307; identification of best practices for patient care at, 279; pathways program at, 280, 282, 286–287, 294–302, 305–307; use of PedsQL by, 213, 229–231

Chronic Care Model (CCM), 52

Chronic illness, children with, 98–100, 215–217. See also Children with special health care needs (CSHCN)

Clinical outliers, **290**

Clinical pathways. See Pathways

Cochrane Library, 284

Coin rubbing, 82, 108

Collaboration, **160**; benefits of, 169; best practices spread by, 12–14;

defining characteristics of, 164; difficulties in implementing, 169–170; evaluation of, 170–172; history of, around child health, 166–169; implications of, for designing CHSR, 172–187; increased, 159–161; need for, 199; stages of, 164–166. *See also* Community-based research (CBR)

Common cause variation, **283**

Commonwealth Fund, 35, 53

Communication: among researchers, policymakers, and practitioners, 319–320; of CHSR, 347–349; and cultural competence, 95–98; with diverse populations, 56–57; and parental competence, 94–95; in pediatric care triad, 93–94; of research, 338–347

Community: complexity of change in, 184–187; defined, **177**; as focus of CHSR, 155–156; moving research out of lab and into, 177–178; needs of, vs. scientific rigor of research, 183–184; reasons for involving, in research, 188–191; shared goals of researchers and, 173–176

Community Care Networks (CCNs), 160

Community health report cards, 49, **132**, 135–140; defined, **130**; examples of projects producing, 138–140; guide to producing, 137

Community Health Status Indicators (CHSI) project, 134–135

Community indicators, 121–150; choosing appropriate, 186–187; defined, **121**; definitions of terms related to, 129–130, 131; descriptive, **140**; examples of applications of, 141–144, 145; factors contributing to growth in use of, 126; federal government's work with, 132–135; foundations' work with, 131–132; future development of, 144, 146–149; history of, 122–128; prescriptive, **140**–141; reasons for

using, 125, 140–141; report card application of, 135–140; theoretical frameworks for, 128–129

Community report cards. *See* Community health report cards

Community Tracking Study, 158

Community-based agencies and organizations (CBOs), 315, 325

Community-based research (CBR), **188**–199; characteristics of, 195–198; history of, 191–193; need for, 199; overview of, 193–195; rationale for, 188–191; ways for initiating, 191

Community-level social indicators, 122, 125, **130**. *See also* Community indicators

Comorbidity, **215**–216, **290**

Competence: cultural, **54**–55, **95**–98; parental, 94–95

Complementary or alternative medicine (CAM), **91**–93

Comprehensive Community Mental Health Services for Children and Their Families program, 167–168

Conceptual models, **243**–246

Construct validity, **227**

Consumer Assessment of Health Plans Study (CAHPS), 32

Continuous quality improvement (CQI), **30**, **280**. *See also* Plan, do, study, act (PDSA) system

Control group, **99**

Conventional medicine, 76

Costs: of child health care, 36; controlling, potential of applied CHSR for, 355; of household-centered care, 103; reducing, by standardizing care, 276–278; savings of, with pathways program, 302

Council of State Governments, 142

Cross-informant variance, **219**

Cross-sectional research design, **99**

Crossing the Quality Chasm (Institute of Medicine), 12, 57, 67–68

Cultural competence, **54**–55, **95**–98

Culture, **54**; change of, with pathways and disease management, 305–306; as consideration in designing CHSR, 176–177; defined, **68**–69; as influence on definition of health problems, 85–86; terms related to, 69–72; understandings of health related to, 87–88, 107–110, 258

Cumulative proportion charts, 290–291

Cupping, 108

D

Data Harbor, Inc., 37

Data Matters, 146

David and Lucile Packard Foundation, 37, 193, 347

Death: causes of, in children, 41; publication of hospital rates of, 30

Decision support (DS) systems, **290**

Demographics: defined, **38**; as difference between children and adults, 43–47, **248**. *See also* Sociodemographic variables

Dependence: defined, **37**; as difference between children and adults, 38–40, **248**

Description, as purpose for using indicators, 125

Descriptive community indicators, **140**

Developmental change: defined, **37**; as difference between children and adults, 38, **248**

Devolution, **158**–159, 315, 322–323

Differential epidemiology: defined, **37**–38; as difference between children and adults, 40–43, 44, 45, **248**

Disabled children, 98–100, 215–217. *See also* Children with special health care needs (CSHCN)

Disease: due to household practices, 83–86; as orientation of HSR, 35; vs. illness, **96**

Disease management (DM): at Children's Hospital and Health Center

(San Diego), 302–307; culture change with implementation of, 305–306; defined, **275**; developing programs for, 302–305; factors needed for success of, 305

Disease-specific measures, **217**–218

Disparities. *See* Health disparities

Dissemination of research information, 339–340

Diversity, 54–57, 177

E

Early and Periodic Screening, Diagnosis and Treatment (EPSDT), 50

Early Head Start program, 330

Effectiveness of health care services, 51

Efficacy of health care services, 51

80–20 rule, 289

Enculturation, **69**

Environmental Justice: Partnerships for Communication Program, 192

Epidemiology: as approach to community indicators, 128; differential, 37–38, 40–43, 44, 45, **248**; first efforts in, **122**; and population health, **17**; social, of injury, 80

Equilibrium model of health, 108–109

Ethnicity, **54**, **70**–71; vs. race, 55, 70

Ethnocentrism, **97**

Ethnography, **182**

Ethnoracial background, 55–56

Evaluation: of collaboration, 170–172; as component of applied CHSR, 6; as purpose for using indicators, 125; of quality of health outcomes, 8–9. *See also* Assessment

F

Falls, 78–79

Family, defined, **73**

Family functioning, 222–223

Family Support Act of 1988, 339, 342

Family-centered care, 100–101

Federal government: community indicator movement role of, 132–135;

community-based research projects
of, 192; health care coverage provided by, 29; health plan monitoring programs of, 32; Medicare
hospital death rates published by,
30; shift of responsibilities of,
158–159, 315, 322–323
Federal Interagency Forum on Child
and Family Statistics, 135, 148, 186
Flexner Report, 28
Flow model of health, 107–108
Folk-sector medicine, 75
Foundation Consortium, 168
Foundation for Accountability
(FACCT), 9, 32, 53
Foundations: community indicator
movement role of, 131–132; community-based research projects
of, 192–193; research communicated by, 346–347. See also specific
foundations
Framing messages, 342
Functional biomedical acculturation,
70, 259–260
Functional status, 209–210
Functional Status Measure (FSII-R),
227–228

G
Generalizability of research, 333–334
Generic measures, 215–217, 218
Geographic information systems
(GISs), 143–144, 145
Goals: set using indicators, 125;
shared by researchers and commu-
nity, 173–176
Government. See Federal government
Government Accounting Office, 50

H
Harvard Family Research Project
(HFRP), 346
Harvard School of Public Health, 195
Head Start, 331; Early, 330
Health: broadened understanding of,
in community-based research, 157,

196; cultural understandings of,
87–88, 107–110, 258; defined, by
WHO, 7, 159, 210–211, 248
Health Belief Model, 89
Health beliefs: as barrier to care,
257–258, 263, 264; culture as influence on, 87–88, 107–110, 258; as
influence on patterns of resort,
89–90, 257
Health care: assessing overuse, underuse, and misuse of, 51–52; as complex adaptive system, 4–5; managed
care system of, 158, 277–278; need
for standardization of, 276–278;
new models of, 278–279; pediatric,
sources of, 74–77
Health Care Financing Administration (HCFA), 33
Health care services. See Health
services
Health Cost and Utilization Project
(HCUP), 49
Health disparities: efforts to reduce,
48; of minority children, 47–48,
248, 250–251
Health Employers Data and Information Set (HEDIS), 32
Health insurance: and access to care,
49–51, 262; number of children
without, 49. See also Medicaid;
State Children's Health Insurance
Program (S-CHIP)
Health Plan Employer Data Information Set (HEDIS), 9, 162
Health problems, culture as influence
on defining, 85–86
Health Resources and Services Administration (HRSA), 134
Health services: challenges to delivery
of, 9–12; Donabedian's model of,
33–34, 251–252; efficacy vs. effectiveness of, 51; utilization of, by
children, 40, 42, 43, 45
Health services research (HSR): defined, 25; early examples of, 26–27;
inception and development of,

33–35. *See also* Applied child health services research (CHSR); Child health services research (CHSR)

Health Services Research (journal), 33, 36

Health status: applied CHSR's potential for improving, 356; defined, **130, 209**

Health-related quality of life (HRQL), 209–232, **243**; benefits of assessment of, 212–215; conceptual model of access to care and, 244–245, 246; defining, 209–211; developmental change considered in, **38**; disease-specific measures of, **217**–218; factors influencing, 220–225; future instruments for measuring, 232, 266–267; generic measures of, **215**–217, 218; model of quality of care and, for vulnerable children, 254–267; pediatric, instruments for measuring, 226–229; rationale for separate model of, for vulnerable children, 246–254; self-report vs. proxy report for assessing, 215, 218–220; uses of instruments measuring, 211–212

Health-Related Quality of Life Questionnaire, 304

Health-seeking process, **88**–89

Healthcare Forum Foundation, 143

Healthcare Matrix, 7–8

Healthy Communities movement, 160

Healthy People initiative, 162

Healthy People 2000 (U.S. Department of Health and Human Services), 134

Healthy People 2010 (U.S. Department of Health and Human Services), 48, 162

Healthy Start Support Services for Children and Families Act (California), 165

Henry J. Kaiser Family Foundation, 35, 49, 257, 262

Hierarchy of resort, **91**

Home visiting, 102, 304

Hospital Research and Educational Trust, journal *Health Services Research* sponsored by, 33

Hospitals: publication of death rates for, 30; standards for, 28–29

Household: communication between health system and, 93–98; defined, **72**–73; designing CHSR focusing on, 103–106; disease and illness due to practices in, 83–86; health-producing, 77–78; impact of chronic illness or disability in children on, 98–100; injury occurring in, 78–83; intersection of health care system with, 74–77; service delivery centered on, 100–103; vs. family, 73

Human capital, **47**

Hypothetical constructs, **244**

I

Illness: chronic, 98–100, 215–217; due to household practices, 83–86; vs. disease, **86**

Indicators, **31**; choosing appropriate, 186–187; defined, **186**; leading health, 162. *See also* Community indicators; Social indicators

Injuries: intentional, 81–83; occurring at home, 78–83; patterns of, 79–80; and risk perception, 80–81; unintentional, 78–81

Inoculation, smallpox, 26–27

Institute for Healthcare Improvement (IHI): Breakthrough Series, 13; plan, do, study, act (PDSA) system promoted by, 280–281

Institute for the Future, 158

Institute of Medicine (IOM), 6, 9, 11, 12, 25, 35, 52, 57, 67, 104, 106, 162, 246, 251, 278; *Crossing the Quality Chasm*, 12, 57, 67–68; *To Err Is Human*, 11

Institute on Race and Poverty, 250

Internal consistency reliability, **226**

J

Jacksonville, Florida, "Quality Indicators for Progress" project, 138–139
John A. Hartford Foundation, 35
Joint Commission on Healthcare Organizations (JCAHO), 28, 355

K

Kids Count initiative, 131–132
Knowledge, gap between practice and, in health care, 10, 51
Knowledge brokering, 348–349

L

Language barriers, 95–96
Latino children: health insurance coverage of, 50, 261; risk of poor health status for, 251. See also Minority children
Leading health indicators, 162
Leapfrog Group, 355
Longitudinal research design, **99**

M

Managed care, 158, **277–278**
Manpower Demonstration Research Corporation, 339
Maternal and Child Health Block Grant program, 162
Maternal and Child Health Bureau, 123
Media, communication of research by, 345
Medicaid, 29, 49–50
Medical audits, 29
Medical education, standardization of, 28
Medical Expenditure Panel Survey (MEPS), 49
Medicare, 29, 30
Microsystem, **11**
Minority children: health disparities for, 47–48, 248, 250–251; increasing number of, 44–46; injured in long falls, 78; living in poverty, 44, 250. See also specific ethnic groups

Models, conceptual, **243–246**
Modular assessment, **218**
Monitoring: child health, as concern of CHSR, 49; as purpose for using indicators, 125
Morbidity, 247
Multiple regression, **321**

N

National Aeronautics and Space Administration (NASA), 124
National Association of Children's Hospitals and Related Institutions (NACHRI), 36, 283
National Center for Health Services Research (NCHSR), 34
National Center for Health Statistics, 47, 133
National Civic League, 160
National Commission on Technology, Automation, and Economic Progress, 123–124, 124
National Committee for Quality Assurance (NCQA), 32, 53, 162
National Heart, Lung, and Blood Institute (NHLBI), 51
National Initiative for Child Health Quality, 13
National Institute of Environmental Health Sciences (NIEHS), 192
National Institutes of Health, 47, 48, 183, 184; and inception of field of health services research, 33; on when to use qualitative methods, 182
National Library of Medicine, 34
National Neighborhood Indicators Partnership, 146
National Quality Forum, 355
Native Americans: congenital hip disease among (Navajos), 85–86; infant mortality rate among, 47; oral tradition of, 176. See also Minority children
Needs assessment, **130**
Noncategorical approach, **253**

Nurses: as champions, 286; training in applied CHSR for, 357

O

Obesity, and household practices, 83–85

Occupation, 72

Operational definitions, 8, **244**

Oregon Benchmarks, 142

Organizations: accrediting and regulatory, potential benefits of applied CHSR for, 354–355; advocacy and professional, communication of research by, 345–346

Outcomes, 3, **34**, **129**, **252**; patient, early effort to track, 27; web of causation for, 178–180

"Outcomes Toolkit," 143

Outcomes-based accountability, 125, 161–163

Outliers, **321**; clinical, **290**

P

Pacific Business Group on Health, 21, 136

Pain, types of, 224–225

Parallel forms, **220**

Parents: competence of, 94–95; impact on, of caring for chronically ill or disabled children, 99; as primary caregivers, 73

Pareto principle, **289**

Partnering. *See* Collaboration

Pathways, **16**, 279–280; at Children's Hospital and Health Center (San Diego), 280, 282, 286–287, 294–302, 305–307; compliance with, 299; cost savings with, 302, culture change with implementation of, 305–306; defined, **275**, 279; factors needed for success of, 305; literature review in development of, 284–285, 298; plan, do, study, act (PDSA) system as process for, **280**–294; sample, 296–297,

300–301; team for developing, 285–287

Patient-centered care, **67**

Patients: in pediatric triad, 39–40; safety of, 11

Patterns of resort: to CAM therapies, 91–93; defined, **89**; health beliefs' influence on, 89–90, **257**; and health-seeking process, 88–89; and hierarchy of resort, 90–91

Pediatric care triad, 39–40, **94**, 104

Pediatric Health Information System (PHIS), 283

Pediatric Quality of Life Inventory (PedsQL), 212, 213; in development of disease management program, 304; oncology clinic's use of, 212, 230–231; overview of, 228–229; rheumatology clinic's use of, 213, 229–230, 547

Performance measures, **130**, **143**

Pew Charitable Trusts, 35

Physical activity, household practices encouraging, 84–85

Physicians: as champions, 286; concepts presented to, by CCHO, 16–17; and pathway development, 280; in pediatric triad, 39–40; training in applied CHSR for, 357; under managed care, 277–278

Plan, do, study, act (PDSA) system, **19**, **280**, **354**; acting stage of, 294; doing stage of, 287–289; planning stage of, 281–287; steps of, 281; studying stage of, 289–294

Policy: changing environment for, 322–323; characteristics of research relevant to, 331–334; perspectives on, 324–326; relationship between research and, 329–331; storytelling in making of, 342–344

Policymakers: beliefs about role of science, 321–322; communicating research information to, 340–341; communication among researchers, practitioners, and, 315–317; defined,

313; how research used by, 329–331; interdependence among researchers, practitioners, and, 315–317; types of, 326–329

Politics: as consideration in designing CHSR, 175; as influence on use of research, 334, 336–337

Popular-sector medicine, 75

Poverty: and children's health, 44, 250; as influence on HRQL, 222

Practice: gap between knowledge and, 10, 51; gap between research and, 313–314, 317–322. See also Best practices

Practitioners: communication among researchers, policymakers, and, 319–320; defined, 313; interdependence among researchers, policymakers, and, 315–317; perspectives of, on policy, 325

Prescriptive community indicators, 140–141

Preventive services, 40, 43

Primary data, 103

Processes, 3, 34, 251–252

Professional-sector medicine, 75

Project D.A.R.E., 334

Promising Practices Network, 346–347

Proposition 10 (California Children and Families Act), 142, 316, 337

Proxy: measures as, 55, 250; report by, in pediatric HRQL instruments, 215, 218–220

Psychometric properties, 217

Public Health Institute, study on beverage contracts in California, 336

Q

Qualitative research methods, 182–183

Quality: defining, in health care, 8–9, 12; difficulty of assessing, of health care services to children, 13–14; evaluation of, of health outcomes, 8–9; history of measuring, in health

care, 29–32; improved consumer choice based on, 354; making business case for, 20–21, 356; potential of applied CHSR for improving, 355–356

Quality of care: as concern of CHSR, 51–54; defined, 251; measuring, for children, 252–254; model of, and HRQL for vulnerable children, 254–267; potential benefit of applied CHSR in measuring, 354–355

Quality of life (QOL), 128, 210. See also Health-related quality of life (HRQL)

R

Race, 54, 70–71; vs. ethnicity, 55, 70

Randomized controlled trials (RCTs), 51, 178; disadvantages of, 180–181, 319, 321

Rapid-cycle improvement, 19, 280; plan, do, study, act (PDSA) system of, 280–294

Recall interval, 230

Redefining Progress, 127, 132, 140, 143, 144

Relevance of research, 318–319, 332–333

Reliability, 218; internal consistency, 226

Report cards. See Community health report cards

Research: action, 191; characteristics of, relevant to policy, 331–334; communication of, 338–347; contextual forces influencing use of, 334–338; gap between practice and, 313–314, 317–322; how policymakers use, 329–331; relevance and usefulness of, 318–319, 332–333. See also Community-based research (CBR)

Research Forum on Children, Families, and the New Federalism, 346

Research methodology: for community-based research, 180–184, 197–198;

qualitative, 182–183; scientific rigor of, 183–184

Researchers: beliefs about role of science, 321–322; communication among policymakers, practitioners, and, 319–320; communication techniques for, 341–344; interdependence among policymakers, practitioners, and, 315–317; partners for communication by, 344–347; policy perspectives of, 325; shared goals of community and, 173–176; shortage of, trained in child HSR, 36; suggestions for, on communicating CHSR, 347–349

Risk adjustment, 30, 104

Risk perception, and injury, 80–81

Robert Wood Johnson Foundation, 32, 37; Child Health Initiative, 132; health services research funding by, 35; Improving Chronic Illness Care program, 52

Run charts, 283, 284, 291

S

San Diego, California: County Child and Family Health and Well-Being Report Card project, 139–140, 149. *See also* Children's Hospital and Health Center (San Diego)

San Diego County Health and Human Services Agency, 138

Secondary data, 103

Self-report, in pediatric HRQL instruments, 218–220

Shewart-Deming cycle, 280. *See also* Plan, do, study, act (PDSA)

Siblings: impact of chronically ill or disabled children on, 99–100; risk of childhood injury for, 79–80

Smallpox inoculation, 26–27

Smoking, illness and disease due to, in household, 83

Social capital, 47, 179

Social indicators: community-level,

122, 125, 130; defined, 122; history of, 123–125. *See also* Community indicators

Social strain, 224

Social support, 223–224

Society, 68

Sociodemographic variables, 221–222. *See also* Demographics

Socioeconomic status (SES), and vulnerability, 249–250. *See also* Poverty

Special cause variation, 283

Stakeholders, 121, 125

State Children's Health Insurance Program (S-CHIP), 50, 316, 335

Storytelling, 342–344

Structure, 3, 34, 251

Substance Abuse and Mental Health Services Administration, 167, 176

Sustainability, 128, 172–173, 196

SWOT analysis, 303

Systems thinking, 10–11

T

Technology, and community indicators, 126, 143

Time: community's vs. researchers' orientation toward, 175–176; and gap between research and practice, 320–321; required for change, 185

To Err Is Human (Institute of Medicine), 11

Total quality management (TQM), 29–30

Training, in applied CHSR, 357

Translators, 96

Tuskegee Syphilis Study, 189

U

United Way of America, 137

Unnecessary variation, 10, 276

Urban Institute, Assessing the New Federalism (ANF) project, 159

U.S. Bureau of the Census, 45

U.S. Consumer Product Safety Commission, 79

U.S. Department of Education, 192
U.S. Department of Health and
  Human Services, 160, 192, 250,
  331; Healthy People initiative, 48,
  134, 162; Office of the Assistant
  Secretary for Planning and Evalua-
  tion, 127, 133
U.S. Department of Housing and
  Urban Development (HUD), 192
U.S. Environmental Protection
  Agency (EPA), 128, 192
U.S. Geological Survey, 143

V

Validity, 218; construct, 227
Value, 14, 31
Variance, cross-informant, 219
Variation: common cause, 283; spe-
  cial cause, 283; unnecessary, 10,
  276
Vermont-Oxford Neonatal network,
  13
Vernacular medicine, 76
Vital statistics, 122

Vulnerability: defined, 249; and ethnicity, 250–251; in model of quality
  of care and HRQL, 255–256, 261;
  and socioeconomic status (SES),
  249–250

W

W. K. Kellogg Foundation, 35, 193
Washington Business Group on
  Health, 21
Welfare reform, 50
White House Office of Science and
  Technology Policy, 192
Woburn, Massachusetts, research on
  childhood leukemia in, 195
Women, as primary caregivers, 100
World Bank, 192
World Health Organization (WHO),
  130, 160, 247; definition of health,
  7, 159, 210–211, 248; Quality of
  Life Group, 210

Y

Youth Action Project, 190–191